T0306117

TREATMENT OF MULTIPLE MYELOMA AND RELATED DISORDERS

Owing to major advances in understanding the biology and pathogenesis of the disease, the management of multiple myeloma is changing rapidly. New diagnostic and prognostic criteria have been introduced, and treatment options are multiplying with high-dose chemotherapy regimens, stem cell transplants, and the development of novel agents and immune-based strategies that target tumor cells directly.

This book is aimed at the practitioner who is looking to put these advances into clinical context. It will serve as an up-to-date resource for treatment of myeloma and related disorders. Chapters are written by international authorities and contain color photos, diagrams, and algorithms outlining preferred treatment strategies. Relevant scientific information is integrated throughout, but the focus here is on providing practical therapeutic guidance for oncologists and hematologists caring for myeloma patients. The book covers all myeloma subtypes and related disorders, including amyloidosis, Waldenström macroglobulinemia, plasmacytoma, MGUS, and POEMS syndrome.

Dr. S. Vincent Rajkumar is Professor of Medicine at Mayo Clinic College of Medicine and Chair of the Mayo Clinic Myeloma, Amyloidosis, and Dysproteinemia Group. He has authored more than 250 papers and book chapters, primarily in the field of myeloma and related plasma cell disorders. He has led several clinical trials investigating the role of new agents in myeloma. Dr. Rajkumar is a member of the American Society of Clinical Oncology Cancer Education Committee as well as the Scientific Advisory Board of the International Myeloma Foundation. Dr. Rajkumar is an associate editor of the Mayo Clinic Proceedings and is on the editorial boards of *American Journal of Oncology Review* and *Leukemia Research*.

Dr. Robert A. Kyle is Professor of Medicine and Laboratory Medicine at Mayo Clinic in Rochester, Minnesota. He served as the William H. Donner Professor of Medicine and Laboratory Medicine and was Section Head and Chairman of the Division of Hematology. Dr. Kyle is one of the most respected authorities in the field of multiple myeloma and related disorders and has authored more than 750 papers and book chapters, primarily in the field of myeloma and related plasma cell disorders. He has led several major clinical trials and epidemiological studies in the field. Dr. Kyle is currently Chairman of the Scientific Advisory Board of the International Myeloma Foundation, Chairman of the Scientific Advisory Committee of the International Waldenström's Macroglobulinemia Foundation, and President of the International Society of Amyloidosis.

During his career, Dr. Kyle has been recognized as the first recipient of the Robert A. Kyle Award for the Waldenstrom's Macroglobulinemia Foundation, first recipient of the Robert A. Kyle Lifetime Achievement Award from the International Myeloma Foundation, recipient of the Mayo Clinic's Henry S. Plummer Distinguished Internist Award, recipient of the Mayo Clinic's Distinguished Clinician Award, and recipient of the Mayo Clinic's Distinguished Alumni Award. He was also recipient of the 2007 David Karnofsky Award and Lecture at ASCO.

TREATMENT OF MULTIPLE MYELOMA AND RELATED DISORDERS

Edited by

S. VINCENT RAJKUMAR
Mayo Clinic College of Medicine

ROBERT A. KYLE
Mayo Clinic College of Medicine

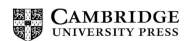

CAMBRIDGE
UNIVERSITY PRESS

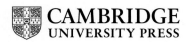

Shaftesbury Road, Cambridge CB2 8EA, United Kingdom

One Liberty Plaza, 20th Floor, New York, NY 10006, USA

477 Williamstown Road, Port Melbourne, VIC 3207, Australia

314–321, 3rd Floor, Plot 3, Splendor Forum, Jasola District Centre, New Delhi – 110025, India

103 Penang Road, #05–06/07, Visioncrest Commercial, Singapore 238467

Cambridge University Press is part of Cambridge University Press & Assessment, a department of the University of Cambridge.

We share the University's mission to contribute to society through the pursuit of education, learning and research at the highest international levels of excellence.

www.cambridge.org
Information on this title: www.cambridge.org/9780521515030

First published 2009

A catalogue record for this publication is available from the British Library

Library of Congress Cataloging-in-Publication data
Treatment of multiple myeloma and related disorders / edited by S. Vincent Rajkumar, Robert A. Kyle.
    p. ; cm.
Includes bibliographical references and index.
ISBN 978-0-521-51503-0 (hardback)
1. Multiple myeloma – Treatment.   2. Multiple myeloma – Diagnosis.
3. Paraproteinemia – Treatment.   4. Paraproteinemia – Diagnosis.   I. Rajkumar,
S. Vincent.   II. Kyle, Robert A., 1928–   III. Title. [DNLM: 1. Multiple
Myeloma – therapy.   2. Multiple Myeloma – diagnosis.   3. Paraproteinemias –
diagnosis.   4. Paraproteinemias – therapy. WH 540 T784 2009]
RC280.B6T73   2009
616.99´418–dc22   2008039651

ISBN   978-0-521-51503-0   Hardback

....

CONTENTS

CONTRIBUTORS

Kenneth C. Anderson, MD
Kraft Family Professor of Medicine
Harvard Medical School
25 Shattuck St.
Boston, MA 02115

Chief, Division of Hematologic Neoplasia
Director, Jerome Lipper Myeloma Center and
    LeBow Institute for Myeloma
    Therapeutics
Dana-Farber Cancer Institute
44 Binney St.
Mayer 557
Boston, MA 02115

William I. Bensinger, MD
Professor of Medicine
University of Washington
1959 NE Pacific
Seattle, WA 98195

Director, Autologous Stem Cell
    Transplantation
Clinical Research Division
Fred Hutchinson Cancer Research Center
1100 Fairview Ave. N
Seattle, WA 98109

P. Leif Bergsagel, MD, FRCPC
Professor of Medicine
Mayo Clinic College of Medicine
13400 E. Shea Blvd.
Scottsdale, AZ 85259

Consultant
Mayo Clinic
13400 E. Shea Blvd.
Scottsdale, AZ 85259

Joan Bladé, MD
Associate Professor of Medicine
University of Barcelona
Casanova 136
08036 Barcelona, Spain

Senior consultant
Department of Hematology
Hospital Clinic
Villarroel, 170
08036 Barcelona, Spain

Meletios A. Dimopoulos, MD
Professor and Chairman
Department of Clinical Therapeutics
University of Athens School of Medicine
80 V. Sofias Ave.
Athens, Greece 115 28

Director
Department of Clinical Therapeutics
Alexandra Hospital
80 V. Sofias Ave.
Athens, Greece 115 28

Angela Dispenzieri, MD
Associate Professor of Medicine
Division of Hematology
Mayo Clinic
200 First St. SW
Rochester, MN 55905

Rafael Fonseca, MD
Professor of Medicine
Division of Hematology–Oncology
Mayo Clinic
200 First St. SW
Rochester, MN 55905

Consultant
Division of Hematology-Oncology
Mayo Clinic
13400 E. Shea Blvd.
Scottsdale, AZ 85259

Morie A. Gertz, MD
Chair and Professor of Medicine
Department of Medicine, Division
    of Hematology
Mayo Clinic
200 First St. SW
Rochester, MN 55905

Consultant
Division of Hematology
Mayo Clinic
200 First St. SW
Rochester, MN 55905

J.-L. Harousseau, MD
Professor
Department of Hematology
1 Place Alexis Ricordeau
Nantes, 44093, France

Head, Department of Hematology
1 Place Alexis Ricordeau
Nantes, 44093, France

Suzanne R. Hayman, MD
Consultant, Division of Hematology
Assistant Professor of Medicine
Mayo Clinic
200 First St. SW
Rochester, MN 55905

Efstathios Kastritis, MD
Professor and Chairman
Department of Clinical Therapeutics
University of Athens School of Medicine
80 V. Sofias Ave.
Athens, Greece 115 28

Director
Department of Clinical Therapeutics
Alexandra Hospital
80 V. Sofias Ave.
Athens, Greece 115 28

Jonathan L. Kaufman, MD
Assistant Professor
Department of Hematology and Medical Oncology
Emory University
1365C Clifton Rd. NE
Atlanta, GA 30322

Robert A. Kyle, MD
Professor of Medicine and Laboratory Medicine
Division of Hematology
Mayo Clinic
200 First St. SW
Rochester, MN 55905

Sagar Lonial, MD
Associate Professor
Department of Hematology and
    Medical Oncology
Emory University
1345 Clifton Rd. NE
Atlanta, GA 30322

Giampaolo Merlini, MD
Full Professor
Department of Biochemistry
University of Pavia
Viale Taramelli, 3/b
Pavia, Italy, 27100

Director
Center for Research and Treatment of
    Systemic Amyloidosis
Fondazione IRCCS Policlinico San Matteo
Viale Golgi, 19
Pavia, Italy, 27100

Marc S. Raab, MD, PhD
Instructor of Medicine
Department of Medicine
University of Heidelberg
INF 410
Heidelberg, 69120, Germany

Staff Physician
Multiple Myeloma Research Center
National Center of Tumor Diseases
INF 350
Heidelberg, 69120, Germany

S. Vincent Rajkumar, MD
Professor of Medicine
Chair, Myeloma Amyloidosis
Dysproteinemia Group
Division of Hematology
Mayo Clinic
200 First St. SW
Rochester, MN 55905

Paul G. Richardson, MD
Associate Professor of Medicine
Harvard Medical School
25 Shattuck St.
Boston, MA 02115

Clinical Director
Jerome Lipper Center for Multiple Myeloma
Dana-Farber Cancer Institute
44 Binney St., Dana 1B02
Boston, MA 02115

G. David Roodman MD, PhD
Professor of Medicine
Department of Hematology-Oncology
University of Pittsburgh
VAMC, University Dr. C, R&D 151U
Pittsburgh, PA 15240

Director, Center for Bone Biology at
    UPMC and Myeloma
    Medicine/Hematology-Oncology
University of Pittsburgh Medical Center
    and University of Pittsburgh Cancer
    Institution

5150 Centre Ave., 5th Floor
Pittsburgh, PA 15232

Laura Rosiñol, MD, PhD
Specialist in Hematology
Department of Hematology
Hospital Clinic
Villarroel, 170
08036 Barcelona, Spain

A. Keith Stewart, MB, ChB
Professor
Division of Hematology-Oncology
Mayo Clinic
13400 E. Shea Blvd.
Scottsdale, AZ 85259

Consultant
Division of Hematology–Oncology
Mayo Clinic
13400 E. Shea Blvd.
Scottsdale, AZ 85259

Steven P. Treon, MD, MA, PhD
Associate Professor
Harvard Medical School
M547, 44 Binney St.
Boston, MA 02115

Director
Bing Center for Waldenström's
    Macroglobulinemia
Dana-Farber Cancer Institute
M547, 44 Binney St.
Boston, MA 02115

1   Diagnosis and Genetic Classification of Multiple Myeloma

Rafael Fonseca and P. Leif Bergsagel

INTRODUCTION

In the past decade we have seen great advances in our understanding of the genetic abnormalities present in multiple myeloma (MM) cells, which is believed to be the culprit in the pathogenesis of this disease.[1] This progress has been, in great part, facilitated by the advent of novel molecular genetic and cytogenetic techniques, as well as the unparalleled power available through the genomic revolution. Furthermore, the continued testing for many of these genetic aberrations in large cohorts of patients has allowed for an increasingly accurate description of oncogenomics using primary patient samples. The translation and testing of this basic knowledge in these patient cohorts has provided clinical relevance that truly spans from the bench to the bedside. While much progress has been made in the understanding of the disease, many questions remain, particularly those capable of addressing progression events from the benign stages and unraveling complex interactions supporting clonal survival and evolution. In this chapter we discuss the knowledge regarding a global overview of genetic aberrations of MM cells, primary genetic lesions, secondary genetic events, and, lastly, their clinical implications.

GLOBAL OVERVIEW OF MM GENETICS

At the top hierarchical level, human MM can be divided into two diseases: hyperdiploid MM (H-MM) and nonhyperdiploid MM (NH-MM).[2,3] The dichotomy separation of MM into these two entities is appealing from the didactic perspective and is clearly substantiated by an extensive body of literature. The biologic basis for the dichotomy is not clear, and enough exceptions exist so that it only reflects a broad distinction to what appears to be different pathogenetic pathways for clonal plasma cell proliferation.

The first observations of this dichotomy were made by Smadja and colleagues through the careful analysis of a series of MM cases with abnormal metaphases.[2] They were able to observe that one-half of MM cases appeared to be close to the diploid karyotype, with some versions exhibiting duplications resulting in the 4N versions of the tumor (originally called hypodiploid and hyperdiploid MM). In contrast, the other half of patients have multiple trisomies resulting in a median chromosome count of 53. Subsequently, Debes-Marun and others identified recurrent patterns of chromosome aberrations being present in these two subsets, confirming some homogeneity between all NH-MM leading to the current designation.[3] Furthermore, our group was the first to show that this dichotomy is largely dictated by the segregation of the recurrent IgH translocations with NH-MM.[4] This close association, in addition to the recurrent patterns of association, has led to the currently accepted model that MM can be divided into these two broad categories[4,5] (Figure 1.1).

It is worth noting at this point that the dichotomy has high relevance for the clinical implications of genetic features in MM; the prognosis overall of H-MM is better than that of NH-MM, although greater precision is required for clinical decision making. This more indolent nature of H-MM, and a presumed greater dependency on the bone marrow microenvironment for growth, has precluded the establishment of human cell lines from H-MM as first proposed by us.[4] This, of course, becomes highly relevant, given the implications for the applicability of preclinical work done using cell lines mostly representing NH-MM.

The two pathways also have implications with regard to baseline clinicopathologic features. While most patients with H-MM have evident bone lesions, a substantial minority of NH-MM [up to 50% of cases with t(4;14)(p16;q32)] have no lytic bone lesions (Table 1.1). This is likely an explanation of why bone lesions, despite being a

TABLE 1.1. Prevalence of bone disease by genetic category in multiple myeloma

Series	N	H-MM (%)	NH-MM (%)	P value
Fonseca	365	35/220 (84)	39/145 (73)	0.012
t(4;14)(p16.3;q32)			62	NS
t(14;16)(q32;q23)			54	NS
t(11;14)(q13;q32)			62	NS
Keats	205			
t(4;14)(p16.3;q32)			19/29 (66)	NS
Bergsagel (MRI)	172	62/70 (89)	74/102 (73)	
t(4;14)(p16.3;q32)			16/28 (57)	0.002
t(14;16)(q32;q23)			6/11 (55)	0.04
t(11;14)(q13;q32)			30/32 (94)	0.02
Stewart	72			
t(4;14)(p16.3;q32)			6/11 (55)	0.72

NS, not significant; MRI, magnetic resonance imaging

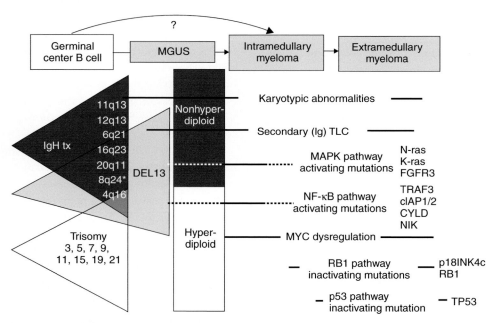

Figure 1.1. Multistep molecular pathogenesis of multiple myeloma (MM). A minimum number of intermediates in the MM pathogenesis pathway are depicted. Horizontal lines indicate the approximate timing of specific oncogenic events, with solid lines indicating the most likely time that these events will occur. MGUS: monoclonal gammopathy of undetermined significance.

sign of advanced disease, have not emerged as an important prognostic factor for MM (i.e., because NH-MM, the more aggressive variant, frequently lacks bone lesions). As one more example, one must remember that plasma cell leukemia, the most aggressive variant of all MM, is rarely associated with bone lesions.[6] Hyperdiploid MM is traditionally associated with a more indolent disease, present in higher frequency in elderly male patients, and with a bias for usage of IgG kappa (κ) monoclonal proteins.[7-10] Again this is likely an explanation of IgA and lambda (λ) monoclonal proteins as negative prognostic factors (being more common in NH-MM).

The dichotomy between H-MM and NH-MM is evident beginning in the very early stages of the disease.[11] Our group demonstrated, using a validated FISH base scoring system, that one-half of the monoclonal gammopathy of undetermined significance (MGUS) and smoldering MM (SMM) cases show evidence of H-MM (or H-MGUS), while the recurrent IgH translocations are more common in cases with NH-MM (or NH-MGUS).[11] This observation further supports the primordial importance of the biology for the two main subgroups. Furthermore, we have recently established, albeit with a limited number of cases studied, that the overall ploidy category does not change over time.[12] That is, the majority (if not all) of the patients with H-MM will remain H-MM throughout the course of the disease.

PRIMARY GENETIC LESIONS

Immunoglobulin (Ig) translocations

Some original karyotype studies had identified the presence of Ig heavy-chain (IgH) translocations in patients with MM.[13-15] However, the recurrent partners to these translocations were not readily identified. The only partner that was evident was chromosome 11q13, a translocation easily visible in informative karyotypes.[16] Because the majority of translocation partners had not been identified, no specific clinical or prognostic associations had been associated with these abnormalities. Initially the t(11;14)(q13;q32) was believed to be associated with more aggressive disease, but this was merely due to the fact that patients with karyotype abnormalities, any abnormality, have a more proliferative clone and greater degree of bone marrow involvement.[16] The notion of IgH translocations driving the pathogenesis of MM was appealing since they have been associated with the pathogenesis of many other B-cell neoplasms.[17]

In 1995 and 1996, seminal papers were published by Bergsagel, Kuehl, and colleagues, in which they were able to demonstrate that the majority of human MM cell lines harbor IgH translocations, involving the switch regions, presumptively occurring at the time of Ig class switching.[18,19] This was the first indication that IgH translocations could be more common in MM than was previously suspected. Subsequent work by their team demonstrated that two previously unrecognized translocations, t(4;14)(p16;q32)

and t(14;16)(q32;q23), were each present in 25% of the human MM cell lines.[20-22] Chesi reported that the genes *FGFR3/MMSET* and *c-MAF* were upregulated respectively in the case of these translocations and by juxtaposition of these genes to the enhancer elements of the IgH genes.[20-22] Nishida and colleagues used a strategy to detect IgH translocations in primary patient samples (without regard to the chromosome partner) and were able to show that up to 75% of cases had this abnormality (a fraction now known to be higher than the usual ~50%).[23]

t(11;14)(q13;q32) and CCND3 translocations

The t(11;14)(q13;q32) is the most common chromosome translocation in MM, present in 15%-18% of cases.[24,25] This translocation results in the upregulation of cyclin D1 (CCND1) with presumptive signaling promoting cell proliferation.[26] The translocation also results in upregulation of another gene *MYEOV*, although the consequences of this have not been fully elucidated.[27] The translocation is present (as are all other translocations) in the premalignant stages of the disease, with studies reporting a prevalence in MGUS of up to 25% of cases.[28,29] This indicates that it is not sufficient to promote malignant transformation of plasma cells. However, the translocation is unique among MM genetic changes in that it can be the sole genetic aberration in karyotypes, and it is associated usually with diploidy, likely indicating the need of few genetic changes allowing clonal evolution.[14,15,30]

The translocation has some unique association with clinicopathologic features such as lymphoplasmacytic morphology, light-chain-only disease, CD20 cell surface expression, and lambda light-chain gene use.[24,25,31] Overall, patients with t(11;14)(q13;q32) seem to have a more favorable outcome, but most series not showing the magnitude of this trend are such that they reach statistical significance.[24,25] However, this group is heterogeneous, with some patients having aggressive disease. One study by gene expression profiling showed two subtypes of t(11;14)(q13;q32) possibly dissecting some that would exhibit more aggressive disease.[32] Another IgH translocation that involves cyclin D3 (CCND3) has been described in 5% of MM cases.[33] While the clinicopathologic implications for this translocation are unknown, it is presumed to be similar to t(11;14)(q13;q32) since at the gene expression level the patterns are nearly identical between the two subgroups.[34]

t(4;14)(p16;q32)

The t(4;14)(p16;q32) is cytogenetically cryptic such that its detection by karyotype is impossible and it requires FISH, RT-PCR, or gene expression profiling for its detection.[20,22,30] Chesi and colleagues discovered this translocation in the human MM cell lines.[20,22] The translocation results in the increased expression of FGFR3 and MMSET.[20,22] In up to 25% of cases the translocation is unbalanced, always with loss of der14 and consequent loss of expression of FGFR3.[35] The translocation is unique in that it is the only one amenable for detection using RT-PCR strategies.[22,35,36] The orientation of the *MMSET* and *IgG* genes results in a hybrid transcript (IgH-MMSET and MMSET-IgH) that can be detected in the bone marrow and blood of patients with t(4;14)(p16;q32).[22,35-38] This assay has been used at the research level for diagnostic and disease-monitoring purposes.[22,35-38]

The t(4;14)(p16;q32) is known to be present in 15% of MM cases and to be associated with more aggressive disease.[24,35,39] Patients with t(4;14)(p16;q32) have not derived benefit from intensive therapy with high doses of melphalan.[24,40-42] Patients with t(4;14)(p16;q32) who undergo a single stem cell transplant will usually experience relapse in less than one year and will usually be refractory to alkylators and steroids.[24,40-42] Only recently, bortezomib has emerged as a possible agent capable of inducing disease control in this subset of the disease.[43-45] The failure with current therapies has led to the development of novel strategies targeting this translocation. A small molecule inhibitor of FGFR3 showed preclinical activity in human MM cell lines with t(4;14)(p16;q32).[46,47] While preliminary analysis did not show clinically significant activity against the disease, this study exemplifies what in all likelihood will be the future of MM treatments: targeted approaches against the driving genetic lesions.

Patients with t(4;14)(p16;q32) in MM cases are enriched with IgA λ usage and have a high prevalence of chromosome 13 deletions/monosomy.[24,35,39,48,49] This has been recently implicated as the reason for the negative associations between chromosome 13 deletions and prognosis: that chromosome 13 deletion is a surrogate (if not perfect) marker for t(4;14)(p16;q32). While the t(4;14)(p16;q32) is also observed in the premalignant stages of the disease, it appears to be less common in patients with MGUS and somewhat more enriched in SMM.[28,29] This would be a possible explanation for the often cited clinical notion (without much supporting evidence) that MM progressing from SMM is more aggressive [perhaps because of the underlying t(4;14)(p16;q32) biology].

t(14;16)(q32;q23) and other MAF translocations

The last main group of IgH translocations involves the family of *MAF* genes.[21,32] The most common translocation, also discovered by Chesi, Bergsagel, and colleagues is the t(14;16)(q32;q23).[21] This translocation is present in 5% of MM cases and is associated with a more aggressive clinical course.[39,50] Two variants exist that involve MAFa and MAFb but are very rare and only involve less than 2% of cases. It is likely (although currently unknown) that these two translocations will also exhibit the same clinical associations described with t(14;16)(q32;q23).[50-52] Like the t(4;14)(p16;q32) patients with MAF, translocations are more frequently associated with IgA λ proteins and have a tendency for enrichment for chromosome 13 deletions.[39,50]

Other translocations

Several other translocations have been implicated in MM pathogenesis, but none of them are present in a sufficient proportion of cases to know what the clinical implications are. Except for those involving MYC (see below), they will not be discussed further in this chapter.

Trisomies

Aneuploidy is common in MM, but specific patterns are evident.[7,11] In particular, trisomies are the hallmark of cases of H-MM. While there is evidence of ongoing genomic instability in MM, demonstrated by monosomies and trisomies of all chromosomes, it is only trisomies that are seen in a significant proportion of cases and reproducibly identified by several studies.[7,11,53] That is, genomic instability alone cannot explain the patterns of predilection for trisomies observed in H-MM.[3] Patients with H-MM have trisomies that involve most of the odd-numbered chromosomes, particularly chromosomes 9, 11, and 15. It is notable that trisomy of chromosome 13 is almost never observed (<1% of cases).[3] What drives the establishment of trisomies as oncogenic events, and how they contribute to MM pathogenesis, remains unknown. It is presumed now that trisomies contribute in a gene dosage fashion in promoting cell

Subtype	Prevalence %	Genetics	CCND upregulated	Prognosis
11q13	15	t(11;14)(q13;q32)	D1	Better
4p16	15	t(4;14)(p16;q32)	D2	Poor
MAF	6	t(14;16)(q32;q23)	D2	Poor
D1	42	H-MM	D1	Better
D1 + D2	10	H-MM ?	D1 + D2	Unknown
D2	10	Unknown	D2	Unknown
None	2	Unknown	None	Unknown

TABLE 1.2. Translocation-cyclin (TC) classification of myeloma

survival and proliferation. It appears that several trisomies are required for the establishment of H-MM, so complex interactions must operate in sustaining the clone.[7]

TRANSLOCATION-CYCLIN CLASSIFICATION

A proposal by Kuehl and Bergsagel has been made that almost all MM cases can be said to have a uniform pattern of upregulation of genes associated with the cell cycle (Table 1.2).[34,51] This classification, the translocation-cyclin (TC) classification, identifies all MM subtypes characterized by a translocation plus evidence of three cyclin D genes upregulation.[34,51] Patients with H-MM are characterized by increased expression of CCND1, at levels substantially lower than those observed in t(11;14)(q13;q32), but CCND1 is not expressed in normal plasma cells.[34,51] Patients with the "high-risk" translocations, t(4;14)(p16;q32) and t(14;16)(q32;q23), have downstream upregulation of CCND2. There are two more ill-defined categories of patients with both CCND1 and CCND2 upregulation and patients with none of the aforementioned abnormalities.[34,51] Provocatively, half of the patients lacking cyclin D expression appear to have no expression of RB (see below), consistent with biallelic deletion, and strongly supporting the role of cyclinD/RB dysregulation in the pathogenesis of MM (Bergsagel, unpublished).

CHROMOSOME 13 DELETION

The first specific genetic lesions associated with prognostic significance in MM were chromosome 13 abnormalities, namely deletions and monosomies. These were identified by the group from the University of Arkansas as associated with shorter survival.[54,55] While previous work by Dewald and others had identified any metaphase abnormalities

with poor prognosis,[15] chromosome 13 abnormalities were the first specific lesions to be identified.

Chromosome 13 deletions are present in roughly one-half of all MM cases.[56-59] It has been subsequently determined that, unlike CLL, MM chromosome 13 abnormalities are mostly monosomies (85% of cases) and less commonly interstitial deletions.[56,57] Fully elucidating the prognostic contribution of chromosome 13 deletions is complicated because of its tight association with high-risk genetic lesions such as t(4;14)(p16;q32). It is assumed now, although not conclusively shown, that the negative prognostic implications of chromosome 13 deletions are due to these associations. Chromosome 13 abnormalities are present in MGUS.[28,60-62]

Many features suggest that indeed chromosome 13 deletions are important in the pathogenesis of MM, including its clonal selection, recurrent nature, high prevalence in some groups such as t(4;14)(p16;q32), and prognostic implications. It is notable that while many chromosomes are trisomic, trisomy of chromosome 13 is exceedingly rare. The area of minimal deletion of 13 is not fully elucidated and is still under investigation.[56,57,63] Others have suggested *TRIM13* as the putative tumor suppressor gene deleted in cases with chromosome 13 abnormalities.[64] In our group we have continued to focus on *Rb* as a putative tumor suppressor gene implicated in chromosome 13 deletions. We have found it to be associated with a level of expression that is dose dependent (R Fonseca, unpublished). We have found that introduction of *Rb* slows down cell growth, while reduction in the level of *Rb* expression results in cell growth acceleration. These and other studies continue to explore the role of other genes located in chromosome 13 as pathogenic in MM (R Fonseca, unpublished).

PROGRESSION GENETIC EVENTS

A number of genetic events are believed to play a significant role in the pathogenesis of MM. As has been discussed, the primary genetic events are present in MGUS, many times in cases without progression for more than a decade. As such, they are insufficient to promote full malignant behavior of the clone. Therefore, it is believed that other factors will facilitate additional cell proliferation or survival.

Most of the factors believed to be secondary will be present across most of the primary genetic subtypes. That is, while, in general, translocations are mutually exclusive, secondary genetic events can be seen in many of the subtypes of the disease, even if clustered or biased for some. It is possible, yet not known, that some genetic events are primarily associated with progression for certain genetic subtypes. For instance, the only factor convincingly believed to be associated with progression from MGUS to MM is *ras* mutational status.[65-68] Most recently, we and others have shown that ras mutations are more common in patients with t(11;14)(q13;q32) and less so in the other "high-risk" translocations subtypes[69] (Chng et al., in press, Leukemia).

Deletions of 17p13 and p53 inactivation

Deletions of 17p13 have emerged as very important prognostic factors for MM.[24,39,41,70-73] Multiple series have shown that patients harboring 17p13 deletions, most of them involving *p53*, have shortened survival and more aggressive disease features.[24,39,41,70-74] Deletions are present in only 10% of cases at the time of diagnosis and are associated with shorter survival, hypercalcemia, extramedullary plasmacytomas, CNS disease, and circulating plasma cells (a feature known to predict for aggressive disease behavior).[24,39,41,70-74] In the majority of cases of MM with 17p13 deletion there is no concurrent mutation of *p53*, yet patients with and without mutations still exhibit aggressive disease behavior.[74] We have recently observed that in almost all cases of plasma cell leukemia there is inactivation of *p53*.[75] We have hypothesized that MM cells are capable of surviving in the absence of bone marrow microenvironment signaling but normally undergo apoptosis upon loss of this signaling in the presence of normal *p53* function. Yet, when cells lose this signaling they become emancipated from the bone marrow signaling, spill into the peripheral blood for circulation, form extramedullary tumoral masses (plasmacytomas), and result in a clinical phenotype of aggressive and nonresponsive disease.

NF-κB abnormalities

We have recently described a series of genetic aberrations whose common consequence is the upregulation of the NF-κB signaling pathway (we think predominantly the noncanonical pathway) (Figure 1.2).[76] Through a number of mechanisms, positive regulators are hyperactive (by amplification or translocation) and negative regulators are downregulated (by deletion or combination of deletion and mutation). The net result is increased signaling of NF-κB, documented by increased processing of p100 to p52, and the survival consequences associated with the transcriptional factor effects associated with NF-κB. While the exact prevalence of these genetic aberrations is not known, we currently believe that up to 25% of MM cases have specific genetic changes leading to the hyperactivation of NF-κB. As one such example we derived, using gene expression profiling data, an index, we believe, indicates the level of NF-κB activity.[76] Using this index we observe that 50% of MM cases exhibit increased NF-κB expression. In half of these cases we find the specific genetic causes for this activation and in the other half they are yet to be determined.

Further studies of the significance of the abnormality have revealed that in human MM cell lines and primary patient samples with the genetic changes, one consistently observes the downstream consequences predicted by these aberrations. Furthermore, in cases with inactivation of these tumor suppressors (e.g., TRAF3 by biallelic deletion), reintroduction of wild-type TRAF3 abrogates the increased processing of p100 to p52. These genetic changes are all distributed evenly across the major genetic subtypes of the disease, implying their acquisition as progression events in the disease. In summary, the cumulative evidence suggests the important role of constitutive NF-κB activation in the pathogenesis of plasma cell neoplasms. Clinically this also may be of importance in predicting the likelihood of response to therapy. Certain therapeutics, but particularly the proteasome inhibitors, are believed to induce apoptosis by deregulating the complex interactions associated with NF-κB survival signaling in MM.[77] Accordingly our hypothesis has been that cases with constitutive NF-κB activation should be more dependent on its continued activation for cell survival, and that disrupting this pathway would be more likely to induce cell apoptosis and death, leading to better clinical outcomes. One opportunity to test this hypothesis existed in the context of a pharmacogenomic study associated with a large phase 3 clinical trial of bortezomib in patients with relapsed/refractory MM.[78] Many patients treated in this clinical trial had samples submitted so that GEP was performed. Since

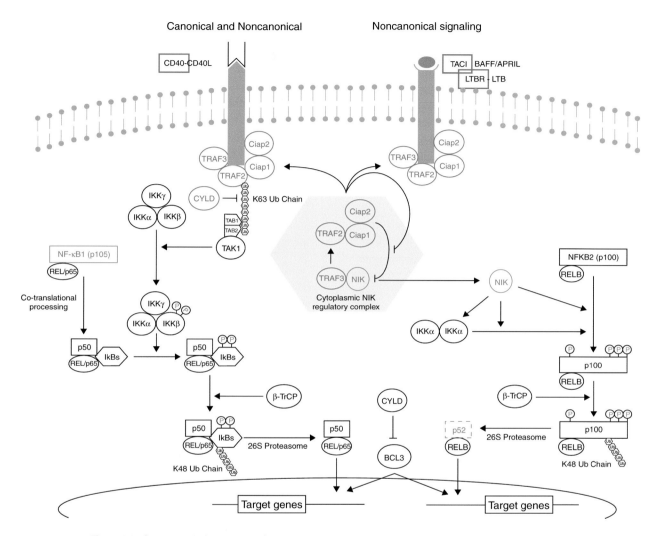

Figure 1.2. Cartoon depicting the genes found by genetic mechanisms contributing to constitutive activation of the NF-κB pathway. Genes depicted in green are those tumor suppressor genes inactivated by deletion and mutation or biallelic deletion. Genes depicted in red are positive regulators of the pathway with increased activity as a consequence of chromosome translocation or amplification. Reproduced with permission from Keats, J et al. *Cancer Cell* 2007; 12(2):131-44.

we did not have DNA available, we could only look at cases with a very low level of TRAF3 as a surrogate for cases with constitutive NF-κB activation.[76] Using an ROI-derived cut-off value for the level of expression of TRAF3 of 0.6, patients were separated into "low" and "normal TRAF3" levels of expression. Patients who had the normal TRAF3 activity exhibited the usual response rate to bortezomib (~35%), while patients with low levels of TRAF3 expression exhibited a 90% response rate. While these studies can only be considered preliminary, they highlight the real potential

for using genetic categories as predictors of clinical benefit of specific therapies.

One of the major challenges in the clinical applicability of these new findings will be their conversion to practical tools to be used with clinical diagnostic samples. In our original studies mutations were detected in at least 14 NF-κB-associated genes (including true mutations, deletions, translocations, amplifications, etc.).[76] Accordingly, a comprehensive genomic approach is not feasible in the clinic. Our aforementioned GEP-derived NF-κB index is not fully validated for clinical use and is awaiting confirmation of larger studies that combine a comprehensive genomic approach of mutation detection alongside gene expression profiling. Furthermore, it is unlikely that GEP will ever be a practical diagnostic tool for MM. It is then that a functional readout of the consequences of increased NF-κB activity is needed. In all cases where we found mutations we found by Western blot an increased processing of p100 to p52. Performing a Western blot with clinical samples will be complicated, given the requirement of cell selection. Thus, we are left with slide or flow-based, single-cell analysis for evidence of hyperactivation of NF-κB. We have tested and published the use of immunohistochemistry and immunofluorescence to detect nuclear localization of NF-κB in MM cells. Potentially, flow-cytometric-based strategies could also be used but can only be done prospectively since they require fresh samples.

MYC abnormalities

Translocations that involve an MYC gene are rare or absent in MGUS but occur in 15% of MM tumors, 44% of advanced tumors, and nearly 90% of HMCL. Mostly, these rearrangements involve c-MYC, but about 2% of primary tumors ectopically express N-MYC (and presumably have N-MYC translocations, as confirmed in some cases), and an L-MYC rearrangement has been identified only in one HMCL. These translocations, often heterogeneous in primary tumors, are usually complex rearrangements or insertions, sometimes involving three different chromosomes.[32,79-81] An Ig locus is involved in 25% of these translocations: The IgH locus is involved somewhat more than the Igλ locus, but the Igκ locus is only rarely involved.[79] Thus MYC rearrangements are thought to represent a progression event that occurs at a time when MM tumors are becoming less stromal cell dependent and/or more proliferative, whereas biallelic c-MYC expression stimulated by IL-6 and other cytokines occurs at earlier phases of tumorigenesis. Important questions about the role of MYC translocations in MM are raised by two observations. First, Avet-Loiseau and his colleagues found that MYC translocations were rare in primary plasma cell leukemia, a surprising result given the high prevalence in advanced primary tumors and HMCL that are derived from primary and secondary plasma cell leukemia.[82] Second, a large study by Avet-Loiseau and colleagues showed no effect of

MYC rearrangements on prognosis.[83] Unfortunately, they were not able to determine if MYC/Ig rearrangements affect prognosis. In contrast, in an analysis of 596 patients at Arkansas for which GEP data was deposited, patients with tumors that express N-MYC (presumably as a result of a translocation) or express very high levels of c-MYC (normalized value > 4) had a significantly poorer survival than the entire group of patients (WM Kuehl, personal communication). In the C57BL/6 strain of mice, that is predisposed to develop MGUS, late activation of a MYC transgene universally leads to MM, indicating a causative role of MYC dysregulation in the progression of MGUS to MM.[84]

Chromosome 1 abnormalities

A number of labs have determined by a combination of FISH, array comparative genomic hybridization (aCGH), and gene expression profiling (GEP) that there is a gain of sequences – and corresponding increased gene expression – at 1q21 in 30%-40% of tumors. These gains are concentrated substantially in those tumors that have a t(4;14) or t(14;16), or have a high proliferation expression index.[85-87] Although not formally proven by examination of paired samples, the gain of chromosome 1q21 sequences may occur de novo in tumors with t(4;14) or t(14;16) translocations, but is associated with tumor progression and an increased proliferative capacity in other tumors. It has been proposed that the increased proliferation in tumors with gain of 1q21 sequences is due to the increased expression of CKS1B as a result of an increased copy number.[88] One might expect to find other mechanisms, such as localized amplification or a translocation, if increased CKS1B expression is a cause of increased proliferation, but there is no evidence for other mechanism to increase CKS1B expression. Furthermore, CKS1B expression correlates closely with the expression of a number of proliferation genes in a wide variety of tumors where it appears to be a consequence rather then a cause of the proliferation. So, it seems prudent to remain skeptical that CKS1B is the gene targeted by gain of 1q21 sequences.

A large study from UAMS established that 1q21 amplification detected by FISH is a significant and independent poor prognostic factor.[87] However, another study from the Mayo Clinic shows that while significantly associated with poor prognosis on univariate analysis, 1q21 gain was not an independent prognostic factor on Cox proportional hazard analysis.[86] The discrepancies in the results from UAMS and the Mayo Clinic in terms of the independent prognostic impact of 1q21 gain by FISH may be related to differences in the factors included in the Cox proportional hazard analysis. In the Mayo Clinic analysis, the prognostic impact of 1q21 gain was no longer significant when the plasma cell labeling index and t(4;14) were included in the modeling, suggesting that much of the prognostic impact of 1q21 gain on univariate analysis is mediated through its close association with poor risk genetics and proliferative disease.[86]

As mentioned earlier, *CKS1B* has been implicated as the candidate gene on 1q21 mediating biological and prognostic impact. However, when the relative prognostic strength of 1q21 copy gain and increase *CKS1B* expression is analyzed in a multivariate model, 1q21 copy gain is the more significant prognostic factor.[86] Therefore, the overall evidence that a critical gene located on 1q21 may be causatively involved in mediating progression and prognosis is weak. Instead, it appears more likely that chromosome 1q amplification is a marker of more clonally advanced and genomically unstable tumors that are more likely to progress. The gains on 1q are frequently associated with deletions of 1p, which has also been associated with a poor prognosis.[89,90]

p16 and p18 abnormalities

It is conceivable and logical that additional hits favoring cell cycle progression could be implicated in the pathogenesis of MM. Inactivation of *p16* via methylation has been observed in up to 50% of MM cases and has been reported as associated in possible familial associations of MM.[91-95] Deletions of *p16* are uncommon.[93] We have recently found that the presence of *p16* methylation confers no significant prognostic association, and thus its role in the pathogenesis of the disease remains unknown.[93] Two recent studies showed that most MM tumors express little or no p16, regardless of whether the gene is methylated.[95,96] This suggests that low expression mostly is not due to methylation, which may be an epi-phenomenon. Despite one example of an individual with a germline mutation and loss of the normal p16 allele in MM tumor cells,[97] it remains unclear if inactivation of p16 is a critical and presumably early event in the pathogenesis of MM.

In contrast, it seems apparent that inactivation of *p18INK4C*, a critical gene for normal plasma cell development, is likely to contribute to increased proliferation. Biallelic deletions of p18 have been observed in 10% of MM

cases and are also believed to be involved in the pathogenesis of the disease.[98-101] Forced expression of p18INK4C by retroviral infection of HMCL that express little or no endogenous p18 substantially inhibits proliferation. Paradoxically, about 60% of HMCL and 60% of the more proliferative MM tumors have increased expression of p18 compared to normal plasma cells. There is evidence that the E2F transcription factor, which is upregulated in association with increased proliferation, increases the expression of p18, presumably as a feedback mechanism. Apart from the lack of a functional RB1 protein in approximately 10% of HMCL, the mechanism(s) by which most HMCL and proliferative tumors become insensitive to increased p18 levels is not yet understood.

High-risk gene expression profiling

The advent of gene expression profiling has allowed further refinements to our ability to prognosticate patients. In particular, the group from the University of Arkansas has been able to identify a genetic signature indicative of "high-risk" disease and present in 15% of MM cases (Figure 1.3).[50] These individuals were characterized by evidence of high proliferative disease and included patients with many of the major genetic categories.[50] The signature initially was derived from a composite analysis of 70 genes but could subsequently be reduced to 17 genes. The conversion of this signature to practical clinical tools could allow identification of cases with more aggressive disease. The correlations of the signature with other validated clinical methods of proliferations assessment such as flow-based S-phase and the plasma cell labeling index would be of great interest. In any case this signature has been internally validated by the same group and others,[102] and identifies cases with more aggressive disease. Other means to identify genetic signatures of aggressive disease such as a centrosome index have also been postulated.[103]

CLINICAL IMPLICATIONS OF GENETIC SUBTYPES

High-risk disease patients have had shorter survival whether treated by conventional forms of alkylator therapy or with high-dose therapy with stem cell support. These observations lead to the recommendations by our group

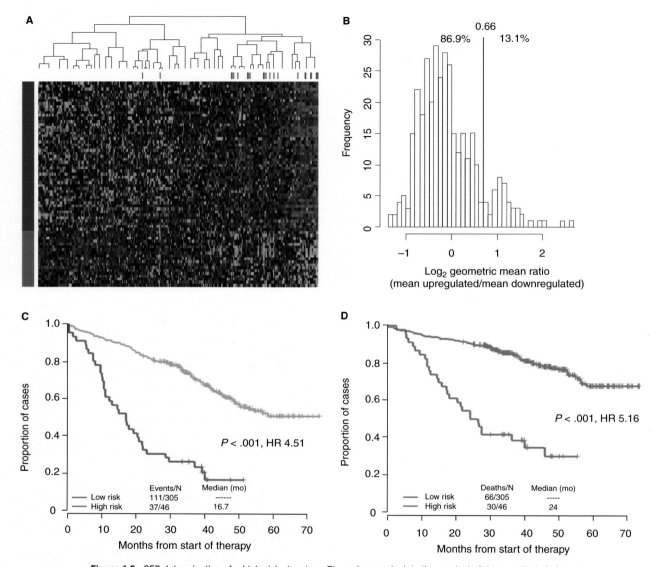

Figure 1.3. GEP determination of a high-risk signature. The red curve depicts the survival of these patients being substantially shorter than that of patients without the signatures. Reproduced with permission from Shaughnessy, JD et al. *Blood* 2007; 109(6):2276-84.

that patients with high-risk MM derive less benefit from the latter intervention and should be considered for alternative management strategies.[104]

Consensus clinical implications: high-risk disease

There is a need to develop clinically applicable tests to identify patients with more aggressive disease.[104] To this effect our

group has proposed the establishment of a molecular cytogenetic classification based high-risk disease (Figure 1.4).[104] This group is composed, at the genetic level, of patients with t(4;14)(p16;q32), t(14;16)(q32;q23) or 17p13 deletions. The group is composed of nearly 25%-30% of MM cases and, traditionally, would have identified groups of patients with a median survival of 2 years or less. We also recognize other means by which a patient can, and should, be identified as being in the high-risk genetic category and include

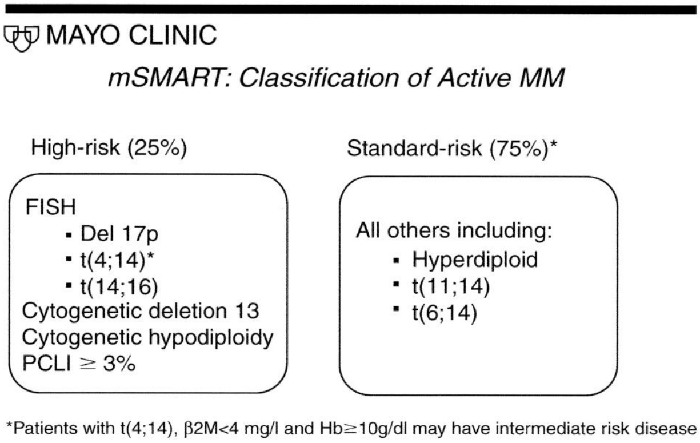

✛ MAYO CLINIC
mSMART: Classification of Active MM

High-risk (25%)   Standard-risk (75%)*

FISH
- Del 17p
- t(4;14)*
- t(14;16)
Cytogenetic deletion 13
Cytogenetic hypodiploidy
PCLI ≥ 3%

All others including:
- Hyperdiploid
- t(11;14)
- t(6;14)

*Patients with t(4;14), β2M<4 mg/l and Hb≥10g/dl may have intermediate risk disease

Figure 1.4. mSMART risk-stratification
Source: Mayo Clinic

hypodiploidy by karyotype, chromosome 13 deletion or monosomy by karyotype, and a high plasma cell labeling index (>3%). The importance of this notion is that the classification not only identifies MM patients with high-risk disease and with greater likelihood of dying earlier, but it does so by identifying clone-specific factors (as opposed to host features).

Based on this classification we now recommend a tailored treatment approach that considers genetic risk at the time of management decision.[105] This algorithm requires early determination of risk category and assumes that stem cell transplant is still a viable option for a subset of patients. In patients who are candidates for stem cell transplant, induction is initiated with while risk category is determined. Patients with standard risk disease can be treated with either standard stem cell transplant or continued on the same induction therapy. In contrast, we believe that patients with high-risk disease should consider early introduction of a bortezomib-containing regimen such as melphalan, prednisone (MP), and bortezomib.[105] In patients who are not stem cell transplant candidates the mainstay of therapy remains based on melphalan and prednisone. However, in cases with low-risk disease one might consider a regimen such as MP plus thalidomide and on patients with high-risk disease one might consider MP plus bortezomib. These two regimens (and others containing lenalidomide) have not been directly compared; these recommendations are based on currently available best data.

The t(11;14)(q13;q32) and MM-associated conditions

Plasma cell leukemia

Patients with plasma cell leukemia can be classified as those who present de novo with the diagnosis (primary plasma cell leukemia) versus those that progress to extramedullary disease after having being diagnosed with MM (secondary plasma cell leukemia).[6,75,106] In both instances we believe a major factor driving the presence of high numbers of circulating plasma cells is the inactivation of *p53*.[75] In a recent study we reported that nearly 75% of cases have some form of *p53* inactivation.[75] In the case of primary plasma cell leukemia we have found that the majority of cases harbor t(11;14)(q13;q32).[75,106] This serves as an example of how, despite normally being more benign, selected cases with t(11;14)(q13;q32) exhibit aggressive clone growth features.[75,106]

Light-chain amyloidosis

Nearly one-half of cases with light-chain amyloidosis (AL) harbor t(11;14)(q13;q32).[107,108] The majority of cases with AL have minimal plasmacytosis, with one-third of patients having no measurable monoclonal proteins.[109]

IgM MM

It has been recently recognized that IgM MM exists as an entity that is distinct from Waldenström macroglobulinemia.[110,111] Avet-Loiseau and colleagues showed that the majority of cases with IgM MM harbor t(11;14)(q13;q32)[111] while we have shown that IgH translocations never occur in the clonal cells of Waldenström macroglobulinemia.[111] In this last entity the only recurrent genomic abnormality is deletion of the long arm of chromosome 6.[111]

Progression from MGUS to MM

Until now no specific prognostic or predictive ability for progression from MGUS to MM has been associated with specific genetic abnormalities. Most of the major genetic aberrations detectable in MM can also been observed in MGUS. Two notable exceptions are deletions of 17p13 and rearrangements of MYC, which appear to be rare in MGUS (R. Fonseca, unpublished). There is still some controversy regarding the prevalence of chromosome 13 deletions in MGUS. Some studies have suggested a similar prevalence in MGUS as in MM,[61] while others showed similar rates in both states.[60,62] More recent data from our group suggests that the prevalence of chromosome 13 deletions is lower in MGUS than in MM.

TABLE 1.3. Testing for high-risk cytogenetic abnormalities

FISH tests	Prognosis	Other value and comments
Minimal genetic testing (Essential tests)		
t(4;14)(p16;q32)	Poor	Delaying HSCT
t(14;16)(q32;q23)	Poor	Delaying HSCT
17p13 deletions	Poor	Delaying HSCT
		Drug resistance and extramedullary disease
Comprehensive panel		
t(11;14)(q13;q32)	Better	Differentiating IgM MM; AL and MM diagnosis.
H-MM	Better	Clinicopathologic features.
		Standard risk defined
Chromosome 13	Intermediate	Good prognostic markers if combined with β_2-microglobulin or PCLI
IgH Trx	Variable	Negative prognosis for H-MM in one study
Test not routinely done		
Other IgH Trx	Presumed poor	Rarity makes testing low yield
1q amplification	Poor	Data regarding prognosis still evolving
MYC aberrations	Poor?	Complex testing strategies needed

HSCT, hematopoietic stem cell transplant; PCLI, plasma cell labeling index; Trx, translocations.

There is still a suggestion that t(11;14)(q13;q32) may be slightly more prevalent among cases with minimal plasmacytosis, most evident in AL.[107,108] Indeed AL represents clonal plasma cell proliferations that become clinically evident because of the induction of complications. Thus the clinical phenotype unmasks states of plasmacytosis normally not detectable. With as many as 50% of AL patients having t(11;14)(q13;q32) this would suggest that the abnormality is negatively selected for progression from earlier states of plasmacytosis. Given it takes 1×10^9 expansion for MGUS to be detectable, it is only logical to speculate that many more individuals harbor clonal plasma cells at levels below current methods for detection (except those having AL complications). It is then that one can hypothesize that many more individuals in the population could harbor t(11;14)(q13;q32) (for instance at levels of expansion of 1×10^7 or less levels). And if indeed t(11;14)(q13;q32) is negatively selected for progression we would suggest that for all states of plasmacytosis this would be by far the most common genetic aberration in MM.

In contrast, there is also a suggestion that t(4;14)(p16;q32) is less common among MGUS cases than in MM.[29,35] In some instances the abnormality has been detected in cases without disease progression for many years. However, it seems that the prevalence is lower in benign clonal plasmacytosis, perhaps even biased in favor of SMM. This would suggest that once acquired a t(4;14)(p16;q32) makes the clone advance further towards malignancy and that overall (considering states of subclinical monoclonal plasmacytosis) the t(4;14)(p16;q32) is far less common than t(11;14)(q13;q32). It is likely that similar principles apply for the t(14;16)(q32;q23) but there is less data in this regard.

Minimal genetic testing

To detect the high-risk genetic features a FISH panel capable of detecting the two translocations plus chromosome 17p13 deletions is recommended (Table 1.3).[104] These assays must be done with cells that are either sorted (such as is done by the IFM) or by scoring FISH in conjunction with immunofluorescence of the cytoplasm (i.e., cIg-FISH). Assays that do not employ this methodology and only score unselected cell nuclei derived from hypotonic preparations are inadequate and lack sensitivity and specificity. At Mayo we employ a more comprehensive panel that also includes detection of H-MM, t(11;14)(q13;q32), chromosome 13 deletions, and IgH translocations (not otherwise specified). While additional testing could identify the less common versions of the IgH translocations they have not been routinely employed, given the very low prevalence of such abnormalities.

Obtaining karyotypes can also be done to ascertain risk category in MM. The main problem still is the lack of sensitivity of the test with informative metaphases only being obtained in 10%-30% of cases. When informative the presence of hypodiploidy[112] or chromosome 13 deletions has already been defined as associated with a more adverse outcome. It becomes less clear how to interpret cases where abnormal metaphases exhibit abnormalities normally associated with a better outcome such as hyperdiploidy. This becomes complicated since obtaining abnormal metaphases is a surrogate of more proliferative clones and greater extent of bone marrow involvement (even when putative favorable markers are identified).[113]

The future clinical testing for risk categories in MM is yet to be defined. The conversion of genomics driven information into practical diagnostic tools could very significantly alter the management of MM in the future. This will require the necessary conversion of these gene signatures into immunohistochemistry panels or flow cytometry panels capable of providing the same information. The issue is particularly complex in MM where the tumor cells coexist with normal marrow hematopoietic elements, necessitating selection (purification) of cells prior to any genomic analysis.

CONCLUSIONS

In conclusion, we have seen great advances in our understanding of the genetic lesions associated with disease initiation and progression. This information is currently being used to make prognostic and therapeutic decisions regarding therapy. Our current therapy algorithms take into primary consideration genetic category to ascertain risk-stratification. Furthermore, this information is now the basis for small molecule targeted therapy development. New findings suggest that a predictive pharmacogenomic approach may be used in the future to select ideal candidates for therapies such as is the case of high response to bortezomib for patients with low TRAF3 levels of expression. Despite this, much progress needs to be made to understand fully the intricate genomic interactions leading to disease pathogenesis. It is only when the picture becomes evident that a comprehensive

genome-drive-targeted therapy will be designed in a complete rational fashion. While much remains to be done, the aforementioned examples highlight the great progress in our understanding of MM biology.

REFERENCES

1. Fonseca R, Barlogie B, Bataille R, et al. Genetics and cytogenetics of multiple myeloma: a workshop report. *Cancer Res* 2004;64(4):1546-58.
2. Smadja NV, Fruchart C, Isnard F, et al. Chromosomal analysis in multiple myeloma: cytogenetic evidence of two different diseases. *Leukemia* 1998;12(6):960-9.
3. Debes-Marun C, Dewald G, Bryant S, et al. Chromosome abnormalities clustering and its implications for pathogenesis and prognosis in myeloma. *Leukemia* 2003;17(2):427-36.
4. Fonseca R, Debes-Marun CS, Picken EB, et al. The recurrent IgH translocations are highly associated with nonhyperdiploid variant multiple myeloma. *Blood* 2003;102(7):2562-7.
5. Smadja NV, Leroux D, Soulier J, et al. Further cytogenetic characterization of multiple myeloma confirms that 14q32 translocations are a very rare event in hyperdiploid cases. *Genes Chromosomes Cancer* 2003;38(3):234-9.
6. Noel P, Kyle RA. Plasma cell leukemia: an evaluation of response to therapy. *Am J Med* 1987;83(6):1062-8.
7. Chng WJ, Ketterling RP, Fonseca R. Analysis of genetic abnormalities provides insights into genetic evolution of hyperdiploid myeloma. *Genes Chromosomes Cancer* 2006;45(12):1111-20.
8. Chng WJ, Santana-Davila R, Van Wier SA, et al. Prognostic factors for hyperdiploid-myeloma: effects of chromosome 13 deletions and IgH translocations. *Leukemia* 2006;20(5):807-13.
9. Chng WJ, Kumar S, Vanwier S, et al. Molecular dissection of hyperdiploid multiple myeloma by gene expression profiling. *Cancer Res* 2007;67(7):2982-9.
10. Greipp PR, Trendle MC, Leong T, et al. Is flow cytometric DNA content hypodiploidy prognostic in multiple myeloma? *Leuk Lymphoma* 1999;35(1-2):83-9.
11. Chng WJ, Van Wier SA, Ahmann GJ, et al. A validated FISH trisomy index demonstrates the hyperdiploid and nonhyperdiploid dichotomy in MGUS. *Blood* 2005;106(6):2156-61.
12. Chng WJ, Winkler JM, Greipp PR, et al. Ploidy status rarely changes in myeloma patients at disease progression. *Leuk Res* 2006;30(3):266-71.
13. Kwong YL, Lie AK, Chan LC. Translocation (11;14)(q13;q32) and partial trisomy 1q in a case of multiple myeloma [letter]. *Am J Hematol* 1993;44(3):212-13.
14. Sawyer JR, Waldron JA, Jagannath S, Barlogie B. Cytogenetic findings in 200 patients with multiple myeloma. *Cancer Genet Cytogenet* 1995;82(1):41-9.
15. Dewald GW, Kyle RA, Hicks GA, Greipp PR. The clinical significance of cytogenetic studies in 100 patients with multiple myeloma, plasma cell leukemia, or amyloidosis. *Blood* 1985;66(2):380-90.

16. Fonseca R, Witzig TE, Gertz MA, et al. Multiple myeloma and the translocation t(11;14)(q13;q32) – a report on 13 cases. *Br J Haematol* 1998;101(2):296-301.

17. Nishida K, Taniwaki M, Misawa S, Abe T. Nonrandom rearrangement of chromosome 14 at band q32.33 in human lymphoid malignancies with mature B-cell phenotype. *Cancer Res* 1989;49(5):1275-81.

18. Bergsagel PL, Chesi M, Brents LA, Kuehl WM. Translocations into IgH switch regions – the genetic hallmark of multiple myeloma. *Blood* 1995;86(10):223-223.

19. Bergsagel PL, Chesi M, Nardini E, Brents LA, Kirby SL, Kuehl WM. Promiscuous translocations into immunoglobulin heavy chain switch regions in multiple myeloma. *Proc Natl Acad Sci USA* 1996;93(24):13931-6.

20. Chesi M, Nardini E, Brents LA, et al. Frequent translocation t(4;14)(p16.3;q32.3) in multiple myeloma is associated with increased expression and activating mutations of fibroblast growth factor receptor 3. *Nature Genet* 1997;16(3):260-4.

21. Chesi M, Bergsagel PL, Shonukan OO, et al. Frequent dysregulation of the c-maf proto-oncogene at 16q23 by translocation to an Ig locus in multiple myeloma. *Blood* 1998;91(12):4457-63.

22. Chesi M, Nardini E, Lim R, Smith K, Kuehl W, Bergsagel P. The t(4;14) translocation in myeloma dysregulates both FGFR3 and a novel gene, MMSET, resulting in IgH/MMSET hybrid transcripts. *Blood* 1998;92:3025-34.

23. Nishida K, Tamura A, Nakazawa N, et al. The Ig heavy chain gene is frequently involved in chromosomal translocations in multiple myeloma and plasma cell leukemia as detected by in situ hybridization. *Blood* 1997;90(2):526-34.

24. Avet-Loiseau H, Attal M, Moreau P, et al. Genetic abnormalities and survival in multiple myeloma: the experience of the Intergroupe Francophone du Myelome. *Blood* 2007;109(8):3489-95.

25. Fonseca R, Harrington D, Oken M, et al. Myeloma and the t(11;14)(q13;q32) represents a uniquely defined biological subset of patients. *Blood* 2002;99(10):3735-41.

26. Chesi M, Bergsagel PL, Brents LA, Smith CM, Gerhard DS, Kuehl WM. Dysregulation of cyclin D1 by translocation into an IgH gamma switch region in two multiple myeloma cell lines. *Blood* 1996;88(2):674-81.

27. Janssen JW, Vaandrager JW, Heuser T, et al. Concurrent activation of a novel putative transforming gene, myeov, and cyclin D1 in a subset of multiple myeloma cell lines with t(11;14)(q13;q32). *Blood* 2000;95(8):2691-8.

28. Avet-Loiseau H, Facon T, Daviet A, et al. 14q32 translocations and monosomy 13 observed in monoclonal gammopathy of undetermined significance delineate a multistep process for the oncogenesis of multiple myeloma. Intergroupe Francophone du Myelome. *Cancer Res* 1999;59(18):4546-50.

29. Fonseca R, Bailey RJ, Ahmann GJ, et al. Genomic abnormalities in monoclonal gammopathy of undetermined significance.[see comment]. *Blood* 2002;100(4):1417-24.

30. Sawyer JR, Lukacs JL, Thomas EL, et al. Multicolour spectral karyotyping identifies new translocations and a recurring

31. Garand R, Avet-Loiseau H, Accard F, Moreau P, Harousseau J, Bataille R. t(11;14) and t(4;14) translocations correlated with mature lymphoplasmocytoid and immature morphology, respectively, in multiple myeloma. *Leukemia* 2003;this issue.

32. Zhan F, Huang Y, Colla S, et al. The molecular classification of multiple myeloma. *Blood* 2006;108(6):2020-8.

33. Shaughnessy J Jr., Gabrea A, Qi Y, et al. Cyclin D3 at 6p21 is dysregulated by recurrent chromosomal translocations to immunoglobulin loci in multiple myeloma. *Blood* 2001;98(1):217-23.

34. Bergsagel PL, Kuehl WM, Zhan F, Sawyer J, Barlogie B, Shaughnessy J Jr. Cyclin D dysregulation: an early and unifying pathogenic event in multiple myeloma. *Blood* 2005;106(1):296-303.

35. Keats JJ, Reiman T, Maxwell CA, et al. In multiple myeloma, t(4;14)(p16;q32) is an adverse prognostic factor irrespective of FGFR3 expression. *Blood* 2003;101(4):1520-9.

36. Perfetti V, Coluccia A, Intini D, et al. Translocation t(4;14) (p16.3;q32) Is a Recurrent Genetic Lesion in Primary Amyloidosis. *Leukemia* 2001;158:1599-603.

37. Stewart JP, Thompson A, Santra M, Barlogie B, Lappin TR, Shaughnessy J Jr. Correlation of TACC3, FGFR3, MMSET and p21 expression with the t(4;14)(p16.3;q32) in multiple myeloma. *Br J Haematol* 2004;126(1):72-6.

38. Stewart AK, Chang H, Trudel S, et al. Diagnostic evaluation of t(4;14) in multiple myeloma and evidence for clonal evolution. *Leukemia* 2007;21(11):2358-9.

39. Fonseca R, Blood E, Rue M, et al. Clinical and biologic implications of recurrent genomic aberrations in myeloma. *Blood* 2003;101(11):4569-75.

40. Chang H, Sloan S, Li D, et al. The t(4;14) is associated with poor prognosis in myeloma patients undergoing autologous stem cell transplant. *Br J Haematol* 2004;125(1):64-8.

41. Chang H, Qi XY, Samiee S, et al. Genetic risk identifies multiple myeloma patients who do not benefit from autologous stem cell transplantation. *Bone Marrow Transplant* 2005;36(9):793-6.

42. Gertz MA, Lacy MQ, Dispenzieri A, et al. Clinical implications of t(11;14)(q13;q32), t(4;14)(p16.3;q32), and −17p13 in myeloma patients treated with high-dose therapy. *Blood* 2005;106(8):2837-40.

43. Mateos MV, Hernandez JM, Hernandez MT, et al. Bortezomib plus melphalan and prednisone in elderly untreated patients with multiple myeloma: results of a multicenter phase I/II study. *Blood* 2006;108(7):2165-72.

44. Jagannath S, Richardson PG, Sonneveld P, et al. Bortezomib appears to overcome the poor prognosis conferred by chromosome 13 deletion in phase 2 and 3 trials. *Leukemia* 2007;21(1):151-7.

45. Chang H, Trieu Y, Qi X, Xu W, Stewart KA, Reece D. Bortezomib therapy response is independent of cytogenetic abnormalities in relapsed/refractory multiple myeloma. *Leuk Res* 2007;31(6):779-82.

46. Trudel S, Ely S, Farooqi Y, et al. Inhibition of fibroblast growth factor receptor 3 induces differentiation and apoptosis in t(4;14) myeloma. *Blood* 2004;103(9):3521-8.

pathway for chromosome loss in multiple myeloma. *Br J Haematol* 2001;112(1):167-74.

47. Trudel S, Li ZH, Wei E, et al. CHIR-258, a novel, multitargeted tyrosine kinase inhibitor for the potential treatment of t(4;14) multiple myeloma. *Blood* 2005;105(7):2941-8.

48. Avet-Loiseau H, Facon T, Grosbois B, et al. Oncogenesis of multiple myeloma: 14q32 and 13q chromosomal abnormalities are not randomly distributed, but correlate with natural history, immunological features, and clinical presentation. *Blood* 2002;99(6):2185-91.

49. Fonseca R, Oken MM, Greipp PR. The t(4;14)(p16.3;q32) is strongly associated with chromosome 13 abnormalities in both multiple myeloma and monoclonal gammopathy of undetermined significance. *Blood* 2001;98(4):1271-2.

50. Shaughnessy JD Jr., Zhan F, Burington BE, et al. A validated gene expression model of high-risk multiple myeloma is defined by deregulated expression of genes mapping to chromosome 1. *Blood* 2007;109(6):2276-84.

51. Bergsagel PL, Kuehl WM. Critical roles for immunoglobulin translocations and cyclin D dysregulation in multiple myeloma. *Immunol Rev* 2003;194:96-104.

52. Shaughnessy JD Jr. Global gene expression profiling in the study of multiple myeloma. [Review] [94 refs]. *Int J Hematol* 2003;77(3):213-25.

53. Carrasco DR, Tonon G, Huang Y, et al. High-resolution genomic profiles define distinct clinico-pathogenetic subgroups of multiple myeloma patients. *Cancer Cell* 2006;9(4):313-25.

54. Tricot G, Barlogie B, Jagannath S, et al. Poor prognosis in multiple myeloma is associated only with partial or complete deletions of chromosome 13 or abnormalities involving 11q and not with other karyotype abnormalities. *Blood* 1995;86(11):4250-6.

55. Tricot G, Sawyer JR, Jagannath S, et al. Unique role of cytogenetics in the prognosis of patients with myeloma receiving high-dose therapy and autotransplants. *J Clin Oncol* 1997;15(7):2659-66.

56. Avet-Loiseau H, Daviet A, Saunier S, Bataille R. Chromosome 13 abnormalities in multiple myeloma are mostly monosomy 13. *Br J Haematol* 2000;111(4):1116-7.

57. Fonseca R, Oken M, Harrington D, et al. Deletions of chromosome 13 in multiple myeloma identified by interphase FISH usually denote large deletions of the q-arm or monosomy. *Leukemia* 2001;15:981-6.

58. Königsberg R, Zojer N, Ackermann J, et al. Predictive role of interphase cytogenetics for survival of patients with multiple myeloma. *J Clin Oncol* 2000;18(4):804-12.

59. Zojer N, Konigsberg R, Ackermann J, et al. Deletion of 13q14 remains an independent adverse prognostic variable in multiple myeloma despite its frequent detection by interphase fluorescence in situ hybridization. *Blood* 2000;95(6):1925-30.

60. Avet-Loiseau H, Li JY, Morineau N, et al. Monosomy 13 is associated with the transition of monoclonal gammopathy of undetermined significance to multiple myeloma. Intergroupe Francophone du Myelome. *Blood* 1999;94(8):2583-9.

61. Fonseca R, Bailey RJ, Ahmann GJ, et al. Genomic abnormalities in monoclonal gammopathy of undetermined significance. *Blood* 2002;100(4):1417-24.

62. Konigsberg R, Ackermann J, Kaufmann H, et al. Deletions of chromosome 13q in monoclonal gammopathy of undetermined significance. *Leukemia* 2000;14(11):1975-9.

63. Walker BA, Leone PE, Jenner MW, et al. Integration of global SNP-based mapping and expression arrays reveals key regions, mechanisms, and genes important in the pathogenesis of multiple myeloma. *Blood* 2006;108(5):1733-43.

64. Elnenaei MO, Hamoudi RA, Swansbury J, et al. Delineation of the minimal region of loss at 13q14 in multiple myeloma. *Genes Chromosomes Cancer* 2003;36(1):99-106.

65. Liu P, Leong T, Quam L, et al. Activating mutations of N- and K-ras in multiple myeloma show different clinical associations: analysis of the Eastern Cooperative Oncology Group Phase III Trial. *Blood* 1996;88(7):2699-706.

66. Bezieau S, Devilder MC, Avet-Loiseau H, et al. High incidence of N- and K-Ras activating mutations in multiple myeloma and primary plasma cell leukemia at diagnosis. *Hum Mutat* 2001;18(3):212-24.

67. Neri A, Murphy JP, Cro L, et al. Ras oncogene mutation in multiple myeloma. *J Exp Med* 1989;170(5):1715-25.

68. Paquette RL, Berenson J, Lichtenstein A, McCormick F, Koeffler HP. Oncogenes in multiple myeloma: point mutation of N-ras. *Oncogene* 1990;5(11):1659-63.

69. Rasmussen T, Kuehl M, Lodahl M, Johnsen HE, Dahl IM. Possible roles for activating RAS mutations in the MGUS to MM transition and in the intramedullary to extramedullary transition some plasma cell tumors. *Blood* 2005;105(1):317-23.

70. Drach J, Ackermann J, Kromer E, et al. Short survival of patients with multiple myeloma and p53 gene deletion: A study by Interphase FISH. *Blood* 1997;90:244a.

71. Drach J, Ackermann J, Fritz E, et al. Presence of a p53 gene deletion in patients with multiple myeloma predicts for short survival after conventional-dose chemotherapy. *Blood* 1998;92(3):802-9.

72. Chang H, Sloan S, Li D, Keith Stewart A. Multiple myeloma involving central nervous system: high frequency of chromosome 17p13.1 (p53) deletions. *Br J Haematol* 2004;127(3):280-4.

73. Chang H, Qi C, Yi QL, Reece D, Stewart AK. p53 gene deletion detected by fluorescence in situ hybridization is an adverse prognostic factor for patients with multiple myeloma following autologous stem cell transplantation. *Blood* 2005;105(1):358-60.

74. Chng WJ, Price-Troska T, Gonzalez-Paz N, et al. Clinical significance of TP53 mutation in myeloma. *Leukemia* 2007;21(3):582-4.

75. Tiedemann RE, Gonzalez-Paz N, Kyle RA, et al. Genetic aberrations and survival in plasma cell leukemia. *Leukemia* 2008;22(5):1044-52.

76. Keats JJ, Fonseca R, Chesi M, et al. Promiscuous mutations activate the noncanonical NF-κB pathway in multiple myeloma. *Cancer Cell* 2007;12(2):131-44.

77. Richardson PG. A review of the proteasome inhibitor bortezomib in multiple myeloma. *Expert Opin Pharmacother* 2004;5(6):1321-31.

78. Mulligan G, Mitsiades C, Bryant B, et al. Gene expression profiling and correlation with outcome in clinical trials of the proteasome inhibitor bortezomib. *Blood* 2007;109(8):3177-88.

79. Avet-Loiseau H, Gerson F, Magrangeas F, Minvielle S, Harousseau JL, Bataille R. Rearrangements of the c-myc oncogene are present in 15% of primary human multiple myeloma tumors. *Blood* 2001;98(10):3082-6.

80. Kuehl WM, Bergsagel PL. Multiple myeloma: evolving genetic events and host interactions. *Nat Rev Cancer* 2002;2(3):175-87.

81. Shou Y, Martelli ML, Gabrea A, et al. Diverse karyotypic abnormalities of the c-myc locus associated with c-myc dysregulation and tumor progression in multiple myeloma. *Proc Natl Acad Sci USA* 2000;97(1):228-33.

82. Avet-Loiseau H, Daviet A, Brigaudeau C, et al. Cytogenetic, interphase, and multicolor fluorescence in situ hybridization analyses in primary plasma cell leukemia: a study of 40 patients at diagnosis, on behalf of the Intergroupe Francophone du Myelome and the Groupe Francais de Cytogenetique Hematologique. *Blood* 2001;97(3):822-5.

83. Avet-Loiseau H, Attal M, Moreau P, et al. Genetic abnormalities and survival in multiple myeloma: the experience of the Intergroupe Francophone du Myelome. *Blood* 2007;109:3489-95.

84. Chesi M, Robbiani DF, Sebag M, et al. AID-dependent MYC activation induces multiple myeloma in a conditional mouse model of post-germinal center malignancies. *Cancer Cell* 2008;(in press).

85. Chang H, Qi X, Trieu Y, et al. Multiple myeloma patients with CKS1B gene amplification have a shorter progression-free survival post-autologous stem cell transplantation. *Br J Haematol* 2006;135(4):486-91.

86. Fonseca R, Van Wier SA, Chng WJ, et al. Prognostic value of chromosome 1q21 gain by fluorescent in situ hybridization and increase CKS1B expression in myeloma. *Leukemia* 2006;20(11):2034-40.

87. Hanamura I, Stewart JP, Huang Y, et al. Frequent gain of chromosome band 1q21 in plasma-cell dyscrasias detected by fluorescence in situ hybridization: incidence increases from MGUS to relapsed myeloma and is related to prognosis and disease progression following tandem stem cell transplantation. *Blood* 2006;108(5):1724-32.

88. Zhan F, Colla S, Wu X, et al. CKS1B, over expressed in aggressive disease, regulates multiple myeloma growth and survival through SKP2- and p27Kip1-dependent and independent mechanisms. *Blood* 2007;109(11):4995-5001.

89. Wu KL, Beverloo B, Lokhorst HM, et al. Abnormalities of chromosome 1p/q are highly associated with chromosome 13/13q deletions and are an adverse prognostic factor for the outcome of high-dose chemotherapy in patients with multiple myeloma. *Br J Haematol* 2007;136(4):615-23.

90. Chang H, Ning Y, Qi X, Yeung J, Xu W. Chromosome 1p21 deletion is a novel prognostic marker in patients with multiple myeloma. *Br J Haematol* 2007;139(1):51-4.

91. Mateos MV, Garcia-Sanz R, Lopez-Perez R, et al. Methylation is an inactivating mechanism of the p16 gene in multiple myeloma associated with high plasma cell proliferation and short survival. *Br J Haematol* 2002;118(4):1034-40.

92. Ribas C, Colleoni GW, Felix RS, et al. p16 gene methylation lacks correlation with angiogenesis and prognosis in multiple myeloma. *Cancer Lett* 2005;222(2):247-54.

93. Gonzalez-Paz N, Chng WJ, McClure RF, et al. Tumor suppressor p16 methylation in multiple myeloma: biological and clinical implications. *Blood* 2007;109:1228-32.

94. Ng MH, Chung YF, Lo KW, Wickham NW, Lee JC, Huang DP. Frequent hypermethylation of p16 and p15 genes in multiple myeloma. *Blood* 1997;89(7):2500-6.

95. Dib A, Barlogie B, Shaughnessy JD Jr., Kuehl WM. Methylation and expression of the p16INK4A tumor suppressor gene in multiple myeloma. *Blood* 2007;109(3):1337-8.

96. Gonzalez-Paz N, Chng WJ, McClure RF, et al. Tumor suppressor p16 methylation in multiple myeloma: biological and clinical implications. *Blood* 2007;109(3):1228-32.

97. Dilworth D, Liu L, Stewart AK, Berenson JR, Lassam N, Hogg D. Germline CDKN2A mutation implicated in predisposition to multiple myeloma. *Blood* 2000;95(5):1869-71.

98. Tasaka T, Berenson J, Vescio R, et al. Analysis of the p16INK4A, p15INK4B and p18INK4C genes in multiple myeloma. *Br J Haematol* 1997;96(1):98-102.

99. Dib A, Peterson TR, Raducha-Grace L, et al. Paradoxical expression of INK4c in proliferative multiple myeloma tumors: biallelic deletion vs increased expression. *Cell Div* 2006;1:23.

100. Drexler HG. Review of alterations of the cyclin-dependent kinase inhibitor INK4 family genes p15, p16, p18 and p19 in human leukemia-lymphoma cells. *Leukemia* 1998;12(6):845-59.

101. Kulkarni MS, Daggett JL, Bender TP, Kuehl WM, Bergsagel PL, Williams ME. Frequent inactivation of the cyclin-dependent kinase inhibitor p18 by homozygous deletion in multiple myeloma cell lines: ectopic p18 expression inhibits growth and induces apoptosis. *Leukemia* 2002;16(1):127-34.

102. Chng WJ, Kuehl WM, Bergsagel PL, Fonseca R. Translocation t(4;14) retains prognostic significance even in the setting of high-risk molecular signature. *Leukemia* 2008;22(2):459-61.

103. Chng WJ, Ahmann GJ, Henderson K, et al. Clinical implication of centrosome amplification in plasma cell neoplasm. *Blood* 2006;107(9):3669-75.

104. Stewart AK, Bergsagel PL, Greipp PR, et al. A practical guide to defining high-risk myeloma for clinical trials, patient counseling and choice of therapy. *Leukemia* 2007;21(3):529-34.

105. Dispenzieri A, Rajkumar SV, Gertz MA, et al. Treatment of newly diagnosed multiple myeloma based on Mayo Stratification of Myeloma and Risk-adapted Therapy (mSMART): consensus statement. *Mayo Clin Proc* 2007;82(3):323-41.

106. Avet-Loiseau H, Daviet A, Brigaudeau C, et al. Cytogenetic, interphase, and multicolor fluorescence in situ hybridization analyses in primary plasma cell leukemia: a study of 40 patients at diagnosis, on behalf of the Intergroupe Francophone du Myelome and the Groupe Francais de Cytogenetique Hematologique. *Blood* 2001;97(3):822-5.

107. Hayman SR, Bailey RJ, Jalal SM, et al. Translocations involving heavy-chain locus are possible early genetic events in patients with primary systemic amyloidosis. *Blood* 2001;98:2266-8.

108. Harrison CJ, Mazzullo H, Ross FM, et al. Translocations of 14q32 and deletions of 13q14 are common chromosomal abnormalities in systemic amyloidosis. *Br J Haematol* 2002;117(2):427-35.

109. Gertz MA, Lacy MQ, Dispenzieri A. Amyloidosis: Recognition, confirmation, prognosis, and therapy [Review]. *Mayo Clin Proc* 1999;74(5):490-4.

110. Avet-Loiseau H, Garand R, Lode L, Harousseau JL, Bataille R. Translocation t(11;14)(q13;q32) is the hallmark of IgM, IgE, and nonsecretory multiple myeloma variants. *Blood* 2003;101(4):1570-1.

111. Schop RF, Kuehl WM, Van Wier SA, et al. Waldenström macroglobulinemia neoplastic cells lack immunoglobulin heavy chain locus translocations but have frequent 6q deletions. *Blood* 2002;100(8):2996-3001.

112. Smadja NV, Bastard C, Brigaudeau C, Leroux D, Fruchart C. Hypodiploidy is a major prognostic factor in multiple myeloma. *Blood* 2001;98(7):2229-38.

113. Rajkumar SV, Fonseca R, Dewald GW, et al. Cytogenetic abnormalities correlate with the plasma cell labeling index and extent of bone marrow involvement in myeloma. *Cancer Genet Cytogenet* 1999;113(1):73-7.

2 Staging and Risk-Stratification of Multiple Myeloma

A. Keith Stewart

INTRODUCTION

Multiple myeloma is heterogeneous with respect to the genetic initiating event underpinning the development of the disease, subsequent responsiveness to chemotherapy, and, particularly, to long-term survival.[1-4] As has been clinically evident over many decades, simple biochemical markers such as the myeloma isotype and the presence or absence of skeletal disease or anemia provided a rough estimate with regard to prognosis. Nevertheless, these crude tools have gradually been supplanted by more sophisticated technologies for estimating prognosis, and a time has now been reached at which routine genetically based prognostication can be performed. When appropriate testing is performed, more accurate estimations of median event-free and overall survival can be provided to the patient, probable response to transplant can be gauged, and the appropriateness of this therapy can be assessed with greater accuracy.[5] It is important to note, however, that even with modern prognostication tools existing data are based on older therapies that have evolved substantially over the past few years such that not all genetic factors that were considered high-risk earlier this decade have maintained such high significance in the presence of more effective chemotherapy. This chapter will review both standard and genetically based prognostic markers with respect to their use and choice in prognosis prediction, in transplant response, and in choice of therapy.

PROGNOSTIC FACTORS ASSOCIATED WITH TUMOR BURDEN

The Durie–Salmon classification for many years was the most widely adopted classification system used to predict outcome for multiple myeloma patients.[4] This revolved around measures of tumor mass as identified by the presence of lytic bone disease, anemia, hypercalcemia, and the level and height of the monoclonal protein spike. A further subclassification by renal function was performed. Although useful for many years, a more recent attempt to improve on this classification system using data from 11 171 patients from American, Asian, and European continents was published.[1] This international staging system (ISS) simplified things down to two blood tests that can be routinely obtained in most centers. These include the β_2-microglobulin and albumin as demonstrated in Table 2.1. This ISS discriminates three risk groups with median survivals of 62, 44, and 29 months, a finding that is independent of age, geography, and standard or transplant therapy.

In other studies that have employed routinely available laboratory markers as predictors of prognosis, the presence of anemia and an immunoglobulin A (IgA) isotype as well as thrombocytopenia and renal insufficiency have also variably been reported to have poor prognostic impact.[6]

While helpful, particularly for those centers without access to genetic-based testing, each of these tools has major limitations with respect to predicting outcome. For example, it has become apparent in recent years that extensive lytic bone disease does not necessarily predict for poor survival, as it is often linked to genetic subtypes of myeloma with less proliferation and longer survival.[7] Thus the presence of lytic bone disease alone, which would place patients in Durie–Salmon stage 3, is no longer felt to be a particularly good marker for clinical outcomes. In contrast, the β_2-microglobulin has maintained its significance in many studies, even in the presence of genetic-based testing, and thus the ISS does appear to have more predictive values.[8,9]

INITIATING GENETIC EVENTS

The strongest independent predictors of clinical outcome yet identified relate to the underlying initial genetic

TABLE 2.1. International prognostic index

Stage	β_2-Microglobulin	Albumin
Stage 1	<3.5	≥3.5
Stage 2	<3.5 or 3.5-5.5	<3.5
Stage 3	>5.5	

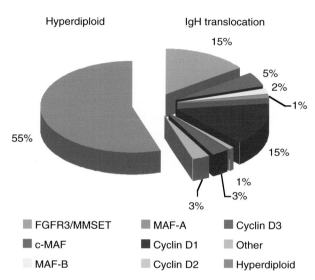

Figure 2.1. Genetic subtypes of myeloma.

event(s) that characterize the myeloma.[7,10] These initiating events involve one of two genetic processes. In the first, a variety of different oncogenes are translocated into the Ig heavy-chain switch region with resulting ectopic over-expression of an oncogene in plasma cells, which then become immortalized.[7,10] In the second major genetic subtype of myeloma, hyperdiploidy (the presence of excess chromosomal copies) is evident, particularly for the odd-numbered chromosomes.[3,11,12] Approximately 40% of patients have an IgH translocation, while approximately 60% of patients are hyperdiploid. These genetic changes are summarized in Figure 2.1 and are discussed in detail in Chapter 1. The different genetic subtypes of myeloma and their clinical relevance are outlined below.

Hyperdiploidy

Hyperdiploid myeloma makes up the majority of patient cases. This can most commonly be detected with the use

of fluorescence in situ hybridization (FISH) technologies.[3,11,12] A number of clinical studies have demonstrated that this abnormality can be found even in the very early stages of monoclonal gammopathies, but is present in 60% of newly diagnosed myeloma patients and is generally associated with an elderly patient population with more bone disease and usually an IgG isotype.[13] Although these are generalizations, as might be predicted, this population tends to have a favorable prognosis compared to other patients. For example, in the French Myeloma Intergroup (IFM) trial of tandem transplantation, patients with hyperdiploid myeloma could be predicted to have median event-free survivals after vincristine, adriamycin, and dexamethasone (VAD) based chemotherapy and tandem transplant in the range of 7-8 years.[9]

t(11;14), t(6;14), and t(6;22)

These three translocations each involve a member of the cyclin D family, D1, D2, and D3.[10] The cyclin D1 translocations are relatively common, affecting 15% of patients; cyclin D2 translocations are very rare, affecting less than 1% of patients; and cyclin D3 translocations affect approximately 4% of patients. Together these translocations affect approximately 18%-20% of patients overall. Interestingly, although other genetic subtypes of myeloma do not directly involve a *cyclin D* gene, in all myeloma patients, a cyclin D is upregulated even if as a downstream consequence of an initiating genetic event. Thus overexpression of a cyclin D is a unifying feature in multiple myeloma.[10] For the translocations involving the *cyclin D* genes outcomes have been, for the most part, favorable for patients; however, it is important to note that almost all plasma cell leukemias arise from a t(11;14) translocation[14] and that amyloidosis[15] is more common in this patient cohort.

t(4;14)

The t(4;14) affects approximately 5% of patients with monoclonal gammopathy of undetermined significance, 14% of multiple myeloma patients, and 26% of human myeloma cell lines.[16] This translocation disrupts two potential oncogenes: fibroblast growth factor receptor 3 (FGFR3) on derivative 14 and MMSET on derivative 4. Interestingly, the expression of FGFR3 is often lost as a progression event in approximately 20% of patients. These translocations can be picked up either using FISH or, in the patients who have retained FGFR3 expression, using flow cytometry or immunohistochemistry.[17] In all studies reported to date, using dexamethasone or VAD-based treatment regimens followed by stem cell transplant and in patients who are not destined for transplant receiving VBMCP (vincristine, carmustine, melphalan, cyclophosphamide, prednisone), the presence of a t(4;14) has generally been associated with a poor outcome.[9,18] This translocation is heavily linked to the presence of IgA isotype, a younger patient population, and frequent deletion of chromosome 13.[19] In fact, the rather poor prognosis associated with the presence of deletion of chromosome 13 by cytogenetics likely reflects its high association with the t(4;14) myeloma. In one study from France, Avet-Loiseau and colleagues[9] show that this poor risk group of myeloma patients could be further subdivided by the presence of a high or low β_2-microglobulin. Patients with no anemia and a low β_2-microglobulin fare relatively well even with the presence of the t(4;14), whereas those with either anemia or a high β_2-microglobulin and the presence of t(4;14) fare poorly with very short event-free survivals after stem cell transplant.

We have previously shown that the poor outcome for this patient population is related to early relapse, and, in fact, the initial response to therapy is actually higher than that for the general population. Probably because these patients have a rather short lead time to development of active clinical disease, bone disease tends to be slightly less common in this patient population.

Because of the very short event-free survival even after tandem transplant, it has generally been considered by our group that the role of transplant is diminished in this population and probably confers little advantage.[20] We therefore currently do not recommend transplant for these patients.

Recent data from Barlogie and colleagues[21] and from a large randomized multicenter phase 3 clinical trial, has suggested that the introduction of bortezomib may have a salutary role in overcoming this high-risk group of patients. Unfortunately, follow-up for these newer studies is still short, and it has certainly been our experience that even with bortezomib therapy these patients tend to relapse quickly; thus more investigational therapeutic regimens need to be employed.

Translocation t(14;16) and t(16;22)

These two translocations disrupt members of the MAF transcription family traditionally involved in T-cell development.[22] These translocations occur in approximately 5%-8% of myeloma patients and are thus rare, but as with the t(4;14) above, tend to confer a rather poor prognosis. Cyclin D2 is often elevated in these patient populations as a downstream consequence of MAF overexpression, as MAF binds the cyclin D2 promoter with its resulting upregulation. Less is known about MAF translocated patients because of its rarity; however, this patient population tends to be younger and enriched for chromosome 13 deletion and high-risk features.[7]

PROGRESSION EVENTS

All of the translocations just described tend to be associated with early stages of disease, and, as is recognized clinically, these patients may live many years without treatment. Progression events are therefore critical in the development of myeloma with end organ damage requiring treatment. Many markers of enhanced proliferation and secondary events confirming more active disease have been described. We will focus just on the more common of these here.

Deletion of Chromosome 13

Deletion of chromosome 13 can be detected by FISH or by cytogenetics.[3] By FISH, deletion of chromosome 13 has been found to be present in approximately 40% of patients, and it has only weakly negative prognostic significance.[23] By conventional cytogenetics, deletion of chromosome 13 has been found in 15% of patients and many of these are linked to the high-risk IgH translocation subtypes described earlier. Given that chromosome 13 deletion tracks closely with the high-risk translocations,[24] it is not surprising that this deletion when detected confers a very poor prognosis. Again, it appears that the use of bortezomib may have some ameliorative effect on these high-risk patients.[25]

Mutation of NF-κB

We have recently described 40% of patients acquiring activation of the nuclear factor-κB (NF-κB) pathway as a consequence of a progression event and most frequently involving a deletion of TRAF3, CYLD, BIRC2/3, or translocation of genes such as *NIK* or *CD40*.[26] The net effect of overexpression of NF-κB is generally negative with some links to high-risk disease but more responsiveness to bortezomib, as might be predicted.

Amplification of chromosome 1

Amplification of chromosome 1 is frequently detected as a progression marker.[27] The exact gene responsible for the excess proliferation of myeloma cells associated with the amplification of chromosome 1 is not known, but it has been postulated to be CKS1B. Amplification of CKS1B or amplification of chromosome 1, in general, tends to be associated with a poor prognosis in most, but not all, series.

Deletion of 17p (p53)

Deletion of p53 is present in 10% of myelomas at diagnosis, 40% of advanced myeloma, and 60% of human myeloma cell lines. Deletion of chromosome 17 and, as a consequence, of p53 is associated with very poor outcome in all series.[28] As one example, 9 of 11 cases of CNS involvement with plasma cells were associated with the deletion of p53,[29] and even using the most sophisticated genetic markers on gene expression profiles yet available the presence of p53 deletion is generally associated with poor outcome despite the therapy employed.[18]

Other genetic changes

Numerous other genetic changes can be identified at progression of multiple myeloma, including deletions of PTEN, mutations of RAS or FGFR3, activation of the STAT3/PRL3 pathway, and complex cytogenetic changes on phenotype. Of these, we would recommend routine testing for only an abnormal karyotype by conventional cytogenetics, as this may identify even those relatively good genetic risk patients who have a poor outcome due to secondary proliferation events.[30]

Other markers of proliferation

Although indirect, other markers of proliferation have been widely employed in different centers, including the plasma cell labeling index, the β_2-microglobulin or lactic dehydrogenase level,[30] and more recently the presence of a high proliferation index on gene expression profiling.[31] In all instances, a proliferative tumor is associated with poor outcome and will identify those patients even with a low-risk initiating genetic event with an average outcome who have converted to high-risk patients.

Gene expression profiling

Recently, sophisticated gene expression profiling has been performed by the University of Arkansas Medical Center, which has been able to tease out a list of 70 genes associated with very poor outcome in myeloma patients.[31] Efforts are now being made to narrow this gene list down further and make it amenable to a clinically proven diagnostic test. Interestingly, this analysis has been able to identify 14% of patients with extremely high-risk multiple myeloma that seems to be present irrespective of the underlying genetic initiating event and is associated with a very poor outcome even in the presence of bortezomib and tandem transplant approaches to therapy.

INFLUENCE OF PROGNOSTIC FACTORS ON TREATMENT OUTCOMES

In previous years, the availability of more accurate prognostic testing was felt to be of little clinical value since treatment did not vary from patient to patient and was generally based on dexamethasone and transplant for younger patients and based on alkylating agent and corticosteroid for elderly patients. With the advent of modern therapeutics including bortezomib, lenalidomide, and thalidomide, the scenario is now changing. It has been further influenced by the ability of the genetic markers identified above to allow more accurate prediction of clinical outcome. We believe strongly that all patients should have routine genetic testing performed at baseline, not only to assist with treatment decision making but also as a stratification factor for clinical trials and, finally, so that the patient can, with more assurance, make informed decisions about quality of life and life planning.

SUMMARY

To summarize the above discussion of high-risk and standard-risk genetics, we have produced Figure 2.2 and placed this on the web (www.msmart.org) for ease of use by clinicians. This describes our classification of myeloma

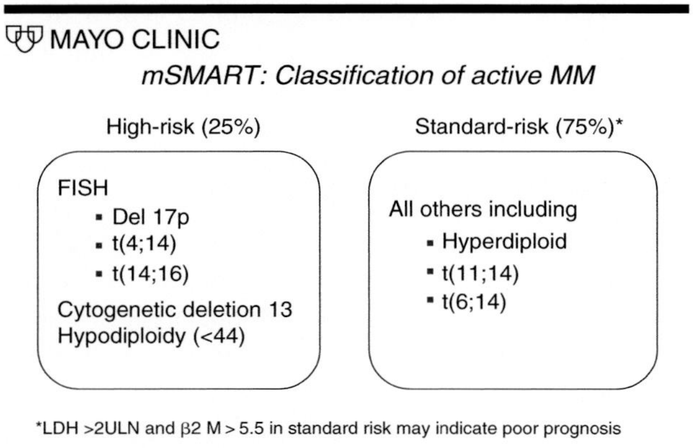

MAYO CLINIC
mSMART: Classification of active MM

High-risk (25%)   Standard-risk (75%)*

FISH
- Del 17p
- t(4;14)
- t(14;16)

Cytogenetic deletion 13
Hypodiploidy (<44)

All others including
- Hyperdiploid
- t(11;14)
- t(6;14)

*LDH >2ULN and β2 M > 5.5 in standard risk may indicate poor prognosis

Figure 2.2. Genetic risk-stratification of multiple myeloma.
Source: Dispenzieri et al. Mayo Clin Proc 2007; 82:323–341; Revised and updated: January 2008.

into 25% of patients with high-risk genetics underpinning their disease and 75% of patients with average risk. Although imperfect, we believe this is a reasonable compromise between test availability, published literature, and pragmatic concerns. It is important, however, for the treating clinician to realize that there will be patients in the low average risk group who will not fare so well; thus additional testing such as β_2-microglobulin, lactate dehydrogenase (LDH), and conventional karyotype cytogenetics can be employed.

THERAPEUTIC IMPLICATIONS OF GENETIC PROGNOSTICATION

Transplant-eligible patients

For patients young enough to undergo the rigors of autologous stem cell transplant, data from over 1500 patients treated with VAD- or dexamethasone-based chemotherapy followed by high-dose melphalan indicates an event-free survival of only 9 months for patients in the high-risk genetic category as defined above.[9,14,32] Given this relatively short outcome, we no longer feel that autologous stem cell transplant can be relied on as definitive therapy in this high-risk patient subgroup. Thus, we recommend that these patients be subjected to more investigational procedures from the outset, including use of new drugs as induction therapy. In contrast, patients with standard-risk

genetics can have a median overall survival of 7-8 years, even with a single autologous transplant,[9] and, thus, we continue to recommend this therapeutic approach for the transplant-eligible patient. In some studies, the poor outcome seen, for example, with the t(4;14) is ameliorated by a normal hemoglobin and low β_2-microglobulin; thus there may be a subset of t(4;14) patients who continue to show some benefit from transplant, although this has not been verified by other trials.

Although allogeneic transplant has been recommended by some for the high-risk genetic subgroup, there is no evidence whatsoever in support of this course. In fact, the only randomized trial that examined high-risk myeloma patients with mini-allotransplant was negative and favored an auto-transplant approach.[33]

Bortezomib

As mentioned above, a number of studies have now suggested a survival advantage to high-risk myeloma patients who received bortezomib[25,34,35]. One word of caution is that follow-up is short and numbers are small in all studies purporting to show an advantage for bortezomib-treated patients, and it must also be remembered that response rates are initially usually higher in this more proliferative tumor. Nevertheless, given the remarkably poor outcomes of VAD- and dexamethasone-based therapies, even with added transplant, the suggestion that bortezomib may have the ability to overcome at least some of the high-risk genetics is certainly encouraging. Probably the most persuasive data to date are from the Little Rock, Arkansas Total Therapy Program, in which Barlogie and colleagues have demonstrated that Total Therapy 3 (which improved upon Total Therapy 2 by the addition of bortezomib) has managed to overcome the high risk associated with the t(4;14) translocation.[21] Thus, we recommend for patients with high-risk myeloma that bortezomib be introduced early and probably in preference to other treatment options.

Thalidomide and lenalidomide

Very little data exist on the role of thalidomide and lenalidomide in high-risk myeloma. Follow-up is too short and

A

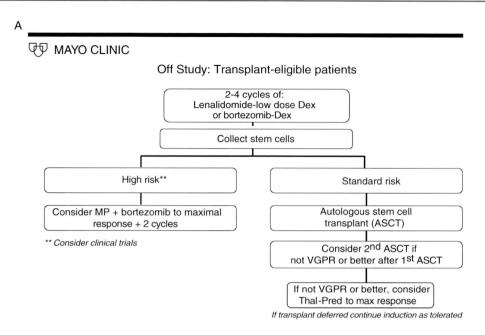

B

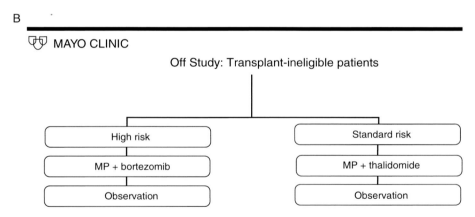

Figure 2.3. (A) Risk-adapted therapy for transplant-eligible patients. (B) Risk-adapted therapy for transplant-ineligible patients.
Source (A, B): Dispenzieri et al. Mayo Clin Proc 2007; 82:323–341; Revised and updated: January 2008.

numbers are too small for any meaningful conclusions to be derived at this time, although such studies are under way.

Treatment of the elderly patient

As with the younger transplant-eligible patient, we believe bortezomib should be employed for elderly patients with high-risk genetics for the reasons mentioned above. Certainly data from the recently reported VISTA trial tend to suggest once more that the use of bortezomib together with melphalan and prednisone is able to abrogate some of the early relapse features associated with high-risk genetics, although follow-up is again short and numbers are too small to be convincing.[34] Our risk-adapted algorithm[20] is summarized in Figure 2.3A and B for transplant-eligible and transplant-ineligible patients, respectively.

SUMMARY

In summary, while standard laboratory testing, including hemoglobin, β_2-microglobulin, albumin, and LDH as well as Ig isotype can provide clues as to the future course of each individual patient's myeloma, these are less accurate, for the most part, than the use of genetic-based prognostication. Our approach is summarized in the earlier figures defining high-risk and standard-risk myeloma, and its influence on our treatment decision pathway is described. Clearly this is a very rapidly evolving field and the one that requires more intense study, but we already believe that the era of risk-adaptive therapy for myeloma has come and should be widely adopted.

REFERENCES

1. Greipp PR, San Miguel J, Durie BG, et al. International staging system for multiple myeloma. *J Clin Oncol* 2005;23:3412-20.

2. Stewart AK, Bergsagel PL, Greipp PR, et al. A practical guide to defining high-risk myeloma for clinical trials, patient counseling and choice of therapy. *Leukemia* 2007;21:529-34.

3. Fonseca R, Barlogie B, Bataille R, et al. Genetics and cytogenetics of multiple myeloma: a workshop report. *Cancer Res* 2004;64:1546-58.

4. Kyle RA, Rajkumar SV. Multiple myeloma. *N Engl J Med* 2004;351:1860-73.

5. Salmon SE, Beckord J, Pugh RP, Barlogie B, Crowley J. α-Interferon for remission maintenance: preliminary report on the Southwest Oncology Group Study. *Semin Oncol* 1991;18:33-6.

6. San Miguel JF, Garcia-Sanz R. Prognostic features of multiple myeloma. *Best Pract Res Clin Haematol* 2005;18:569-83.

7. Bergsagel PL, Kuehl WM. Molecular pathogenesis and a consequent classification of multiple myeloma. *J Clin Oncol* 2005;23:6333-8.

8. Rajkumar SV, Fonseca R, Lacy MQ, et al. Beta-2-microglobulin and bone marrow plasma cell involvement predict complete responders among patients undergoing blood cell transplantation for myeloma. *Bone Marrow Transplant* 1999;23:1261-6.

9. Avet-Loiseau H, Attal M, Moreau P, et al. Genetic abnormalities and survival in multiple myeloma: the experience of the Intergroupe Francophone du Myelome. *Blood* 2007;109:3489-95.

10. Bergsagel PL, Kuehl WM, Zhan F, Sawyer J, Barlogie B, Shaughnessy J Jr. Cyclin D dysregulation: an early and unifying pathogenic event in multiple myeloma. *Blood* 2005;106:296-303.

11. Chng WJ, Santana-Davila R, Van Wier SA, et al. Prognostic factors for hyperdiploid-myeloma: effects of chromosome 13 deletions and IgH translocations. *Leukemia* 2006;20:807-13.

12. Chng WJ, Van Wier SA, Ahmann GJ, et al. A validated FISH trisomy index demonstrates the hyperdiploid and nonhyperdiploid dichotomy in MGUS. *Blood* 2005;106:2156-61.

13. Fonseca R, Bailey RJ, Ahmann GJ, et al. Genomic abnormalities in monoclonal gammopathy of undetermined significance. *Blood* 2002;100:1417-24.

14. Gertz MA, Lacy MQ, Dispenzieri A, et al. Clinical implications of t(11;14)(q13;q32), t(4;14)(p16.3;q32), and -17p13 in myeloma patients treated with high-dose therapy. *Blood* 2005;106:2837-40.

15. Fonseca R, Ahmann GJ, Jalal SM, et al. Chromosomal abnormalities in systemic amyloidosis. *Br J Haematol* 1998;103:704-10.

16. Bergsagel PL, Kuehl WM. Chromosome translocations in multiple myeloma. *Oncogene* 2001;20:5611-22.

17. Stewart AK, Chang H, Trudel S, et al. Diagnostic evaluation of t(4;14) in multiple myeloma and evidence for clonal evolution. *Leukemia* 2007;21:2358-9.

18. Gertz MA, Lacy MQ, Dispenzieri A, et al. Clinical implications of t(11;14)(q13;q32), t(4;14)(p16.3;q32), and -17p13 in myeloma patients treated with high-dose therapy. *Blood* 2005;106:2837-40.

19. Jaksic W, Trudel S, Chang H, et al. Clinical outcomes in t(4;14) multiple myeloma: a chemotherapy-sensitive disease characterized by rapid relapse and alkylating agent resistance. *J Clin Oncol* 2005;23:7069-73.

20. Dispenzieri A, Rajkumar SV, Gertz MA, et al. Treatment of newly diagnosed multiple myeloma based on Mayo Stratification of Myeloma and Risk-adapted Therapy (mSMART): consensus statement. *Mayo Clin Proc* 2007;82:323-41.

21. Barlogie B, Anaissie E, van Rhee F, et al. Incorporating bortezomib into upfront treatment for multiple myeloma: early results of total therapy 3. *Br J Haematol* 2007;138:176-85.

22. Chesi M, Bergsagel PL, Shonukan OO, et al. Frequent dysregulation of the c-maf proto-oncogene at 16q23 by translocation to an Ig locus in multiple myeloma. *Blood* 1998;91:4457-63.

23. Fonseca R, Oken MM, Harrington D, et al. Deletions of chromosome 13 in multiple myeloma identified by interphase FISH usually denote large deletions of the q arm or monosomy. *Leukemia* 2001;15:981-6.

24. Fonseca R, Oken MM, Greipp PR. The t(4;14)(p16.3;q32) is strongly associated with chromosome 13 abnormalities in both multiple myeloma and monoclonal gammopathy of undetermined significance. *Blood* 2001;98:1271-2.

25. Jagannath S, Richardson PG, Sonneveld P, et al. Bortezomib appears to overcome the poor prognosis conferred by chromosome 13 deletion in phase 2 and 3 trials. *Leukemia* 2007;21:151-7.

26. Keats JJ, Fonseca R, Chesi M, et al. Promiscuous mutations activate the noncanonical NF-kappaB pathway in multiple myeloma. *Cancer Cell* 2007;12:131-44.

27. Shaughnessy J. Amplification and overexpression of CKS1B at chromosome band 1q21 is associated with reduced levels of p27Kip1 and an aggressive clinical course in multiple myeloma. *Hematology* 2005;10(suppl 1):117-26.

28. Chang H, Qi C, Yi QL, Reece D, Stewart AK. p53 gene deletion detected by fluorescence in situ hybridization is an adverse prognostic factor for patients with multiple myeloma following autologous stem cell transplantation. *Blood* 2005;105:358-60.

29. Chang H, Sloan S, Li D, Keith Stewart A. Multiple myeloma involving central nervous system: high frequency of chromosome 17p13.1 (p53) deletions. *Br J Haematol* 2004;127:280-4.

30. Barlogie B, Shaughnessy JD Jr. Early results of total therapy II in multiple myeloma: implications of cytogenetics and FISH. *Int J Hematol* 2002;76(suppl 1):337-9.

31. Zhan F, Barlogie B, Mulligan G, Shaughnessy JD Jr, Bryant B. High-risk myeloma: a gene expression based risk-stratification model for newly diagnosed multiple myeloma treated with high-dose therapy is predictive of outcome in relapsed disease treated with single-agent bortezomib or high-dose dexamethasone. *Blood* 2008;111:968-9.

32. Chang H, Qi XY, Samiee S, et al. Genetic risk identifies multiple myeloma patients who do not benefit from autologous stem cell transplantation. *Bone Marrow Transplant* 2005;36:793-6.

33. Facon T, Avet-Loiseau H, Guillerm G, et al. Chromosome 13 abnormalities identified by FISH analysis and serum beta-2-microglobulin produce a powerful myeloma staging system for patients receiving high-dose therapy. *Blood* 2001;97:1566-71.

34. Mateos MV, Hernandez JM, Hernandez MT, et al. Bortezomib plus melphalan and prednisone in elderly untreated patients with multiple myeloma: results of a multicenter phase I/II study. *Blood* 2006;108:2165-72.

35. Chang H, Trieu Y, Qi X, Xu W, Stewart KA, Reece D. Bortezomib therapy response is independent of cytogenetic abnormalities in relapsed/refractory multiple myeloma. *Leuk Res* 2006; 31:779-82.

3 Treatment of Newly Diagnosed Multiple Myeloma

S. Vincent Rajkumar and Robert A. Kyle

INTRODUCTION

The treatment of newly diagnosed multiple myeloma (MM) is rapidly evolving.[1-4] The median survival of patients with symptomatic myeloma until recently was approximately 3 years with oral chemotherapy with melphalan and prednisone (MP),[5] and approximately 5 years with high-dose therapy with autologous stem cell transplantation (ASCT).[6] More recently, thalidomide,[7] bortezomib,[8,9] and lenalidomide[10,11] have emerged as effective agents in the treatment of myeloma. As a result, the survival of patients with MM has improved significantly.[12] Although each of the new drugs first showed activity in patients with advanced relapsed refractory disease, they have now been successfully incorporated into initial therapy. This chapter reviews the current therapeutic options for newly diagnosed myeloma and provides a risk-based approach to the treatment of these patients.

TRANSPLANT ELIGIBILITY AND RISK-STRATIFICATION

The first step in the treatment of myeloma is to establish that the diagnosis is indeed MM. Monoclonal gammopathy of undetermined significance (MGUS) and smoldering MM (SMM) are two entities that do not require any therapy that must be excluded (see Chapter 13). There is no evidence that early treatment of patients with SMM prolongs survival compared to therapy at the time of symptoms.[13,14] However, clinical trials are ongoing to determine whether newer agents can delay the progression of SMM to myeloma.

The next step is to determine whether the patient is a potential candidate for SCT. Transplant eligibility is

Supported in part by Grants CA62242, CA85818, CA93842, and CA100080 from the National Cancer Institute, Bethesda, MD.

determined by a variety of factors such as age, performance status, and comorbidities. In many countries, age 65 is considered as the upper limit for ASCT, and patients who are older are typically treated as nontransplant candidates. On the other hand, in the United States, a greater emphasis is placed on physiological age rather than chronological age to determine transplant eligibility.

Once the determination of transplant eligibility is made, the next step is risk-stratification.[2,15] Risk-stratification is critical in determining choice of initial therapy and the overall approach to therapy. The specific risk factors used to stratify patients at the Mayo Clinic into high-risk and standard-risk myeloma are deletion 13 or hypodiploidy on metaphase cytogenetic studies, deletion 17p or immunoglobulin heavy-chain (IgH) translocations t(4;14) or t(14;16), or plasma cell labeling index of 3% or higher. Presence of any one or more of the above high-risk factors classifies a patient as having high-risk myeloma. High-risk myeloma accounts for approximately 25% of patients, and has a median overall survival (OS) of less than 2-3 years even with tandem SCT compared to more than 6-7 years in patients with standard-risk MM.[2]

The approach to the treatment of symptomatic newly diagnosed MM is outlined in Figure 3.1. Table 3.1 lists the most common regimens used in the treatment of newly diagnosed myeloma. Although we make standard recommendations for therapy, at every step of the treatment clinical trials if available are preferred. Table 3.2 lists the major trials in myeloma that have over the years made a major impact on the treatment of the disease.[6,9,16-25]

INITIAL TREATMENT OF PATIENTS ELIGIBLE FOR TRANSPLANTATION

It is important to avoid protracted melphalan-based therapy in patients with newly diagnosed myeloma who

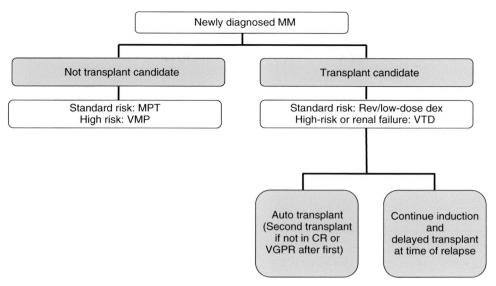

Figure 3.1. Approach to the treatment of newly diagnosed multiple myeloma (MM).
Abbreviations: CR, complete response; MPT, melphalan-prednisone-thalidomide; Rev/low-dose Dex, lenalidomide plus low-dose dexamethasone; VGPR, very good partial response; VMP, bortezomib-melphalan-prednisone; VTD, bortezomib-thalidomide-dexamethasone.

are considered eligible for ASCT, as it can interfere with adequate stem cell mobilization, regardless of whether an early or delayed transplant is contemplated. Thus, the determination of SCT eligibility influences the decision on whether to use melphalan-based therapy. Patients who are determined to be candidates for ASCT are typically treated with 2-4 cycles of non-melphalan-containing induction therapy followed by stem cell harvest. Stem cell harvest is performed early in the disease course in this manner both in patients who pursue upfront ASCT and those who wish to reserve ASCT as a delayed option for relapsed refractory disease.

Vincristine, adriamycin, dexamethasone (VAD)

VAD was used for many years as pretransplant induction therapy for patients considered candidates for ASCT. However, owing to many reasons, including the neurotoxicity of vincristine, which can limit the future use of thalidomide and bortezomib, VAD has fallen out of favor and is rarely used today.[26] Further, most of the activity of VAD is from the high-dose dexamethasone component. In a matched case-control study of 200 patients, response rates with VAD were significantly lower compared to

thalidomide-dexamethasone (Thal/Dex); 76% versus 52%, respectively.[27] Preliminary results from a randomized trial from France confirm these findings.[28] VAD is not recommended anymore as initial therapy.

High-dose dexamethasone

High-dose pulsed dexamethasone as a single agent was used as an induction therapy in the past as an alternative to intravenous VAD.[29] Objective response rates are approximately 45%,[30,31] significantly lower compared to newer induction regimens. In randomized trials, the early mortality rate associated with high-dose dexamethasone is more than 10% in the first 4 months of therapy, reflecting the toxicity and ineffectiveness of this regimen. Its efficacy even in the newly diagnosed setting is limited, with a time to progression (TTP) of only 6-12 months.[31,32] Consequently, single-agent dexamethasone is no longer recommended as initial therapy.

Thalidomide-dexamethasone

Thalidomide as a single agent has a response rate of 25% in heavily pretreated patients with relapsed refractory

TABLE 3.1. Regimens for the treatment of newly diagnosed multiple myeloma

Regimen	Response rate (%)	Usual dosing schedule*
Melphalan-prednisone (MP) (7-day schedule)	50	Melphalan: 8-10 mg, oral, days 1-7 Prednisone: 60 mg/day, oral, days 1-7 Repeated every 6 weeks until plateau
Thalidomide-dexamethasone (Thal/Dex)	65	Thalidomide: 200 mg, oral, days 1-28 Dexamethasone: 40 mg, oral, days 1, 8, 15, 22 every 28 days Repeated every 4 weeks × 4 cycles as pretransplant induction therapy
Lenalidomide-dexamethasone (Rev/low-dose Dex)	70	Lenalidomide: 25 mg, oral, days 1-21 every 28 days Dexamethasone: 40 mg, oral, days 1, 8, 15, 22 every 28 days Repeated every 4 weeks × 4 cycles as pretransplant induction therapy, or continued till plateau or progression if used as primary therapy
Bortezomib-Dex (Vel/Dex)	75	Bortezomib: 1.3 mg/m², intravenous, days 1, 4, 8, 11 Dexamethasone: 40 mg, oral, days 1-4, 9-12 Reduce dexamethasone to days 1-4 after first 2 cycles Repeated every 3 weeks × 4 cycles as pretransplant induction therapy
Melphalan-prednisone-thalidomide (MPT)	70	Melphalan: 0.25 mg/kg, oral, days 1-4 Prednisone: 2 mg/kg, oral, days 1-4 Thalidomide: 100-200 mg, oral, days 1-28 Repeated every 6 weeks × 12 cycles
Bortezomib-melphalan-prednisone (VMP)	70	Melphalan: 9 mg/m², oral, days 1-4 Prednisone: 60 mg/m², oral, days 1-4 Bortezomib: 1.3 mg/m², intravenous, days 1, 4, 8, 11, 22, 25, 29, 32 Repeated every 42 days × 4 cycles followed by maintenance therapy as given below: Melphalan: 9 mg/m², oral, days 1-4 Prednisone: 60 mg/m², oral, days 1-4 Bortezomib: 1.3 mg/m², intravenous, days 1, 8, 15, 22 Repeated every 35 days × 5 cycles
Melphalan-prednisone-lenalidomide (MPR)	80	Melphalan: 0.18 mg/kg, oral, days 1-4 Prednisone: 2 mg/kg, oral, days 1-4 Lenalidomide: 10 mg, oral, days 1-28 Repeated every 4-6 weeks × 9 cycles
Bortezomib-thalidomide-dexamethasone (VTD)	90	Bortezomib: 1.3 mg/m², intravenous, days 1, 4, 8, 11 Thalidomide: 100-200 mg, oral, days 1-21 Dexamethasone: 20 mg/m², oral, days 1-4, 9-12, 17-20 Reduce dexamethasone to days 1-4 after first 2 cycles Repeated every 4 weeks × 4 cycles as pretransplant induction therapy

*Starting and subsequent doses need to be adjusted for performance status, renal function, blood counts, and other toxicities.

disease.[7] Response rates in relapsed disease are approximately 50% with thalidomide plus corticosteroids and more than 65% with a three-drug combination of thalidomide, corticosteroids, and alkylators. It is usually given orally in a dose of 100-200 mg daily. After a response is achieved the dose is adjusted to the lowest dose that can achieve and maintain a response in order to minimize long-term toxicity.

In the past few years, Thal/Dex has emerged as the most commonly used induction regimen for the treatment of newly diagnosed myeloma in the United States, with a response rate of approximately 65%-75%.[33-35] An

TABLE 3.2. Results of selected randomized trials that have had a major impact on myeloma therapy

Trial	Disease stage	Treatment comparison	Total number of patients studied	CR/VGPR (%)	Median PFS (months)	Median OS (months)	Comments
Stem cell transplantation							
IFM 90[6]	Newly diagnosed	Conv. chemo	100	13	18	44	Established role of ASCT
		ASCT	100	38	28	57	
MRC VII[16]	Newly diagnosed	Conv. chemo	201	8	20	42	Confirmed role of ASCT
		ASCT	200	44	32	54	
MAG 90[17]	Newly diagnosed	Delayed ASCT	94	21	13	65	Demonstrated delayed ASCT as an alternative
		Early ASCT	91	32	39	64	
United States Intergroup S9321[18]	Newly diagnosed	Delayed ASCT	255	15*	21	64	Demonstrated delayed ASCT as an alternative; dampened enthusiasm for allogeneic SCT
		Early ASCT	261	17*	25	58	
		Allogeneic SCT	36	17*	NR	–6	
IFM 94[19]	Newly diagnosed	Single ASCT	199	42	25	48	Established role of tandem ASCT if CR/VGPR not achieved with first ASCT
		Double ASCT	200	50	30	58	
PETHEMA[20]	Postinduction (responding patients only)	Conv. chemo	83	11*	33	66	Demonstrated that ASCT may have limited value in patients responding well to induction
		ASCT	81	30*	42	61	
Italian[21]	Newly diagnosed	Tandem ASCT	82	N/A	29	54	Demonstrated efficacy of single ASCT followed by nonmyeloablative SCT in selected patients
		Single ASCT followed by nonmyeloablative SCT	80	N/A	35	80	
New therapies							
Italian GIMEMA group[22]	Newly diagnosed	MP	126	12	27	64% at 3 years	Demonstrated potential value of MPT over the classic MP regimen
		MPT	129	36	54	80% at 3 years	

(continued)

TABLE 3.2 (*continued*)

Trial	Disease stage	Treatment comparison	Total number of patients studied	CR/VGPR (%)	Median PFS (months)	Median OS (months)	Comments
IFM 99-06[23]	Newly diagnosed	MP	196	7	18	33	Changed standard of care in elderly
		MPT	125	47	28	52	to MPT (after three decades of MP)
		Tandem intermediate-dose ASCT	126	43	19	38	
APEX[9]	Relapsed, refractory (1–3 prior therapies)	Bortezomib	333	13†	6**	NR	Led to full approval of bortezomib in the United States
		Dex	336	2†	–3**	NR	
MM-010[24]	Relapsed, refractory (1–3 prior therapies)	Len/Dex	176	24†	11**	Not reached	Pivotal trial establishing role of lenalidomide
		Placebo/Dex	175	5†	–5**	21	
MM-009[25]	Relapsed, refractory (1–3 prior therapies)	Len/Dex	177	24†	11*	30	Led to approval of lenalidomide in the United States
		Placebo/Dex	176	2†	–5*	20	

ASCT, autologous hematopoietic stem cell transplantation; Conv. chemo, conventional chemotherapy; CR, complete response; Dex, dexamethasone; ECOG, Eastern Cooperative Oncology Group; GIMEMA, Gruppo Italiano Malattie Ematologiche dell'Adulto; IFM, InterGroupe Francophone du Myélome; Len, Lenalidomide; MAG, Myélome Autogreffe; MM, multiple myeloma; MP, melphalan plus prednisone; MPT, melphalan, prednisone, thalidomide; MRC, Medical Research Council; NR, not reported; OS, overall survival; PETHEMA, Programa para el Estudio y Tratamiento de las Hemopatias Malignas; PFS, progression-free survival; SCT, stem cell transplantation; VGPR, very good partial response.

*CR only; VGPR not reported. †CR or near CR; **PFS data not available; numbers reflect median time to progression.

Source: This table was originally published in *Blood*. Kyle RA, et al., Multiple myeloma. *Blood*. 2008; 111: 2962-2972 © the American Society of Hematology.

Eastern Cooperative Oncology Group (ECOG) randomized trial compared Thal/Dex with dexamethasone in 207 patients.[30] The best response within four cycles of therapy was significantly higher with Thal/Dex compared to dexamethasone alone (63% versus 41%, respectively, p = 0.0017). Stem cell harvest was successful in 90% of patients in each arm. Deep vein thrombosis (DVT) was more frequent with Thal/Dex (17% vs. 3%). Overall, grade 3 or higher nonhematologic toxicities were seen in 67% of patients within four cycles with Thal/Dex and 43% with dexamethasone alone (p < 0.001). Early mortality (first 4 months) was 7% with Thal/Dex and 11% with dexamethasone alone. On the basis of this trial, the U.S. Food and Drug Administration (FDA) has granted accelerated approval for Thal/Dex for the treatment of newly diagnosed myeloma.

Another study, an international randomized, double-blind, placebo-controlled trial compared Thal/Dex versus dexamethasone alone as a primary therapy in 470 patients with newly diagnosed MM.[31] Among 470 patients enrolled, response rate and TTP were significantly higher with Thal/Dex compared to placebo/Dex (p < 0.001). As in the ECOG trial, DVT is a major problem with Thal/Dex, and other grade 3 and 4 events are more frequent with Thal/Dex compared to dexamethasone alone.

Lenalidomide-dexamethasone (Rev/Dex)

Lenalidomide belongs to a class of thalidomide analogues termed immunomodulatory drugs (IMiDs). Overall response rate with single-agent lenalidomide in relapsed, refractory myeloma is approximately 20%.[11] Two large phase 3 trials have shown significantly superior TTP with Rev/Dex compared to placebo plus dexamethasone in relapsed myeloma.[24,25] On the basis of these studies, Rev/Dex is currently approved by the FDA for the treatment of myeloma in patients who have failed one prior therapy.

In newly diagnosed myeloma, a phase 2 trial conducted at the Mayo Clinic demonstrated remarkably high activity with the Rev/Dex regimen. Of the 34 patients (91%), 31 achieved an objective response, including 2 (6%) achieving complete response (CR) and 11 (32%) meeting criteria for very good partial response (VGPR).[10] Lacy et al.[36] recently updated the results of this study. With longer follow-up, 56% of patients in this trial achieved VGPR or better. In the subset of 21 patients receiving Rev/Dex as

primary therapy without ASCT, 67% achieved VGPR or better. Approximately 50% of patients experienced grade 3 or higher nonhematologic toxicity, similar to rates seen with dexamethasone alone.

An ECOG randomized trial compared Rev/high-dose Dex (dexamethasone: 40 mg, days 1-4, 9-12, 17-20 every 28 days) with Rev/low-dose Dex (dexamethasone: 40 mg, once weekly) in newly diagnosed myeloma in 445 patients.[37,38] Preliminary results show CR plus VGPR rate of 52% with Rev/high-dose Dex versus 42% with Rev/low-dose Dex. Overall survival was significantly superior with Rev/low-dose Dex compared to Rev/high-dose Dex; 1-year survival was 96% versus 87%, respectively. The 1-year survival rate and the early mortality rate in the Rev/low-dose Dex arm are the best results reported in any large phase 3 newly diagnosed trial in which enrollment was not restricted by age or eligibility for SCT. On the basis of this Rev/low-dose Dex is currently the regimen of choice in the Mayo Stratification for Myeloma and Risk-adapted Therapy (mSMART) protocol for the treatment of standard-risk myeloma in patients who are candidates for ASCT outside the setting of a clinical trial.

Recently, Kumar and colleagues[39] have found a lower stem cell yield with Rev/Dex induction, with a small proportion of patients not collecting adequate stem cells for transplantation with growth factor mobilization. Others have not found any problems with stem cell mobilization.[38,40] Patients failing to mobilize with growth factor alone can usually collect successfully with a second attempt using either cyclophosphamide or AMD 3100.

Bortezomib-based regimens

Bortezomib is a novel proteasome inhibitor approved for the treatment of patients with relapsed and refractory MM. In 202 patients with relapsed/refractory MM, approximately one-third responded to single-agent bortezomib therapy, with an average response duration of 1 year.[8] In a recent randomized trial, progression-free survival (PFS) was superior with bortezomib compared to dexamethasone alone in patients with relapsed, refractory MM.[9] Bortezomib is currently approved by the FDA for the treatment of myeloma in patients who have failed one prior therapy.

In newly diagnosed myeloma, response rates of approximately 70%-90% have been observed with bortezomib plus dexamethasone (Vel/Dex),[41,42] Harousseau and colleagues[43] recently reported preliminary results of a randomized trial comparing VAD versus Vel/Dex as pretransplant induction therapy in 482 patients. The CR plus VGPR rates were higher with Vel/Dex compared to VAD before ASCT (47% vs. 19%) and persisted after ASCT as well (62% vs. 42%, p < 0.001). The 1-year PFS and OS rates were 90% and 95% with VAD, and 93% and 97% with Vel/Dex, respectively. No adverse effect on stem cell mobilization has been noted with bortezomib therapy. The most common grade 2 or higher adverse events in one study were sensory neuropathy (31%), constipation (28%), myalgia (28%), and fatigue (25%).[41]

Bortezomib-thalidomide-dexamethasone (VTD) has shown high activity in relapsed refractory myeloma and in newly diagnosed disease. Cavo and colleagues[44] compared Thal/Dex with VTD in a randomized controlled trial in 256 patients. As pretransplant induction therapy, the CR plus VGPR rate was significantly higher with VTD compared to Thal/Dex (60% vs. 27%, respectively, p < 0.001). The VTD regimen was well tolerated and permitted adequate stem cell collection.

In general, the main drawback of bortezomib-based regimens is the need for intravenous therapy. However, bortezomib-based regimens may be of value in patients with renal failure and in patients with high-risk myeloma.

Other induction regimens

Several other induction regimens have been evaluated, for example, liposomal doxorubicin, vincristine, dexamethasone, thalidomide (DVD-T); liposomal doxorubicin, vincristine, dexamethasone, lenalidomide (DVD-R); bortezomib, adriamycin, dexamethasone (PAD); and clarithromycin, lenalidomide, dexamethasone (BiRd).[40] The role of pretransplant induction regimens containing doxorubicin or liposomal doxorubicin need to be weighed in terms of the added side effects that can affect quality of life. Similarly, the value of adding clarithromycin to Rev/Dex in the BiRd regimen is not clear, and more studies are needed. Two randomized trials are also ongoing, investigating bortezomib, lenalidomide, low-dose dexamethasone (VRd) in newly diagnosed myeloma. These regimens should be considered investigational until future studies show that the addition of these agents improves long-term outcome compared to the regimens discussed above.

Summary recommendations for initial therapy in transplant candidates

Most of the regimens discussed above are associated with high response rates. The main choices are Thal/Dex-, Rev/Dex-, and bortezomib-based regimens. Thal/Dex and Rev/Dex have the advantage of oral administration. But both are associated with an increased risk of DVT, necessitating routine thromboprophylaxis (see below). Further, the use of Rev/Dex is not recommended in renal failure. Rev/low-dose Dex is our preferred choice and can be administered both as pretransplant induction therapy as well as chronic, primary therapy following stem cell harvest in patients who choose delayed ASCT.[15] Vel/Dex or VTD are our preferred choices in patients presenting with renal failure. We recommend initial therapy for about 2-4 cycles, followed by stem cell harvest; we do not recommend prolonged therapy or revising therapy to achieve CR prior to stem cell harvest.

INITIAL TREATMENT OF PATIENTS NOT ELIGIBLE FOR TRANSPLANTATION

Patients who are not transplant candidates are treated with standard melphalan-based therapy. For decades, MP has been used as the standard regimen for this group of patients.[1] Over the years, despite better response rates, no survival benefit has been reported with any of the more aggressive combination chemotherapy regimens compared to MP. Recently, two new combinations have emerged with significantly superior survival compared to MP: melphalan, prednisone, thalidomide (MPT); and bortezomib, melphalan, prednisone, bortezomib (MPV).

Melphalan, prednisone

MP has been used in the treatment of MM for more than 40 years.[3,5] The response rate with MP is approximately 50%. The median survival is approximately 3-4 years. A meta-analysis of 26 randomized trials found superior response rates but no survival benefit with combination chemotherapy regimens compared with MP prior to the arrival of thalidomide and bortezomib.[5] MP is well tolerated, but responses can sometimes take 6 months to occur. The substitution of dexamethasone in place of prednisone improves response rate and the speed of response but does not improve OS.

Melphalan, prednisone, thalidomide

Four randomized trials have compared MP with MPT.[22,45,46] Palumbo et al.[22] randomized compared MP for 6 months versus MPT for 6 months followed by maintenance thalidomide. Overall response rates were significantly higher with the MPT compared to MP (76% vs. 48%) as was the CR plus near CR rate (28% vs. 7%). MPT resulted in superior 2-year PFS rates (54% vs. 27%, p < 0.001), and a trend toward an improved 3-year OS. Facon et al.[23] randomized 447 patients (ages 65-75) to MP versus MPT versus tandem ASCT with reduced dose melphalan (Mel 100 mg/m^2). PFS was superior with MPT compared to either MP or tandem MEL100 groups (median PFS: 28 months, 18 months, and 19 months, respectively, p < 0.001). There was also a significant survival advantage with MPT; median OS was 52 months, 33 months, and 38 months, respectively. Early (first 3 months) mortality rate was 8% with MP compared to 3% with MPT.

Hulin et al.[47] confirmed a survival advantage with MPT compared to MP in a randomized trial in 232 patients over the age of 75 (median survival of 45 vs. 28 months, respectively, p = 0.03). This trial showed that the benefit of MPT over MP persists in patients up to at least age 85, but it is important to note that patients received a lower dose of thalidomide of 100 mg/day. In contrast to the three MPT randomized trials discussed so far, Waage and colleagues[48] found no benefit with MPT compared to MP in a randomized placebo-controlled trial. The reasons for this discrepancy are not clear but may be related to the use of high doses of thalidomide (400 mg) in an elderly patient population resulting in increased early mortality particularly among those over the age of 75.

DVT and neuropathy are important concerns with MPT therapy. Grade 3 neuropathy occurs in 6%-8% of patients receiving MPT.[22,23] Overall, grade 3 and 4 adverse events occur in approximately 50% of patients treated with MPT compared to 25% with MP.[22]

Bortezomib, melphalan, prednisone

In a phase 2 trial, Mateos et al.[49] found a response rate of 89%, with a remarkably high CR rate of 32% with the VMP regimen. Impressively, approximately 50% of the patients with CR had no residual bone marrow plasma cells by immunophenotypic studies. A recent randomized trial compared VMP with MP in 682 patients (median age: 71 years).[50] In this trial, VMP had a significantly superior response rate compared to MP (71% vs. 35%, p < 0.001), as well as a superior CR rate (30% vs. 4%). TTP was significantly superior with VMP compared to MP (24 vs. 17 months, respectively, p < 0.001). The 2-year OS rate was 83% with VMP versus 70% with MP, respectively (p < 0.001). Importantly, VMP appeared to overcome adverse cytogenetic features; there was no significant difference in TTP or OS with VMP in patients with and without high-risk myeloma. Neuropathy is a significant risk with VMP therapy; grade 3 neuropathy occurred in 13% of patients.

Melphalan, prednisone, lenalidomide

Palumbo and colleagues[51] tested MPR in 54 newly diagnosed patients older than 65 years of age. At the maximum tolerated dose, the overall response rate was 81%, with 48% of patients achieving at least VGPR or better, and 24% of patients achieving CR. An ECOG randomized trial is comparing MPR with MPT. Major grade 3 and 4 adverse events were neutropenia and thrombocytopenia. All patients received prophylactic aspirin, and using this approach, DVT was found to be uncommon, occurring in only three patients, including two after aspirin discontinuation. On the basis of this trial, MPR appears to be a very effective oral regimen for the treatment of elderly patients with MM who are not candidates for SCT. Another phase 2 trial of MPR is ongoing at the Mayo Clinic. An ECOG randomized trial is comparing MPR with MPT in the United States.

Summary recommendations for initial therapy in transplant candidates

Both MPT and VMP are associated with high response rates, and both regimens are significantly better than MP in terms of OS. MPT has the advantage of oral administration. On the other hand, VMP has the advantage of not increasing the risk of DVT, and there are data that it can overcome the adverse prognostic effect of high-risk cytogenetic abnormalities. MPT is our preferred regimen for standard-risk patients who are not candidates for transplantation, especially given the ease of oral administration and strength of evidence from two peer-reviewed publications.[15,45,51] VMP would be our preferred regimen for high-risk patients who are not candidates for transplantation. We need randomized studies before MPR can be recommended. MP retains a role in patients who lack access to new drugs, are unable to tolerate therapy with these agents, have poor performance status, and in many patients over the age of 85.

TREATMENT OF HIGH-RISK MYELOMA

Patients with high-risk myeloma tend to do poorly with median OS of approximately 2 years even with tandem ASCT. There are three options for these patients.[15] The first option is to treat patients according to transplant eligibility as described above but follow such therapy with long-term maintenance therapy (e.g. lenalidomide or lenalidomide/dexamethasone) given the high risk of relapse.

The second option is novel therapeutic strategies that incorporate bortezomib early in the disease course and reserve SCT for relapsed disease.[2] In several studies, bortezomib appears to overcome the adverse effect of deletion 13.[49,52,53]

The third option is to consider ASCT followed by non-myeloablative allogeneic transplantation in selected patients. A recent IFM 99 trial in patients with deletion 13 and high β_2-microglobulin levels did not show significant benefit with this strategy compared to tandem ASCT.[54] However, in another randomized trial, a significant survival advantage was seen with ASCT followed by a reduced intensity conditioning (RIC) allogeneic SCT compared to tandem ASCT. On an intent-to-treat basis, the median overall and event-free survival were longer with ASCT followed by an RIC compared to tandem ASCT (80 months vs. 54 months, p = 0.01; and 35 months vs. 29 months, p = 0.02, respectively).[21]

Clearly, clinical trials and new agents specifically designed for high-risk myeloma are needed.

DVT PROPHYLAXIS

DVT is a major complication of thalidomide- and lenalidomide-based therapy.[55,56] The incidence of DVT is 1%-3% in patients receiving single-agent thalidomide or lenalidomide but increases to approximately 20% in patients receiving either drug in combination with high-dose dexamethasone and over 25%-30% in patients receiving the agents in combination with doxorubicin or liposomal doxorubicin. The risk of DVT with Thal/Dex and Rev/Dex can be significantly lowered by using low-dose dexamethasone (40 mg once a week) instead of high-dose dexamethasone. MPT and MPR are also associated with a risk of DVT. There is a significant (20%) risk of DVT with MPT in the absence of thromboprophylaxis. However, this rate drops to approximately 3% with the use of thromboprophylaxis (e.g. enoxaparin). Erythropoietin use appears to increase the risk of DVT with ImiD-based therapy.[57]

The International Myeloma Working Group has recently published detailed guidelines on DVT prophylaxis that are based on risk.[56] We recommend that DVT prophylaxis be administered as detailed in these guidelines. For most patients with newly diagnosed myeloma receiving thalidomide- or lenalidomide-based therapy, aspirin alone can be used as DVT prophylaxis as long as patients are receiving low-dose corticosteroids (e.g. dexamethasone 40 mg once a week or prednisone), provided no concomitant erythropoietic agents are used. On the other hand, patients receiving thalidomide or lenalidomide in combination with high-dose steroids or doxorubicin need higher intensity thromboprophylaxis with coumadin (target INR 2-3) or low-molecular weight heparin (equivalent of enoxaparin 40 mg once daily).

RECOMMENDED DOSE OF DEXAMETHASONE IN NEWLY DIAGNOSED MYELOMA

The recent ECOG randomized trial is the only study so far to compare the benefits and risks of high versus low dose of dexamethasone in a randomized study.[37,38] The trial showed that low-dose dexamethasone (40 mg once a week) is safer and more effective than high-dose dexamethasone. We believe that these findings apply to all regimens using high-dose dexamethasone for newly diagnosed myeloma. Thus, we recommend that the dose of dexamethasone with Rev/Dex, Thal/Dex, VTD, and other regimens in newly diagnosed disease be no more than 40 mg once a week.

REFERENCES

1. Kyle RA, Rajkumar SV. Multiple myeloma. *N Engl J Med* 2004;351:1860-73.

2. Rajkumar SV, Kyle RA. Multiple myeloma: diagnosis and treatment. *Mayo Clin Proc* 2005;80:1371-82.

3. Kyle RA, Rajkumar SV. Multiple myeloma. *Blood* 2008;111:2962-72.

4. Rajkumar SV, Kyle RA. Plasma cell disorders. In: Goldman L, Ausiello D, eds. *Cecil Textbook of Medicine*, 23rd ed. Philadelphia, PA: Saunders, 2007;1426-37.

5. Myeloma Trialists' Collaborative Group. Combination chemotherapy versus melphalan plus prednisone as treatment for multiple myeloma: an overview of 6,633 patients from 27 randomized trials. *J Clin Oncol* 1998;16:3832-42.

6. Attal M, Harousseau JL, Stoppa AM, et al. A prospective, randomized trial of autologous bone marrow transplantation and chemotherapy in multiple myeloma. Intergroupe Francais du Myelome. *N Engl J Med* 1996;335:91-7.

7. Singhal S, Mehta J, Desikan R, et al. Antitumor activity of thalidomide in refractory multiple myeloma [see comments]. *N Engl J Med* 1999;341:1565-71.

8. Richardson PG, Barlogie B, Berenson J, et al. A phase 2 study of bortezomib in relapsed, refractory myeloma. *N Engl J Med* 2003;348:2609-17.

9. Richardson PG, Sonneveld P, Schuster MW, et al. Bortezomib or high-dose dexamethasone for relapsed multiple myeloma [see comment]. *N Engl J Med* 2005;352:2487-98.

10. Rajkumar SV, Hayman SR, Lacy MQ, et al. Combination therapy with lenalidomide plus dexamethasone (Rev/Dex) for newly diagnosed myeloma. *Blood* 2005;106:4050-3.

11. Richardson PG, Blood E, Mitsiades CS, et al. A randomized phase 2 study of lenalidomide therapy for patients with relapsed or relapsed and refractory multiple myeloma. *Blood* 2006;108:3458-64.

12. Kumar SK, Rajkumar SV, Dispenzieri A, et al. Improved survival in multiple myeloma and the impact of novel therapies. *Blood* 2007;111:2516-20.

13. Hjorth M, Hellquist L, Holmberg E, Magnusson B, Rodjer S, Westin J. Initial versus deferred melphalan-prednisone therapy for asymptomatic multiple myeloma stage I—a randomized study. Myeloma Group of Western Sweden. *Eur J Haematol* 1993;50:95-102.

14. Grignani G, Gobbi PG, Formisano R, et al. A prognostic index for multiple myeloma. *Br J Cancer* 1996;73:1101-7.

15. Dispenzieri A, Rajkumar SV, Gertz MA, et al. Treatment of newly diagnosed multiple myeloma based on Mayo stratification of myeloma and risk-adapted therapy (mSMART): Consensus Statement. *Mayo Clin Proc* 2007;82:323-41.

16. Child JA, Morgan GJ, Davies FE, et al. High-dose chemotherapy with hematopoietic stem-cell rescue for multiple myeloma. *N Engl J Med* 2003;348:1875-83.

17. Fermand JP, Ravaud P, Chevret S, et al. High-dose therapy and autologous peripheral blood stem cell transplantation in multiple myeloma: up-front or rescue treatment? Results of a multicenter sequential randomized clinical trial. *Blood* 1998;92:3131-6.

18. Barlogie B, Kyle RA, Anderson KC, et al. Standard chemotherapy compared with high-dose chemoradiotherapy for multiple myeloma: final results of phase III US Intergroup Trial S9321. *J Clin Oncol* 2006;24:929-36.

19. Attal M, Harousseau JL, Facon T, et al. Single versus double autologous stem-cell transplantation for multiple myeloma [see comment]. *N Engl J Med* 2003;349:2495-502.

20. Blade J, Rosinol L, Sureda A, et al. High-dose therapy intensification compared with continued standard chemotherapy in multiple myeloma patients responding to the initial chemotherapy: long-term results from a prospective randomized trial from the Spanish cooperative group PETHEMA. *Blood* 2005;106:3755-9.

21. Bruno B, Rotta M, Patriarca F, et al. A comparison of allografting with autografting for newly diagnosed myeloma. *N Engl J Med* 2007;356:1110-20.

22. Palumbo A, Bringhen S, Caravita T, et al. Oral melphalan and prednisone chemotherapy plus thalidomide compared with melphalan and prednisone alone in elderly patients with multiple myeloma: randomised controlled trial. *Lancet* 2006;367:825-31.

23. Facon T, Mary JY, Hulin C, et al. Melphalan and prednisone plus thalidomide versus melphalan and prednisone alone or reduced-intensity autologous stem cell transplantation in elderly patients with multiple myeloma (IFM 99-06): a randomised trial. *Lancet* 2007;370:1209-18.

24. Dimopoulos M, Spencer A, Attal M, et al. Lenalidomide plus dexamethasone for relapsed or refractory multiple myeloma. *N Engl J Med* 2007;357:2123-32.

25. Weber DM, Chen C, Niesvizky R, et al. Lenalidomide plus dexamethasone for relapsed multiple myeloma in North America. *N Engl J Med* 2007;357:2133-42.

26. Rajkumar SV. The death of VAD as initial therapy for multiple myeloma. *Blood* 2005;106:2-3.

27. Cavo M, Zamagni E, Tosi P, et al. Superiority of thalidomide and dexamethasone over vincristine-doxorubicin-dexamethasone (VAD) as primary therapy in preparation for autologous transplantation for multiple myeloma. *Blood* 2005;106:35-9.

28. Fermand J-P, Jaccard A, Macro M, et al. A randomized comparison of dexamethasone + thalidomide (Dex/Thal) vs Dex + Placebo (Dex/P) in patients (pts) with relapsing multiple myeloma (MM). *Blood* 2006;108:3563.

29. Alexanian R, Dimopoulos MA, Delasalle K, Barlogie B. Primary dexamethasone treatment of multiple myeloma. *Blood* 1992;80:887-90.

30. Rajkumar SV, Blood E, Vesole DH, Fonseca R, Greipp PR. Phase III clinical trial of thalidomide plus dexamethasone compared with dexamethasone alone in newly diagnosed multiple myeloma: a clinical trial coordinated by the Eastern Cooperative Oncology Group. *J Clin Oncol* 2006;24:431-6.

31. Rajkumar SV, Rosiñol L, Hussein M, et al. A multicenter, randomized, double-blind, placebo-controlled study of thalidomide plus dexamethasone versus dexamethasone as initial therapy for newly diagnosed multiple myeloma. *J Clin Oncol* 2008;26: 2171-7.

32. Facon T, Mary J-Y, Pegourie B, et al. Dexamethasone-based regimens versus melphalan-prednisone for elderly multiple myeloma patients ineligible for high-dose therapy. *Blood* 2006;107:1292-8.

33. Rajkumar SV, Hayman S, Gertz MA, et al. Combination therapy with thalidomide plus dexamethasone for newly diagnosed myeloma. *J Clin Oncol* 2002;20:4319-23.

34. Weber DM, Gavino M, Delasalle K, Rankin K, Giralt S, Alexanian R. Thalidomide alone or with dexamethasone for multiple myeloma. *Blood* 1999;94(suppl 1):604a (A2686).

35. Cavo M, Zamagni E, Tosi P, et al. First-line therapy with thalidomide and dexamethasone in preparation for autologous stem cell transplantation for multiple myeloma. *Haematologica* 2004;89:826-31.

36. Lacy MQ, Gertz MA, Dispenzieri AA, et al. Long-term results of response to therapy, time to progression, and survival with lenalidomide plus dexamethasone in newly diagnosed myeloma. *Mayo Clin Proc* 2007;82:1179-84.

37. Rajkumar SV, Jacobus S, Callander N, Fonseca R, Vesole D, Greipp P. A randomized phase III trial of lenalidomide plus high-dose dexamethasone versus lenalidomide plus low-dose dexamethasone in newly diagnosed multiple myeloma (E4A03): a trial coordinated by the Eastern Cooperative Oncology Group. *Blood* 2006;108:799.

38. Rajkumar SV, Jacobus S, Callander N, et al. A randomized trial of lenalidomide plus high-dose dexamethasone (RD) versus lenalidomide plus low-dose dexamethasone (Rd) in newly diagnosed multiple myeloma (E4A03): a trial coordinated by the Eastern Cooperative Oncology Group. *ASH Annual Meeting Abstracts* 2007;110:74.

39. Kumar S, Dispenzieri A, Lacy MQ, et al. Impact of lenalidomide therapy on stem cell mobilization and engraftment post-peripheral blood stem cell transplantation in patients with newly diagnosed myeloma. *Leukemia* 2007;21:2035-42.

40. Niesvizky R, Jayabalan DS, Christos PJ, et al. BiRD (Biaxin(R) [clarithromycin]/Revlimid(R)[lenalidomide]/dexamethasone) combination therapy results in high complete- and overall-response rates in treatment-naive symptomatic multiple myeloma. *Blood* 2007;111:1101-9.

41. Jagannath S, Durie BG, Wolf J, et al. Bortezomib therapy alone and in combination with dexamethasone for previously untreated symptomatic multiple myeloma. *Br J Haematol* 2005;129:776-83.

42. Harousseau J, Attal M, Leleu X, et al. Bortezomib plus dexamethasone as induction treatment prior to autologous stem cell transplantation in patients with newly diagnosed multiple myeloma: results of an IFM phase II study. *Haematologica* 2006;91:1498-505.

43. Harousseau JL, Mathiot C, Attal M, et al. VELCADE/dexamethasone (Vel/D) versus VAD as induction treatment prior to autologous stem cell transplantation (ASCT) in newly diagnosed multiple myeloma (MM): updated results of the IFM 2005/01 trial. *ASH Annual Meeting Abstracts* 2007;110:450.

44. Cavo M, Patriarca F, Tacchetti P, et al. Bortezomib (Velcade(R))-Thalidomide-Dexamethasone (VTD) vs Thalidomide-Dexamethasone (TD) in preparation for autologous stem-cell (SC) transplantation (ASCT) in newly diagnosed multiple myeloma (MM). *ASH Annual Meeting Abstracts* 2007;110:73.

45. Facon T, Mary JY, Hulin C, et al. Melphalan and prednisone plus thalidomide versus melphalan and prednisone alone or reduced-intensity autologous stem cell transplantation in elderly patients with multiple myeloma (IFM 99-06): a randomised trial. *Lancet* 2007;370:1209-18.

46. Hulin C, Virion J, Leleu X, et al. Comparison of melphalan-prednisone-thalidomide (MP-T) to melphalan-prednisone (MP) in patients 75 years of age or older with untreated multiple myeloma (MM). Preliminary results of the randomized, double-blind, placebo controlled IFM 01-01 trial. *J Clin Oncol* (Meeting Abstracts) 2007;25:8001.

47. Hulin C, Facon T, Rodon P, et al. Melphalan-prednisone-thalidomide (MP-T) demonstrates a significant survival advantage in elderly patients ≥75 years with multiple myeloma compared with melphalan-prednisone (MP) in a randomized, double-blind, placebo-controlled trial, IFM 01/01. *ASH Annual Meeting Abstracts* 2007;110:75.

48. Waage A, Gimsing P, Juliusson G, Turesson I, Fayers P. Melphalan-prednisone-thalidomide to newly diagnosed patients with multiple myeloma: a placebo controlled randomised phase 3 trial. *ASH Annual Meeting Abstracts* 2007;110:78.

49. Mateos M-V, Hernandez J-M, Hernandez M-T, et al. Bortezomib plus melphalan and prednisone in elderly untreated patients with multiple myeloma: results of a multicenter phase 1/2 study. *Blood* 2006;108:2165-72.

50. San Miguel JF, Schlag R, Khuageva N, et al. MMY-3002: a phase 3 study comparing bortezomib-melphalan-prednisone (VMP) with melphalan-prednisone (MP) in newly diagnosed multiple myeloma. *ASH Annual Meeting Abstracts* 2007;110:76.

51. Palumbo A, Falco P, Corradini P, et al. Melphalan, prednisone, and lenalidomide treatment for newly diagnosed myeloma: a report from the GIMEMA Italian Multiple Myeloma Network. *J Clin Oncol* 2007;25:4459-65.

52. Jagannath S, Richardson PG, Sonneveld P, et al. Bortezomib appears to overcome the poor prognosis conferred by chromosome 13 deletion in phase 2 and 3 trials. *Leukemia* 2006;21:151-7.

53. Sagaster V, Ludwig H, Kaufmann H, et al. Bortezomib in relapsed multiple myeloma: response rates and duration of response are independent of a chromosome 13q-deletion. *Leukemia* 2006;21:164-8.

54. Garban F, Attal M, Michallet M, et al. Prospective comparison of autologous stem cell transplantation followed by dose-reduced allograft (IFM99-03 trial) with tandem autologous stem cell transplantation (IFM99-04 trial) in high-risk de novo multiple myeloma. *Blood* 2006;107:3474-80.

55. Rajkumar SV. Thalidomide therapy and deep venous thrombosis in multiple myeloma [comment]. *Mayo Clin Proc* 2005;80:1549-51.

56. Palumbo A, Rajkumar SV, Dimopoulos MA, et al. Prevention of thalidomide- and lenalidomide-associated thrombosis in myeloma. *Leukemia* 2007;22:414-23.

57. Knight R, Delap RJ, Zeldis JB. Lenalidomide and venous thrombosis in multiple myeloma. *N Engl J Med* 2006;354:2079-80.

4 Maintenance Therapy in Multiple Myeloma

Sagar Lonial and Jonathan L. Kaufman

SUMMARY

The role of maintenance therapy in the treatment of patients with multiple myeloma is currently under extensive evaluation. Maintenance therapy is defined as the addition of chronically applied therapy, following induction in responding or stable patient, with the goal of prolonging survival (ASH:FDA Workshop). Prolonged conventional chemotherapy has not only proven to be ineffective as maintenance therapy, but it is also associated with an increased risk of secondary myelodysplastic syndromes. Interferon α and corticosteroids have also been evaluated as maintenance therapy, but these treatments demonstrated marginal benefit at the cost of excessive toxicity. Recent studies have evaluated the role of maintenance thalidomide with hints that for certain subsets there may be a significant benefit. Additional studies are ongoing, testing the combination of thalidomide and corticosteroids, lenalidomide, and bortezomib in the maintenance setting. Future studies will need to identify not only the relative benefit for these agents in the maintenance setting but also the role cytogenetic risk groups play on the relative benefit of maintenance approaches.

INTRODUCTION

Multiple myeloma is an incurable malignancy characterized by the accumulation of malignant plasma cells. Treatment options for patients with myeloma have utilized alkylator-based therapy in conjunction with corticosteroids, and more recently, the widespread use of high-dose therapy and autologous transplant has improved overall survival (OS) for many of these patients. These improvements in OS have been associated with improving the rate of complete remission, a disease state not known to be associated with a cure but with superior long-term outcomes. Given this improvement in outcomes, many groups have tried to "maintain" patients in a good remission status following initial therapy, and thus the concept of maintenance therapy was born. True maintenance therapy presumes that patients are in complete remission, and that the therapy in question keeps the disease status as such. However, more modern approaches to this definition include therapy for patients who have not achieved complete remission, and are being given "ongoing" therapy in an effort to either drive tumor burden lower or to keep the disease stable at low levels. Both maneuvers are considered maintenance therapy, and this is the spirit in which the current chapter addresses maintenance therapy.

Maintenance therapy for myeloma should, at a minimum, prolong remission duration without significant toxicity. But the ultimate goal of maintenance therapy should also be to prolong OS. That is, an optimal maintenance therapy will result in better outcomes compared to that same therapy delivered at relapse in patients who have not had maintenance therapy. Patients with myeloma have varying clinical courses (indolent vs. aggressive). These differences in disease behavior are the result of underlying differences in myeloma biology. Defining the optimal maintenance strategy will depend on identifying risk groups based on cytogenetics and remission status and applying the use of our currently available agents in a "tailored" way to optimize the benefit of maintenance therapy while minimizing potential toxicity. The following represents a review of maintenance strategies tested previously, current research in the field, and potential future maintenance approaches.

CONVENTIONAL THERAPY

The first attempts at maintenance therapy were to prolong the remission duration following the use of alkylating

TABLE 4.1. Results of maintenance trials using conventional chemotherapy, interferon, or corticosteroids

Study	References	Therapy (n)	PFS/EFS/DOR	Overall survival	Notes
Conventional chemotherapy					
SWOG*	(1)	MP[†] (37) CP[‡] (32) No treatment (27)	Median: 18 months DOR no difference (p > 0.4)	No difference between groups (p > 0.2)	See also Refs (2–7)
Interferon					
MTCG[§]	(8)	Interferon (767) No treatment (776)	27% at 3 years 19% at 3 years (p < 0.00001)	Median: 40 months Median: 36 months (p = 0.01)	Survival measured for both induction and maintenance
Meta-analysis	(9)	Interferon (789) No treatment (826)	4.4-Month increase in EFS for interferon (p < 0.01)	7.0-Month increase in OS for interferon (p < 0.01)	
U.S. intergroup trial S9321	(10)	Interferon (121) No treatment (121)	Median PFS: 23 months 18 months (p = 0.18)	Median OS: 69 months 62 months (p = 0.90)	Post autologous PBSCT or standard therapy
Corticosteroids					
SWOG* 9210	(11)	Prednisone 50 mg QOD Prednisone 10 mg QOD	Median PFS: 15 months 5 months (p = 0.003)	Median OS: 37 months 26 months (p = 0.05)	Post VAD based induction
MY-7[‖]	(12)	Dex. 40 mg 4 days[¶] No treatment	Median PFS: 2.8 years 2.1 years (p = 0.0002)	Median OS: 4.1 years 3.8 years (p = 0.4)	Post MP or M-Dex induction

EFS, event-free survival; DOR, duration of remission; PFS, progression-free survival.
* Southwest Oncology Group.
[†] Melphalan 10 mg/m^2/day for 4 days and prednisone 60 mg/m^2 for 4 days every 6 weeks.
[‡] Carmustine 150 mg/m^2 i.v. on day 4 and prednisone 60 mg/m^2 for 4 days every 6 weeks.
[§] Myeloma Trialists' Collaborative Group.
[‖] National Cancer Institute of Canada Clinical Trials Group MY-7 trial.
[¶] Dexamethasone 40 mg/day for 4 days every 28 days until progression of dose-limiting toxicity.

agent–based induction therapy. The Southwest Oncology Group study randomized 96 patients, all of whom had responded to melphalan and prednisone (MP) based therapy, to one of three arms: continued MP, BCNU plus prednisone, or no further therapy.[1] There was no difference in relapse rate, remission duration, or OS between the three randomized arms, with median remission duration from the time of randomization of 18 months (p > 0.4). In the patients receiving ongoing chemotherapy, more infections, including herpes zoster reactivation and pneumonia, were noted. One patient in the maintenance chemotherapy arm died from acute myelogenous leukemia (AML), whereas no patients in the control arm

developed AML. The investigators concluded that there was no benefit for continued alkylating agent–based therapy following best response to induction therapy.[1] Despite these findings, several other clinical trials were performed assessing the relative benefit for various combinations of chemotherapy and immunosuppressive agents.[2-7] Maintenance chemotherapy provided no clear survival advantage for patients in remission compared with retreatment upon progression (Table 4.1). On the basis of these findings along with the risk of infection and secondary leukemia associated with ongoing alkylating agent chemotherapy, the use of maintenance conventional chemotherapy is no longer recommended.

INTERFERON

Interferon has been extensively studied as maintenance therapy following both low-dose conventional therapy and high-dose therapy. A meta-analyses of the use of interferon both as maintenance and as part of initial induction therapy was reported from the Myeloma Trialists' Collaborative Group.[8] Progression-free survival (PFS) and response duration were improved compared with no maintenance. In addition, patients allocated to interferon maintenance did have a 7-month OS advantage compared with those patients allocated to no maintenance therapy; however, survival after progression was shorter for patients receiving interferon as maintenance therapy (p = 0.007). The magnitude of benefit for interferon was noted to be the largest in smaller trials, with no clear benefit seen from larger trials. In a separate analysis by Fritz and Ludwig,[9] 1615 patients across 13 different trials were evaluated. In their analysis, there was a small benefit in both PFS and OS for those patients receiving interferon as maintenance therapy that was associated with moderate toxicity. More recently, the U.S. Intergroup trial S9321 compared the use of interferon after either high-dose therapy and autologous transplant or standard chemotherapy with VBMCP. The median PFS for the interferon group was 23 months versus 18 months for the control arm (p = 0.18). In addition, there was no difference in survival between the two randomized arms (median OS being 69 months in the interferon group vs. 62 months in the no maintenance group; p = 0.90).[10] On the basis of a lack of clinical benefit as seen in large randomized trials as well as significant morbidity associated with the use of maintenance interferon, interferon maintenance is not routinely recommended for use outside of large randomized clinical trials.

CORTICOSTEROIDS

Corticosteroids are an integral part of treatment for patients with myeloma, both as a part of induction therapy and in the relapse setting. Several investigators have subsequently assessed the role of steroids as maintenance therapy. The strongest data to date comes from the SWOG 9210 clinical trial.[11] Patients were originally randomized to receive VAD plus prednisone versus VAD plus prednisone and quinine. After remission induction patients were then rerandomized to either prednisone 10 mg or 50 mg, both administered every other day until progression. There was no difference in response rate, PFS, or OS between the two initial induction schedules. Of the 250 patients originally on this trial, only 126 participated in the second randomization for maintenance therapy. Among subjects receiving 50 mg prednisone every other day, PFS (14 vs. 5 months; p = 0.003) and OS (37 vs. 26 months; p = 0.05) were significantly longer, when compared with those receiving 10 mg every other day. The toxicities at these schedules were comparable, with only one patient in the high-dose prednisone group who had therapy discontinued early and similar grade 3 or worse toxicity (21% for the 10 mg schedule and 26% for the 50 mg schedule). The actual benefit from the initial induction therapy was quite limited; thus, patients randomized to the higher dose of steroids were likely benefiting from additional therapy as both arms received inadequate induction, and patients in the low-dose prednisone arm did not receive this benefit. While appropriate as a proof of principal study, the clinical utility of this study in the modern era is limited as most patients do receive VAD as initial therapy, and salvage therapy approaches are significantly better than at the time of this study.[11]

The NCIC CTG MY.7 trial assessed dexamethasone maintenance compared with placebo after induction therapy with MP or melphalan and dexamethasone (M-Dex).[12] Of the 585 patients randomized to the initial induction phase (MP vs. MD), 292 did not have disease progression during induction and were thus eligible for the maintenance part of the study. A total of 145 patients were randomized to observation versus 40 mg of dexamethasone for four days every month. Patients treated with dexamethasone maintenance were noted to experience increased toxicity, including hyperglycemia and infections. While median PFS was higher with maintenance dexamethasone (Dex – 2.8 years vs. no Dex – 2.1 years; p = 0.0002), there was no difference in OS (Dex – 4.1 years vs. no Dex – 3.8 years; p = 0.4).[12] While not positive in terms of improving OS benefit, these studies have laid the foundation for the use of corticosteroids in the maintenance setting because of the PFS advantage. Given the toxicity of high-dose corticosteroids overall, and the goal of less toxic maintenance therapy, the utility of corticosteroids alone is likely limited, but in lower dose may be of benefit in conjunction with other agents in the maintenance setting.

THALIDOMIDE

Thalidomide is clearly an active agent both for relapsed and newly diagnosed myeloma. Given its ease of administration and potential use over prolonged periods of time, thalidomide represents an excellent option for clinical investigation in the maintenance setting. Alexanian and colleagues[13] assessed the role of thalidomide with dexamethasone for patients who achieve a partial remission after high-dose therapy and autologous transplant. An improvement in the depth of response from partial response (PR) to at least a very good partial response (VGPR) (>90% reduction in the serum protein) was noted in 57% of the patients. Toxicity of the regimen was manageable and included the commonly observed toxicities of thalidomide such as constipation, fatigue, and peripheral neuropathy. In order to assess the optimal dose of thalidomide when used after high-dose therapy and transplant, Stewart and colleagues[14] in Canada randomized patients to receive either thalidomide 200 mg/day or 400 mg/day, both administered with prednisone 50 mg every other day (NCIC MY-9 trial). The primary endpoint of this trial was to assess the proportion of patients discontinuing or reducing therapy owing to treatment-related toxicity within the first 6 months of maintenance treatment. After a median follow-up of 36.8 months 31% of patients in the 200 mg arm and 69% in the 400 mg arm either discontinued therapy or had a dose modification due to side effects. The percentage of patients remaining on maintenance therapy after 18 months was 76% in the 200 mg vs. 41% in the 400 mg arm. Peripheral neuropathy was the most common reason for discontinuation of thalidomide in both treatment groups. Grade 3 or 4 nonhematological toxicities were observed in 36% and 27% of patients in the 400 mg and 200 mg dose arms, respectively. The occurrence of symptomatic venous thrombosis was 7.5% for all patients, with no difference between the groups. There was also no difference between the two arms in the frequency or rate of discontinuation of prednisone during the study. While there was no formal comparison of PFS, the median post-transplant PFS for both arms analyzed in aggregate was 32.3 months. The authors concluded that 200 mg was the recommended dose for a randomized phase 3 trial comparing thalidomide and prednisone with placebo as maintenance after transplant.[14]

In another trial whose goal was to determine the optimal dose of single-agent thalidomide as maintenance therapy after high-dose therapy and autologous transplant, the U.K. Medical Research Council (MRC) initiated a pilot study comparing different dose levels of thalidomide. The primary endpoint for this study was toxicity and duration of remission after transplant. The long-term tolerance of thalidomide was assessed at five dose levels: 50 mg, 100 mg, 200 mg, 250 mg, and 300 mg. After an initial report with a median follow-up of 6 months in 2003, the MRC recently published the final results of the study.[15,16] With a median follow-up of 32.3 months, 77% (77/100) of patients discontinued thalidomide, 23 owing to progression of disease, and 53 owing to toxicities.[16] Peripheral neuropathy was the most frequent side effect occurring in 72% of the population. Two patients experienced a thrombotic event. The observed lower thrombosis rate is in contrast with the 7.5% thrombosis rate when thalidomide was combined with prednisone as maintenance.[14] No difference in PFS between the difference dose levels was noted. Patients assigned to doses less than 150 mg daily were able to remain on their assigned dose longer and with fewer side effects than patients who were assigned higher doses. Of particular interest is the observation that 15 patients improved their response from PR to complete response (CR) at median of over 13 months. This suggests that the benefit to thalidomide maintenance may not be in maintaining response but in improving the depth of response for patients who did not have an adequate response to initial therapy.

In a retrospective analysis by Brinker et al.,[17] a total of 112 patients who had received maintenance therapy with interferon, thalidomide, or observation, following high-dose chemotherapy and autologous transplant were reviewed. Patients who received thalidomide at any point after transplant had improved median survival (79.6 months) compared to patients who did not (39.6 months). In a multivariate analysis of this patient group taking into account response to transplant, stem cell source, and other factors that may influence outcomes following transplant, the significant predictors for OS were age and use of thalidomide anytime after transplant (p = 0.09). While this analysis only indirectly addresses maintenance therapy (one-half of the thalidomide group were treated as maintenance, with the rest receiving thalidomide at the time of relapse), patients who received maintenance

Title	References	Design	N	PFS	p Value	OS	p Value
IFM 99 02	(18)	Tandem AHSCT	597	Progression free at 3 years	0.003	4 Years	0.04
		Arm 1: no maintenance	200	38%		77%	
		Arm 2: pamidronate	196	39%		74%	
		Arm 3: Thal 400 mg and pamidronate	201	51%		87%	
ALLG MM6	(21,22)	Single AHSCT	243	Progression free at 3 years	0.0003	3 Years	0.02
		Arm 1: Thal 200 mg/Pred	114	35		86%	
		Arm 2: Pred	129	25		75%	
NCIC MY 9	(14)	Single AHSCT	67	Median follow-up: 32 months		4 Years 75%	
		Arm 1. Thal 200/Pred	45	(nr)		nr	
		Arm 2: Thal 400/Pred	22	(nr)		nr	
Tunisian MMSG	(19)	Entire cohort: Single AHSCT	195	Progression free at 3 years	0.02	3-Year survival	0.04
		Second AHSCT	97	57%		65%	
		Maintenance thalidomide	98	85%		85%	

TABLE 4.2. Efficacy of thalidomide as maintenance therapy

AHSCT, autologous hematopoietic stem cell transplantation; nr, not reported; OS, overall survival; PFS, progression-free survival; Pred, prednisone; Thal, thalidomide.

thalidomide had an improved OS compared to patients treated with thalidomide at the time of relapse (p = 0.05).

The IFM 99 02 study was the first randomized study to compare single-agent thalidomide with no maintenance after high-dose therapy and autologous transplant (Tables 4.2 and 4.3). The trial was initiated to assess the impact of thalidomide maintenance on the duration of response after transplant among a group of low-risk patients (zero- or one-risk factor as defined by the IFM of an elevated β_2-microglobulin (β_2M) or deletion 13 by fluorescent in situ hybridization (FISH) analysis. A total of 780 patients less than 65 years old were enrolled to receive VAD induction followed by tandem autologous transplant prepared with melphalan (first transplant 140 mg/m^2; second transplant 200 mg/m^2). Patients with stable disease or better 2 months after the second transplant were randomized to one of three maintenance therapy arms.

At the time of final analysis, 593 of the 780 patients were randomized to receive (1) observation, (2) pamidronate 90 mg/month, or (3) thalidomide 100 mg/day + pamidronate 90 mg/month as maintenance therapy. At approximately 29-month median follow-up from randomization, patients randomized to thalidomide had improvement in event-free survival compared to those patients randomized to no treatment or pamidronate alone (52% [Thal/Pam] vs. 36% [observation] and 37% [Pam only]; p = 0.002).[18] In addition, there was a substantial improvement in OS for the patients randomized to receive maintenance thalidomide compared with the other two arms (87% [Thal/Pam] vs. 77% [observation] and 74% [Pam only]; p = 0.04). Importantly, the survival after relapse was no different between the three arms, suggesting that maintenance thalidomide does not result in the development of highly resistant disease. While the population as a whole

TABLE 4.3. Toxicity of thalidomide as maintenance therapy

Title	References	Design	N	Thal dose	Thrombosis (%)	Neuropathy % (%grad 3–4)
IFM 99 02	18	Tandem AHSCT	597			
		Arm 1: no maintenance	200	0	2	8 (1)
		Arm 2: pamidronate	196	0	1	15 (2)
		Arm 3: Thal 400 mg and pamidronate	201	200 mg (mean)	4	68 (7)
ALLG MM6	21, 22	Single AHSCT	243		nr	nr
		Arm 1: Thal 200 mg/Pred	114	100 mg (median)	nr	nr
		Arm 2: Pred	129	0	nr	nr
NCIC MY 9	14	Single AHSCT	67		7.5	54 (25)
		Arm 1: Thal 200/Pred	45	133 mg (median)	nr	24% grade3/4
		Arm 2: Thal 400/Pred	22	320 mg (median)	nr	27% grade3/4
Tunisian MMSG	19	Single AHSCT	195			
		Second AHSCT	97	0	nr	nr
		Maintenance thalidomide	98	100 mg	0	4% (nr)

AHSCT, autologous hematopoietic stem cell transplantation; nr, not reported; Pred, prednisone; Thal, thalidomide.

had an improvement in event-free survival, relapse-free survival, and OS, there were two subsets of patients who did not appear to benefit from maintenance thalidomide. Patients with deletion 13 (as determined by FISH) and patients who had achieved a VGPR following high-dose therapy derived no improvement in event-free survival when randomized to maintenance thalidomide. In fact, the lack of benefit for the patients with deletion 13 was independent of response. These data further support the ongoing investigation of maintenance thalidomide but suggest that separate maintenance strategies need to be developed for patients with deletion 13 or other adverse prognostic features. This study also questions the role of maintenance thalidomide as a single agent in patients who have achieved a very good PR or better following high-dose therapy.

While the IFM 99 02 study addressed maintenance thalidomide after tandem autologous transplants, the Tunisian group asked whether 6 months of maintenance thalidomide after a single autologous transplant conditioned with melphalan 200 mg/m² was superior to tandem autologous transplant with a total of planned melphalan dose of 400 mg/m² and no maintenance thalidomide.[19] A total of 195 patients were randomly assigned to one of the two treatment arms. All patients received induction therapy with thalidomide and dexamethasone followed by collection of stem cell after cyclophosphamide mobilization. At diagnosis and 3 months after the first autologous transplant the patient characteristics were similar between the two groups. Approximately 40% of patients achieved at least a VGPR following the first transplant. Response was assessed 6 months after the second autologous transplant for patients in arm A (tandem transplant) and after 6 months of maintenance thalidomide for patients in arm B (single transplant and maintenance thalidomide). The proportion of patients who achieved a VGPR or better rate was 51% for arm A compared to 67% for arm B (p = 0.024). The improved VGPR rate translated into improved PFS and OS (Table 4.2). In findings similar to other studies, patients who had achieved a VGPR after the first transplant did not benefit from single-agent thalidomide maintenance. Because of the low dose of thalidomide used for the patients in this study, toxicity was limited with only a 4% thrombosis rate. This study concluded that a single cycle of high-dose therapy and 6 months of maintenance thalidomide was superior to tandem autologous transplant.[19]

However, all the information regarding the use of maintenance therapy is not clearly beneficial. Barlogie and colleagues[20] recently published their experience with the use of thalidomide as maintenance in combination with dexamethasone and interferon as part of the total therapy program. In this study, patients were treated in a uniform manner of induction chemotherapy followed by tandem autologous transplant conditioned with melphalan 200 mg/m², followed by further intensive maintenance

TABLE 4.4. Ongoing randomized trials of maintenance therapy

Title	Study design	Control arm	Experimental arm
NCIC/ECOG MY10	Single AHSCT Melphalan 200 mg/m²	No maintenance	Thalidomide 200 mg and prednisone 50 mg every other day
BMT CTN 0102	Tandem AHSCT Melphalan 200 mg/m² two times	No maintenance	Thalidomide 200 mg and dexamethasone 40 mg for days 1-4 in a 28-day cycle
MRC Myeloma IX	Single AHSCT Melphalan 200 mg/m²	No maintenance	Thalidomide 50 mg to 100 mg
CALGB 100104	Single AHSCT Melphalan 200 mg/m²	No maintenance	Lenalidomide 10 mg daily
IFM 2005 02	Single AHSCT Melphalan 200 mg/m² VGPR or better	No maintenance	Lenalidomide

AHSCT, autologous hematopoietic stem cell transplantation; VGPR, very good partial response.

chemotherapy for an additional four cycles. All patients who had not progressed and could tolerate further therapy received maintenance with interferon (3 million U/m²) three times a week and 4 days of pulse dexamethasone three times a month every 3 months for 1 year followed by interferon alone for subsequent years. Patients were initially randomized to receive thalidomide or no thalidomide throughout the entire course of treatment. CR measured after each phase of treatment was higher in the thalidomide arm, which translated into an improvement in 5-year event-free survival from 44% to 56% (p = 0.01) in the thalidomide treatment group. But, in contradiction to the IFM study, there was no survival advantage with the addition of thalidomide. This was because the OS after relapse or progression was significantly lower in the thalidomide-treated patients (1.1 years) compared to patients randomized to no thalidomide (2.7 years; p = 0.001).[20] While this study involved the use of more than maintenance thalidomide, it does raise the possibility that the use of thalidomide may change the phenotype of the disease, thus impacting the sensitivity and response rate of disease once it relapses. Given the complexity of the total therapy regimen and the numerous other agents administered in conjunction with thalidomide, it is difficult to draw too many conclusions regarding the use of thalidomide as maintenance therapy, but clearly there may be biological implications of ongoing therapy that need to be considered as we design future clinical trials in the maintenance setting.

The Australian Leukaemia and Lymphoma Group (ALLG) recently reported results from a randomized trial of thalidomide maintenance following high-dose therapy and autologous transplant. Thalidomide was started at 200 mg/day in combination with prednisone 50 mg every other day (arm 1; n = 114) or prednisone 50 mg every other day alone (arm 2; n = 129).[21,22] Thalidomide was administered for no longer than 12 months, and the prednisone was administered until progression in both arms. The percentage of patients in an immunofixation negative CR following transplant was similar between the two arms (arm 1 = 9% vs. arm 2 = 11%). The percentage of patients maintaining a PR or better at 12 months was improved in arm 1 compared to arm 2 (83% vs. 53%; p < 0.01). PFS was improved for arm 1 compared to arm 2 at 1 year (91% vs. 69%), 2 years (65% vs. 36%), and 3 years (35% vs. 25%) after randomization. In addition, OS at 3 years was improved for patients receiving thalidomide with prednisone compared to prednisone alone (86% vs. 75%; p = 0.02).[22] The full published report of this study including toxicity and differences among cytogenetic risk categories is currently pending but again suggests that thalidomide with steroids may offer significant benefit for subsets of patients.

Clearly, further studies are needed to address the overall role of maintenance thalidomide, both as a single agent and in combination with corticosteroids. Detailed analyses of these studies with subgroup analysis incorporating depth of remission, stage at diagnosis, and cytogenetics are critical. Ongoing studies including this study will be critical in understanding the role of thalidomide as maintenance (Table 4.4).

FUTURE DIRECTIONS

In addition to thalidomide, several investigators are actively assessing the role of other novel therapeutics as maintenance therapy after both conventional and high-dose therapy. Single-agent bortezomib administered at a dose of 1.3 mg/m^2 once weekly 4 out of 5 weeks after a single cycle of high-dose therapy and autologous transplant has been studied. In this small trial, long-term efficacy data are not available. The investigators did note a 39% varicella zoster reactivation rate.[23] In a phase 1/2 study, bortezomib was administered at doses of 1.0, 1.3, and 1.6 mg/m^2 once weekly 3 out of 4 weeks. The maximum tolerated dose was 1.3 mg/m^2, and efficacy results have not yet been reported. The main observed toxicities were diarrhea, fatigue, nausea, peripheral neuropathy, and again varicella zoster reactivation.[24] A third group also assessed bortezomib at a dose of 1.0 mg/m^2 and 1.3 mg/m^2. Two of the twenty patients have a conversion of response from VGPR to CR during treatment. Again, varicella zoster reactivation was noted. The investigators modified the protocol to include prophylaxis with acyclovir in order to minimize this potential complication, and this has now been recognized as a recommendation for all patients receiving bortezomib-based therapy.[25,26] More studies are needed to determine the optimal dose and long-term response of bortezomib as maintenance. Low-dose lenalidomide is being tested by the CALGB and the IFM in post-transplant randomized placebo-controlled maintenance trials. Since myelosuppression is one of the concerns with lenalidomide-based therapy, careful monitoring of cytopenias in the post-transplant period will be critical. Ongoing clinical trials assessing the role of these novel therapeutics in the maintenance setting are necessary if we are to improve outcomes for patients with myeloma.

CONCLUSION

The FDA and the American Society of Hematology held a workshop to define endpoints in clinical trials for patients with myeloma. The Maintenance Therapy workshop recommended the following triad as the optimal goals of clinical trials evaluating maintenance therapies: (1) improvement of complete response rate; (2) improved PFS; and (3) acceptable toxicity profile as measured by quality of life parameters. Current evidence does not support the use of interferon as maintenance therapy because of its lack of significant improvement in survival and unacceptable toxicity. The scant data that are available do not justify the recommendation of corticosteroids as maintenance therapy for all patients. Conflicting evidence exists for the use of thalidomide as maintenance treatment. Current data are promising, but further randomized

trials are needed to verify its effectiveness and those who will most likely benefit from maintenance thalidomide.

The discovery of targets in myeloma and the development of novel therapeutics are rapidly changing the treatment options for patients with myeloma. Improvements in the basic understanding of plasma cell biology and identification of subsets of myeloma patients that may harbor either good risk (hyperdiploid) or poor risk [del 17p, t(4:14), t(14:16)] biology is also critically important as we design our future maintenance approaches. Rather than a one-size-fits-all approach, perhaps patients with high-risk disease should receive maintenance with active novel agents known to be effective in this disease setting, while patients with good risk disease may be observed, as they have indolent disease and will not ultimately benefit from maintenance therapy. Building treatment programs that maximize survival while maintaining quality of life remain the goal of maintenance treatments for patients with myeloma, and with an improved understanding, we can hope to tailor our therapies in the future to maximize benefit while minimizing long-term toxicity.

REFERENCES

1. Alexanian R, Balcerzak S, Gehan E, Haut A, Hewlett J. Remission maintenance therapy for multiple myeloma. *Arch Intern Med* 1975;135(1):147-52.
2. Alexanian R, Salmon S, Bonnet J, Gehan E, Haut A, Weick J. Combination therapy for multiple myeloma. *Cancer* 1977;40(6):2765-71.
3. Salmon SE, Haut A, Bonnet JD, et al. Alternating combination chemotherapy and levamisole improves survival in multiple myeloma: a Southwest Oncology Group Study. *J Clin Oncol* 1983;1(8):453-61.
4. Alexanian R, Dreicer R. Chemotherapy for multiple myeloma. *Cancer* 1984;53(3):583-8.
5. MacLennan IC, Cusick J. Objective evaluation of the role of vincristine in induction and maintenance therapy for myelomatosis. Medical Research Council Working Party on Leukaemia in Adults. *Br J Cancer* 1985;52(2):153-8.
6. Cohen HJ, Bartolucci AA, Forman WB, Silberman HR. Consolidation and maintenance therapy in multiple myeloma: randomized comparison of a new approach to therapy after initial response to treatment. *J Clin Oncol* 1986;4(6):888-99.
7. Belch A, Shelley W, Bergsagel D, et al. A randomized trial of maintenance versus no maintenance melphalan and prednisone in responding multiple myeloma patients. *Br J Cancer* 1988;57(1):94-9.
8. Myeloma Trialists' Collaborative Group. Interferon as therapy for multiple myeloma: an individual patient data overview of 24 randomized trials and 4012 patients. *Br J Haematol* 2001;113(4):1020-34.

9. Fritz E, Ludwig H. Interferon-alpha treatment in multiple myeloma: meta-analysis of 30 randomised trials among 3948 patients. *Ann Oncol* 2000;11(11):1427-36.

10. Barlogie B, Kyle RA, Anderson KC, et al. Standard chemotherapy compared with high-dose chemoradiotherapy for multiple myeloma: final results of phase III US Intergroup Trial S9321. *J Clin Oncol* 2006;24(6):929-36.

11. Berenson JR, Crowley JJ, Grogan TM, et al. Maintenance therapy with alternate-day prednisone improves survival in multiple myeloma patients. *Blood* 2002;99(9):3163-8.

12. Shustik C, Belch A, Robinson S, et al. A randomised comparison of melphalan with prednisone or dexamethasone as induction therapy and dexamethasone or observation as maintenance therapy in multiple myeloma: NCIC CTG MY.7. *Br J Haematol* 2007;136(2):203-11.

13. Alexanian R, Weber D, Giralt S, Delasalle K. Consolidation therapy of multiple myeloma with thalidomide-dexamethasone after intensive chemotherapy. *Ann Oncol* 2002;13(7):1116-19.

14. Stewart AK, Chen CI, Howson-Jan K, et al. Results of a multi-center randomized phase II trial of thalidomide and prednisone maintenance therapy for multiple myeloma after autologous stem cell transplant. *Clin Cancer Res* 2004;10(24):8170-6.

15. Feyler S, Graham J, Rawstron A, EL-Sherbiny Y, Snowden J, Johnson R. Thalidomide maintenance following high dose therapy in multiple myeloma: A UK Myeloma Forum Phase 2 Study. *Blood* 2003;102(11):Abstract 2558.

16. Feyler S, Rawstron A, Jackson G, Snowden JA, Cocks K, Johnson RJ. Thalidomide maintenance following high-dose therapy in multiple myeloma: a UK myeloma forum phase 2 study. *Br J Haematol* 2007;139(3):429-33.

17. Brinker BT, Waller EK, Leong T, et al. Maintenance therapy with thalidomide improves overall survival after autologous hematopoietic progenitor cell transplantation for multiple myeloma. *Cancer* 2006;106(10):2171-80.

18. Attal M, Harousseau JL, Leyvraz S, et al. Maintenance therapy with thalidomide improves survival in patients with multiple myeloma. *Blood* 2006;108(10):3289-94.

19. Abdelkefi A, Ladeb S, Torjman L, et al. Single autologous stem cell transplantation followed by maintenance therapy with thalidomide is superior to double autologous transplantation in multiple myeloma: results of a multicenter randomized clinical trial. *Blood* 2007;111:1805-10.

20. Barlogie B, Tricot G, Anaissie E, et al. Thalidomide and hematopoietic-cell transplantation for multiple myeloma. *N Engl J Med* 2006;354(10):1021-30.

21. Spencer A, Prince M, Roberts AW, Bradstock KF, Prosser IW. First analysis of the Australasian Leukaemia and Lymphoma Group (ALLG) trial of thalidomide and alternate day predni-solone following autologous stem cell transplantation (ASCT) for patients with multiple myeloma (ALLG MM6). *ASH Annual Meeting Abstracts* 2006;108(11):58.

22. Spencer A, Prince HM, Robert A, Bradstock K, Prosser I. Thalidomide improves survival when used following ASCT. *Haematologica* 2007;92(suppl 2):41-2.

23. Peles S, Fisher NM, Devine SM, Tomasson MH, DiPersio JF, Vij R. Bortezomib (velcade) when given pretransplant and once weekly as consolidation therapy following high dose chemotherapy (HDCT) leads to high rates of reactivation of varicella zoster virus (VZV). *ASH Annual Meeting Abstracts* 2005;106(11):3237.

24. Schiller GJ, Sohn JP, Malone R, et al. Phase I/II trial of bort-ezomib maintenance following autologous peripheral blood progenitor cell transplantation as treatment for intermediate- and advanced-stage multiple myeloma. *ASH Annual Meeting Abstracts* 2006;108(11):5433.

25. Knop S, Hebart H, Kunzmann V, Angermund R, Einsele H. Bortezomib once weekly is well tolerated as maintenance therapy after less than a complete response to high-dose mel-phalan in patients with multiple myeloma. *ASH Annual Meeting Abstracts* 2006;108(11):5099.

26. Chanan-Khan AA, Sonneveld P, Schuster MW, et al. Analysis of varicella zoster virus reactivation among bortezomib-treated patients in the APEX study. *ASH Annual Meeting Abstracts* 2006;108(11):3535.

5 Treatment of Relapsed and Relapsed/Refractory Multiple Myeloma

Marc S. Raab, Paul G. Richardson, and Kenneth C. Anderson

INTRODUCTION

Despite recent advances in therapy, relapsed and refractory multiple myeloma (MM) remains a significant challenge and an area of unmet medical need. Median survival and responses to treatment are characteristically short. Relapsed and refractory MM is defined as patients who achieve at least a minor response (MR) or better followed by relapse and then progress on salvage therapy, or experience progression within 60 days of their last therapy.[1] Successive treatment regimens typically result in progressively shorter response durations, which reflects emerging drug resistance. The observed decrease in response duration may also reflect changes in disease biology within each patient, with tumor cells expressing a more aggressive phenotype, higher proliferative thrust, and lower apoptotic rates.[1]

Although several prognostic factors have been identified for newly diagnosed myeloma, factors that retain prognostic value in the context of relapsed/refractory disease remain to be comprehensively defined. Nonetheless, patients with poor risk include those with t(4;14) or t(14;16), deletion 17 or deletion 13, hypodiploidy, high-β_2-microglobulin, light-chain disease, immunoglobulin A (IgA) isotype, and low serum albumin; clinical challenges in the relapsed/refractory population include renal failure, extramedullary disease, hyposecretory myeloma, and advanced bone disease.[1]

The advent of novel therapies targeting disease biology and tumor microenvironment has significantly improved the prognosis for patients with relapsed and refractory disease. Bortezomib, a first-in-class proteasome inhibitor, and the immunomodulatory agents thalidomide (Thal) and lenalidomide now constitute "backbone" agents in this setting. Bortezomib reflects a paradigm of drug development where accelerated approval emerged from

studies in the relapsed/refractory patient population in 2003, followed by full approval in the relapsed setting in 2005. To further improve outcome in relapsed/refractory patients, combinations of these novel agents with each other, with conventional anti-MM agents, and with newer experimental compounds are currently under investigation. This broad array of agents and targets promises to overcome resistance to both conventional and novel agents and thus ultimately yet further prolonging survival.

TREATMENT OPTIONS

Conventional therapies

Dexamethasone

In 1986, a phase 2 study of Alexanian et al.[2] compared patients resistant to previous treatments with responsive patients and observed favorable response rates of 27% versus 21%, respectively, after administration of intermittent high-dose dexamethasone (Dex) of 40 mg/day for 4 consecutive days beginning on days 1, 9, and 17 of a 28-day cycle. This regimen has since served as a standard arm for several recent randomized trials evaluating novel therapies for relapsed/refractory MM.

Conventional chemotherapy

In order to improve response rates in relapsed/refractory patients compared to those receiving high-dose Dex alone, various chemotherapeutic agents were added and used in combination. Barlogie et al.[3] combined doxorubicin (Dox) and vincristine with pulsed high-dose Dex (VAD) and were able to achieve response rates of up to 65% and improved survival in heavily pretreated patients. These results were confirmed by other studies.[4-7] Since then, Dox/Dex has been used as a platform for combinations with other agents, including melphalan, cyclophosphamide, carmustine, etoposide, and Thal.[8-11] However, the major concerns about Dox are an increased risk for development of cardiomyopathy and its potential for tissue toxicity requiring a central venous line for administration. These issues were addressed by a newly developed pegylated formulation of Dox with lower risk of cardiomyopathy, lower tissue toxicity, and less alopecia. While its activity in combination with Dex is modest, this formulation of Dox has shown great promise when combined versus bortezomib.[12,13] This led to a randomized phase 3 trial comparing pegylated Dox in combination with bortezomib with bortezomib alone in relapsed and relapsed/refractory MM patients, resulting in improved response duration [with a median time to progression (TTP) of 9.3 vs. 6.5 months] and prolonged survival.[14] On the basis of this trial, this combination regimen was approved by the U.S. Food and Drug Administration (FDA) in 2007 for the treatment of bortezomib-naive MM patients after at least one prior therapy.

Hematopoietic stem cell transplant

High-dose chemotherapy rescued by autologous stem cell transplantation (ASCT) is currently considered a standard treatment for younger newly diagnosed patients. However, this treatment approach was first introduced to overcome resistance of MM to conventional chemotherapy and was initially evaluated in patients with refractory disease, resulting in improved response rates,[15-17] but to date, this has not been evaluated prospectively as part of a randomized trial in the relapsed, and/or relapsed/refractory setting. Nonetheless, phase 2 trials have suggested benefit in patients with primary refractory disease,[18] with rates of partial response (PR) of 92% and complete response (CR) of 20%;[19] and in patients with relapsed, chemosensitive disease, PR rates of 75% with CR of 10%-15% have been seen with a median relapse-free and overall survival (OS) of 2 and 3 years, respectively.[20] Interestingly, in relapsed and refractory MM, high-dose therapy and ASCT have been able to achieve progression-free survival (PFS) and OS times of 11 months and 19 months, respectively, but at the cost of substantial toxicity and even treatment-related mortality.[15,21] An increasingly important group of patients with relapse after frontline SCT may benefit from second SCT, in at least a subset of patients with favorable prognostic factors, including prolonged interval (>3 years) from prior transplant.[22]

However, there remains debate as to the optimal time for SCT. Before the ascent of novel agents, one randomized trial compared SCT up-front versus its use as salvage therapy in first relapse. While a higher quality-of-life score for early SCT was reported together with superior PFS, OS did not show any significant difference.[23] This has now to be re-evaluated in the era of novel agents and targeted therapy.

Allogeneic transplantation (allo-SCT) after myeloablative induction/consolidation had been considered a potentially curative approach with a tumor-free graft and graft-versus-myeloma effect with alloreactive donor lymphocytes potentially eradicating the neoplastic clone. While this treatment approach may have been able to achieve durable response rates,[22,24,25] it was linked to an unacceptably high treatment–related mortality of approximately 40%-50%, and therefore was largely discarded as a viable treatment option for most MM patients. Nonmyeloablative regimens, however, offer a lower rate of treatment-related mortality while maintaining the promises of the graft-versus-myeloma effect. For primary refractory or in first-line induction therapy relapsed patients, a sequential high-dose therapy with SCT followed by nonmyeloablative allo-SCT from HLA-identical siblings showed encouraging results.[26] Thus, patients in first relapse after SCT might benefit from a salvage SCT/nonmyeloablative allo-SCT regimen if carefully selected.[27,28] However, heavily pretreated or relapsed/refractory patients have shown poor outcomes with this approach.[29] At present, it is currently recommended that allo-SCT in MM should be performed within controlled clinical trials, exploiting graft-versus-myeloma effects while seeking to minimize attendant toxicity.

Novel agents

Thalidomide

Originally developed as a sedative, Thal entered the field of cancer treatment when the concept of angiogenesis in tumor growth was discovered to be a potentially valuable therapeutic target.[30] Given the increased microvascular density in bone marrow samples of MM patients with active disease when compared with myeloma gammopathy of undetermined significance (MGUS), Thal was one of the first novel agents to be evaluated in MM.[31] In this context, Thal and its analogs (lenalidomide/Revlimid® and CC-4013/Actimid®) formed a new class of anti-MM agents termed immunomodulatory drugs (IMiDs), which share substantial overlap

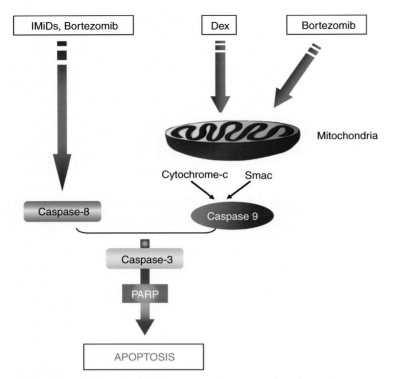

Figure 5.1. Schematic representation of main caspase-mediated pathways for the direct anti-MM effect of proteasome inhibitors, immunomodulatory thalidomide derivatives (IMiDs) and Dex. (From Richardson et al., Hematology 2007:317–323.)

in their biological and clinical functions, but have critical differences in potency and side-effect profiles.[32] Besides their antiangiogenic effects, IMiDs also trigger apoptosis of MM cells via caspase 8 (Figure 5.1); suppress interleukin-6 (IL-6) secretion within the bone marrow microenvironment; sensitize MM cells to therapeutic agents that predominantly utilize the caspase 9–related apoptotic pathway (e.g. Dex or bortezomib); and augment immunologic responses by activating T cells and NK cells.[33,34] Thal alone and in combination has since been extensively studied as therapy for relapsed MM, as induction treatment for newly diagnosed MM, and as maintenance after high-dose melphalan and ASCT. It was FDA approved for the treatment of newly diagnosed MM in combination with Dex in 2006.

Thalidomide monotherapy

The activity of single-agent treatment with Thal in relapsed/refractory MM patients was first described by Singhal et al.[35] and later updated by Barlogie et al.,[36] with

doses ranging from 200 to 800 mg/day (Table 5.1). Most patients were in relapse after ASCT. Thal was able to achieve an overall response rate of 37% (MR+PR+CR) and PR+CR of 30%, with a 2-year event-free survival (EFS) and OS of 20% and 48%, respectively. The role of Thal in relapsed/ refractory MM patients was confirmed in other multiple trials, with overall response rates ranging from 28% to 66% within the first 4 months of treatment [reviewed in Ref. (37)]. A recent systematic review of 42 phase 2 studies reported a PR+CR rate of 29%,[38] with Thal alone associated with relatively low rates of deep venous thrombosis (DVT) of 5% or less.[35,39,40]

Although in some studies higher cumulative doses of Thal have correlated with improved response rates,[35,39] dose escalation beyond 400 mg/day did not further improve response rates and clearly increased side effects. The most common adverse events associated with Thal treatment include constipation, fatigue, DVT, and peripheral neuropathy (PN), which limits dose and duration of treatment.[41] In a phase 2 Mayo Clinic trial, 56% of patients developed symptoms of PN after treatment with Thal, and in only 27% of patients were symptoms reversible, with or without change in treatment.[42] In addition, duration of treatment longer than 6 months seems to dramatically increase the risk of neurotoxicity.[43]

Thalidomide with dexamethasone

Since in vitro data showed that Thal enhanced the anti-MM activity of Dex, this combination has been evaluated extremely in the clinical setting.[44] Initial studies showed responses of 45% in relapsed/refractory patients, including 30% of patients refractory to single-agent Thal.[45] These promising results were confirmed in other trials, summarized in a systematic review, with response rates for Thal-Dex of 51% compared to 29% for Thal alone.[46] In addition, time to response to the combination was significantly shorter with lower doses of Thal (200 mg/day), resulting in less neurotoxicity, sedation, and constipation, while,

TABLE 5.1. Selected studies of thalidomide and lenalidomide

Author N/n	Regimen	Response rate (CR + PR)	Time-to-event data	Key toxicities
Barlogie[35] 169/169	Thal 200-800 mg/day	30% CR: 2%	2-year EFS: 20% 2-year OS: 48%	Grade > 2: CNS 25%, gastrointestinal 16%, peripheral neuropathy 9%
Palumbo[49] First relapse 62/62	Thal 100 mg/day continuously	56%	PFS: 17 months 3-year OS rate: 60%	Tingling and numbness 19%; constipation 18%; sedation 13%
Second relapse and beyond 58/58	Dex 40 mg days 1-4 of each month	46%	PFS: 11 months OS: 19 months	
Offidani[54] 50/50	Six 4-week cycles Thal 100 mg/day Liposomal doxorubicin 40 mg/m^2 day 1 Dex 40 mg days 1-4, 9-12	76% CR/nCR: 32%	EFS: 17 months PFS: 22 months OS: not reached	Grade ≥ 3: neutropenia 16%; nonhematologic toxicities 12% venous thromboembolic disease 12% severe infection 16%
Moehler[53] 56/50	Three 4-week cycles Thal 400 mg/day; Dex 40 mg/day for days 1-4 Cyclophosphamide 400 mg/m^2 and etoposide 40 mg/m^2 cont. infusion on days 1-4	65% CR: 4%	PFS: 16 months OS: not reached	Grade ≥3: infectious complications 36% cardiovascular events 7%
Dimopoulos[55] 53/53	Three to six 4-week cycles Thal 400 mg/day and Dex 20 mg/day days 1-5, 14-18 Cyclophosphamide 150 mg/m^2 every 12 h for days 1-5	60% CR/nCR: 5%	TTP: 8.2 months OS: 17.5 months	Grade 3/4: neutropenia 18/8%
Richardson[62] 67 (once daily) 35 (twice daily)	4-week cycles Len 30 mg once daily or 15 mg twice daily, days 1-21 Dex 40 mg for 4 days every 14 days for suboptimal response	18% CR/nCR: 6% (once daily) 14% CR/nCR: 0% (twice daily)	DOR: 19 months (once daily), 23 months (twice daily) PFS: 4.6 months (combined) OS: 27 months (combined)	Grade 3/4 (once daily): neutropenia 49/12%; thrombocytopenia 15/16%; leukopenia 36/2%; lymphopenia 31/6%; anemia 15/2% Grade 3/4 (twice daily): neutropenia 57/11%; thrombocytopenia 26/17%; leukopenia 34/0%; lymphopenia 31/9%; anemia 11/3%
Weber[63] 171	4-week cycles Len 25 mg days 1-21 Dex 40 mg days 1-4 and 9-12, 17-20 (cycles 1-4)	61% CR: 14.1%	TTP: 11.1 months OS: 29.6 months	Grade ≥ 3: neutropenia 41.2%; DVT/PE 14.7%; thrombocytopenia 12%; anemia 12%; pneumonia > 10%; atrial fibrillation 6%; fatigue 6%; diarrhea 5%
Dimopoulos[64] 176	As above	60% CR/nCR: 15.9%	TTP: 11.3 months OS: not reached	Grade ≥ 3: neutropenia 27%; DVT 11.4%; thrombocytopenia 10%; anemia 6%

however, Thal-Dex increases the risk for DVT, with rates of up to 10%.[47-50] Thus, prophylaxis with therapeutic doses of warfarin or low-molecular-weight heparin (LMWH) are recommended when Thal is given in combination with other agents, including Dex.[51] Given the limited number of controlled trials, a recently published consensus paper summarized the available data and experiences of many experts in the field. Aspirin prophylaxis was recommended for patients receiving IMiD with not more than one risk factor for thrombosis, but if additional factors, such as age, a central catheter, diabetes, cardiac disease, immobilization, MM-related hyperviscosity, and other prothrombotic factors were present, LMWH was recommended, as well as for all patients treated with combinations of Thal (or lenalidomide) with Dex or chemotherapy, and especially Dox.[52]

Thalidomide with other agents

Given the significant improvement of response rates with the combination of Thal and Dex with minimal myelosuppression, Thal-Dex has been incorporated into several other combination regimens to achieve higher response rates and, therefore, an attempt to improve outcome. Thal/Dex with cyclophosphamide and etoposide,[53] liposomal Dox,[54] or multiple agents such as Dox, cisplatin, cyclophosphamide, and etoposide (DT-PACE)[10] achieve response rates of 32%-76% in relapsed/refractory patients. Other trials have explored Thal-Dex with oral cyclophosphamide[55,56] and idarubicin,[57] resulting in similar response rates (Table 5.1).

Lenalidomide

The first member of the new class of immunomodulatory analogs of Thal to be approved by the FDA in 2006 for the second-line treatment of MM patients in combination with Dex was lenalidomide (CC-5013, Revlimid®), originally developed as an inhibitor of tumor necrosis factor-α (TNF-α). The mechanisms of action and its biological profile are very similar to Thal, but it is more potent and has a distinct toxicity profile without the sedative and neurotoxic adverse effects of Thal.[32,58]

Lenalidomide monotherapy

In the lead phase 1 study in MM, lenalidomide was used in doses up to 50 mg/day in a heavily pretreated group of patients, many of whom had been treated with previous high-dose therapy and ASCT or Thal-containing regimens.[59] Clinical responses were seen predominantly in the dose range of 25-50 mg/day, with a best paraprotein response of MR or better in 71% and PR or better in 29% of patients. Importantly, 68% of patients with previous Thal treatment responded to lenalidomide. The profile of side effects was favorable and did not include significant somnolence, constipation, or PN. Dose-limiting toxicity was in fact myelosuppression, leading to a recommended dose of 25 mg/day for subsequent trials.[59] Similar results were reported in a second phase 1 study by Zangari et al.[60] Subsequently, a randomized, single-center phase 2 study comparing lenalidomide 25 mg/day given on 21 days out of a 28-day cycle with 50 mg/day on 10 out of 28 days as post-transplant salvage therapy showed higher cumulative response rates to the former,[61] and, importantly, cytogenetic abnormalities did not affect PFS or OS in this trial.

A parallel multicenter, randomized phase 2 trial compared two dosing schedules of lenalidomide in 101 heavily pretreated patients: 30 mg once daily versus 15 mg twice daily on 21 days out of a 28-day cycle.[62] Previous therapies included ASCT (62%), Thal (53%), and bortezomib (8%), with relapsed/refractory disease in 53%. Since a significant increase in grade 3 and 4 myelosuppression was noted in the twice daily arm at interim analysis, this treatment schedule was stopped after the first 70 patients and a second cohort of 31 patients was enrolled given once daily lenalidomide. Dex at intermediate dose was added in 67% of patients achieving less than MR after two cycles or subsequent progressive disease, and 29% responded. There was no significant difference in response or survival between the two lenalidomide-dosing regimens. Significant PN or DVT occurred in only 3% of all patients, and, importantly, DVT was seen only after the addition of Dex.[62]

Lenalidomide with Dex

On the basis of the observations above, the combination of lenalidomide plus high-dose Dex in patients with relapsed/refractory MM was then investigated in two large, randomized, multicenter, double-blind, placebo-controlled phase 3 trials. The North American MM-009 and the European/Australian MM-010 trials included more than 700 patients who had progressed after at least one previous treatment.[63,64] In both trials, patients received either placebo or lenalidomide 25 mg/day (21 days out of a 28-day cycle). All patients also received Dex 40 mg/day on days 1-4, 9-12, 17-20 out of a 28-day cycle for four cycles, and thereafter Dex 40 mg/day on days 1-4 of each cycle. The recently published results of these trials showed that the combination of lenalidomide with Dex significantly increased response rates and survival of patients with MM. The response rates (at least PR) were higher in patients who received lenalidomide (MM-009: 61%; MM-010: 60%) than in the placebo group (MM-009: 19%; MM-010: 24%). CRs were achieved in 14.1% and 15.9% of patients, respectively, receiving the combination, compared to 0.6% and 3.4% of patients with high-dose Dex alone. The median TTP with lenalidomide was 11.1 and 11.3 months versus 4.7 and 4.7 months, respectively, in the placebo group. Most importantly, median OS increased from 20.2 and 20.6 months with Dex to 29.6 months in the U.S. trial and had not yet been reached with lenalidomide and Dex in the European study. Most recently, updated and pooled results demonstrated an increased OS from 31 months with Dex alone to 35 months after combination therapy despite crossover,[65] similar to the results seen in the APEX trial. In both studies a high number of patients had pretreatment with Thal-containing regimens (MM-009: 43%; MM-010: 35%), and more than 50% of these patients responded to the lenalidomide-containing regimen. However, the North American trial patients in the lenalidomide arm with previous Thal treatment showed a significantly shorter TTP (8.5 months) than those without Thal-containing pretreatment (14.2 months) and a higher DVT rate with prior Thal exposure.

In both trials, the main grade 3 or 4 toxicities were neutropenia (MM-009: 41.2%; MM-010: 29.5%) and thromboembolic events (MM-009: 14.7%; MM-010: 11.4%) in the lenalidomide group compared to the placebo arm of the study (MM-009: 4.6%; MM-010: 2.3%; and MM-009: 3.4%; MM-010: 4.6%). Both trials did not require prophylactic antithrombotic therapy but concluded that such precautions including the use of aspirin should be taken for combination therapies with lenalidomide, as discussed previously.[63,64]

Lenalidomide with other agents

The success of lenalidomide together with Dex prompted a series of trials investigating the addition of chemotherapeutic agents to this combination. In a phase 1/2 trial published in 2006, liposomal Dox and vincristine were combined with lenalidomide and Dex.[66] In a heavily pretreated patient group, this regimen achieved an impressive overall response rate of 75% with 29% of patients in CR or near CR (nCR). However, dose-limiting toxicity included

neutropenic sepsis, and the maximum tolerated dose for lenalidomide was only 10 mg/day. Another study combined conventional Dox with lenalidomide/Dex including 25 mg/day of lenalidomide and achieved an overall response rate of 87%, with CR and nCR in 23% and 60% of 30 patients, respectively, with more manageable toxicity.[67] Cyclophosphamide has also been used in combination with lenalidomide/Dex, achieving a promising CR+PR rate of 65%, with a side-effect profile consisting mainly of neutropenia and DVT, but it limited other nonhematologic toxicity.[68]

Bortezomib

The boronic dipeptide bortezomib is the first-in-class inhibitor of intracellular protein degradation that inhibits a subunit of the proteasome, thereby leading to cell cycle arrest, induction of stress response, antiangiogenic effects, and ultimately to the apoptosis of MM cells [reviewed in Ref. (69)]. Bortezomib triggers both caspase 8–mediated apoptosis and activation of caspase 9–dependent apoptotic pathways (Figure 5.1). Its rapid translation from bench to bedside, with accelerated and then full approval by the FDA within 5 years, has provided a paradigm of drug development in MM.[1,37]

Bortezomib alone or with Dex

In a first phase 1 trial in advanced hematologic malignancies, bortezomib showed impressive activity especially in MM patients, as all eight MM patients enrolled responded.[13] Following these encouraging results as well as a comprehensive preclinical evaluation of this agent in MM, bortezomib was tested in two multicenter phase 2 clinical trials for relapsed/refractory MM patients. In both the SUMMIT and the CREST trials bortezomib was given twice weekly i.v. for the first 2 weeks of a 3-week cycle.

In the larger SUMMIT trial, 202 patients received 1.3 mg/m² bortezomib for up to eight cycles. Oral Dex 20 mg/day together with bortezomib and the following day was added in patients with suboptimal response.[70] More than 90% of all patients had at least three lines of previous therapy and were refractory to their last regimen. Response rates were 35%, including 12% CR/nCR in this heavily pretreated group of patients. The median OS was significantly better than expected at 16 months, with a duration of response (DOR) of 12 months and a median TTP of 7 months.[70]

Comparing two doses of bortezomib (1.0 or 1.3 mg/m²) in 53 patients, the CREST trial suggested the higher dose to be more effective by achieving response rates (CR+PR) with bortezomib alone of 30% and 38%, and in combination with Dex of 37% and 50%, respectively,[71] although importantly activity of the lower dose was confirmed with less toxicity. Interestingly, a recently updated survival analysis showed a median OS of 27 months for lower dose and 60 months for higher dose bortezomib for all patients.[72] On the basis of the results of this phase 2 program of bortezomib, it was approved both by the FDA and EMEA for the treatment of relapsed and refractory MM in 2005.

The international, randomized phase 3 APEX trial followed and compared bortezomib monotherapy versus high-dose Dex in relapsed MM patients who had received 1-3 previous lines of therapy (Table 5.2). In that trial, patients receiving single-agent bortezomib had significantly longer TTP, higher response rate, and improved survival compared to the high-dose Dex arm.[73] An updated analysis of the APEX trial with extended follow-up (median 22 months) revealed a median OS of 29.8 months with bortezomib versus 23.7 months with high-dose Dex. This benefit was seen despite the fact that 62% of the patients on the high-dose Dex arm crossed over to receive bortezomib. The overall response rate (43%) and CR/nCR rate (15%) with bortezomib monotherapy were also higher in the updated analysis than at initial analysis.[74] Bortezomib is, at present, the only agent that has been shown to provide survival benefit and the highest overall response rate (PR+CR) as a single agent in the setting of relapsed MM. Results from the APEX trial also indicate that bortezomib is more active when used earlier in the relapsed setting, with improvement in TTP, DOR, and OS among patients with only one prior therapy compared with those with two or three prior lines of therapy. Finally, these results led to full FDA approval in 2005 for the treatment of patients in first relapse and beyond.

These three trials revealed that the most common side effects associated with bortezomib include fatigue, gastrointestinal events, and PN. The most commonly reported grade ≥ 3 adverse events were PN, thrombocytopenia, neutropenia, and anemia. Bortezomib-induced PN is a key side effect, because it may limit dose and duration of treatment and therefore limit the clinical benefit that patients with bortezomib-responsive MM might otherwise achieve. On the basis of the experience from the SUMMIT and CREST trials, specific management guidelines have been proposed.[75] These guidelines were prospectively tested in the APEX trial: PN occurred in 30% of patients, which was mild to moderate and reversible in the majority of cases and with very little grade 3 PN seen, suggesting that the dose reduction

algorithm is effective.[76] Of note, bortezomib-related PN also resolved or improved in 71% of patients in the SUMMIT and CREST trials who had grade ≥ 3 PN and/or neuropathy requiring discontinuation, with similar reversibility seen in APEX.[75] The hematologic side effects caused by bortezomib are primarily transient thrombocytopenia and neutropenia, which in most cases is reversible and cyclical. For instance, bortezomib is associated with decreased platelet count, and subsequent recovery that occurs in a predictable pattern during each treatment cycle, without any evidence of cumulative toxicity,[77] although low platelet count at baseline ($<70 \times 10^9$/L) is associated with increased risk of grade ≥ 3 thrombocytopenia. In the APEX trial, whilst a higher incidence of grade ≥ 3 thrombocytopenia was observed in the bortezomib arm versus the high-dose Dex arm, the incidence of clinically significant bleeding events (including grade ≥ 3 bleeding events, serious bleeding, and cerebral hemorrhage) did not differ significantly between the two arms.[78]

Bortezomib with conventional agents

It has been shown in preclinical studies that bortezomib sensitizes MM cells to a variety of conventional chemotherapeutic agents including Dox or melphalan, even in MM cells resistant to conventional therapeutics.[79] These studies provided the rationale for a series of clinical trials with bortezomib in combination with Dox, liposomal Dox, melphalan, or cyclophosphamide.

Early-phase clinical trials for bortezomib with liposomal Dox in advanced hematologic malignancies led to a response rate of 73% of 22 evaluable patients, including CR and nCR in 36% of these patients.[13] More recently, a large phase 3 trial comparing bortezomib (1.3 mg/m²; on day 1, 4, 8, and 11 of a 21-day cycle) and pegylated liposomal Dox (30 mg/m²; on day 4) with bortezomib in 646 patients showed significant improvement of the TTP (9.4 vs. 6.5 months), a superior 15-month survival rate (76% vs. 65%), and an increased DOR from 7.0 to 10.2 months for the combination versus bortezomib-alone treatment[14] (Table 5.2). Major adverse events included neutropenia and thrombocytopenia with the combination regimen. Importantly, patients who had previously failed therapy including anthracycline-containing regimens benefited from this combination, consistent with the above-mentioned preclinical data, suggesting that bortezomib can sensitize MM cells to chemotherapy.[79] The improvement in TTP with the combination therapy was independent of the number of prior lines of therapy.[80] These results were the basis for the approval of

TABLE 5.2. Selected studies of bortezomib

Author N/n	Regimen	Response rate (CR + PR)	Time-to-event data	Key toxicities
Richardson[73,74] 333/315	Eight 3-week cycles Btz 1.3 mg/m^2 days 1, 4, 8, 11 Three 5-week cycles days 1, 8, 15, 22	43% CR/nCR: 15%	TTP: 6.2 months OS: 29.8 months DOR: 7.8 months	Grade 3/4: thrombocytopenia 26/4%; neutropenia 12/2%; anemia 9/1%; peripheral neuropathy 7/1%; diarrhea 7/0%; fatigue 5/<1%; dyspnea 5/<1%
Orlowski[14] 322/310	Eight 3-week cycles Btz 1.3 mg/m^2 days 1, 4, 8, and 11 PLD 30 mg/ m^2 day 4	48% CR/nCR 14%	TTP: 9.4 months DOR: 10.2 months	Grade 3/4: neutropenia 30%; thrombocytopenia 22%; anemia 9%; diarrhea 7%; asthenia 6%; fatigue 5%; hand foot syndrome 5%
324/303	Eight 3-week cycles Btz 1.3 mg/m^2 days 1, 4, 8, and 11	43% CR/nCR 11%	TTP: 6.5 months DOR: 7 months	Grade 3/4: thrombocytopenia 15%; neutropenia 14%; anemia 9%; peripheral neuropathy 9%; neuralgia 5%
Berenson[12] 35/34	Eight 4-week cycles Btz 0.7–1.0 mg/m^2 days 1, 4, 8, and 11 Melphalan 0.025–0.25 mg/kg days 1–4	47% CR/nCR: 15%	PFS: 8 months	Grade 3/4: neutropenia 34/6%; thrombocytopenia 37/3%; anemia 23/6%; hypocalcemia 6/0%
Zangari[84] 85/85	Eight 3-week cycles Btz 1.0–1.3 mg/m^2 days 1, 4, 8, and 11 Thal 50–200 mg/day from cycle 2 Dex 20 mg day of/day after btz for suboptimal response after three cycles	55%b CR/nCR: 16%	EFS: 9 months OS: 22 months	Most common grade 3/4 toxicities were thrombocytopenia and neutropenia
Palumbo[88] 30/30	Six 5-week cycles Btz 1–1.6 mg/m^2 days 1, 4, 15, and 22 Melphalan 6 mg/m^2 and prednisone 60 mg/m^2 days 1–5 Thal 100 mg daily	67% CR/nCR: 17%	NR	Grade 3/4: thrombocytopenia; febrile neutropenia; fatigue; anemia; pneumonia; vasculitis; infections; sensory neuropathy
Terpos[89] 44/41	Four 4-week cycles Btz 1.0 mg/m^2 days 1, 4, 8, and 11 Melphalan 0.15 mg/kg days 1–4 Dex 12 mg/m^2 days 1–4, 17–20 Thal 100 mg/day	66% CR/nCR: 37%	PFS: 9.6 months	Grade ≥3: thrombocytopenia 20%; neutropenia 8%; anemia 7%; peripheral neuropathy 6%
Richardson[90] 24/21	Eight 3-week cycles Btz 1.0–1.3 mg/m^2 days 1, 4, 8, and 11 Len 5–20 mg days 1–14 Dex 20 mg day of/day after btz for PD	58% CR/nCR: 6%	NR	Grade 3/4: thrombocytopenia; neutropenia; hyponatremia
Richardson[95] 30/25	3-week cycles Btz 0.7–1.3 mg/m^2 and KOS-953 100–275 mg/m^2 days 1, 4, 8, and 11	32% CR/nCR: 12%	NR	Dose-limiting: grade 3/4 hepatotoxicity; grade 3 pancreatitis Other grade 3/4 events included thrombocytopenia and elevated ALT (manageable with ursodiol)

this combination regimen in 2007 for the treatment of MM patients who have not previously received bortezomib and have received at least one prior line of anti-MM therapy.

Preclinical studies also showed promising activity of the combination of bortezomib with melphalan. Bortezomib was evaluated in dose-escalation trials and achieved response rates of 47% (15% CR/nCR) with oral melphalan[12] and 78% with low-dose i.v. melphalan (34% CR/nCR), including the addition of Dex for patients with suboptimal response.[81] In both trials, improved clinical activity was correlated with higher melphalan doses. High response rates and manageable toxicity profiles have also been reported for bortezomib combined with cyclophosphamide or idarubicin and Dex (CVD and VIM).[82,83]

The different molecular mechanisms of action of bortezomib, compared to conventional chemotherapy, corticosteroids, Thal, or IMiDs, result in synergistic potency when combined with these agents in preclinical models.[33,34] Furthermore, bortezomib alone has been shown to be active even in Thal-refractory MM patients.[70,73] Therefore, numerous clinical trials have aimed to evaluate the addition of Thal to bortezomib-containing regimens.

A phase 1/2 trial tested Thal (50 mg/day) together with bortezomib (1.0 mg/m^2) and Dex in 85 refractory but bortezomib-naive patients (VTD regimen). Thal could be increased up to 200 mg/day and bortezomib up to 1.3 mg/m^2, while Dex was added if response was less than PR.[84] Owing to PN and other toxicities including fatigue, a final dose schedule of bortezomib 1.0 mg/m^2, Thal 200 mg/day, and Dex 40 mg was proposed for further investigation. This regimen achieved a 55% PR (or better) rate, with 16% CR/nCR. Median EFS and OS were 9 months and 22 months, respectively, and were not influenced by prior Thal treatment and/or cytogenetic abnormalities. Importantly, low-dose Thal (<100 mg/day) proved as effective as higher doses but with less toxicity.

To enhance the promising results of bortezomib/Dox, other studies investigated the addition of Thal[85] or Thal and Dex[86] to this regimen: overall response rates were 65% with 25% CR/nCR even in patients previously treated with these agents. Early data suggest that these response rates might be further improved by the combination of bortezomib, Thal, and Dex with liposomal Dox.[87]

The addition of Thal (50 mg/day) to the bortezomib/melphalan combination together with prednisone (VMPT) has also further improved response rates, with 67% of 30 patients achieving a PR or better.[88] Similar results were reported for the addition of intermittent Thal (100 mg/day for days 1-4) and Dex.[89] Although neurotoxicity is a concern with the combination of bortezomib and Thal, it has not been a major limitation, likely due to the relatively low doses of Thal and short treatment duration used, although over time cumulative rates of PN of up to 50% have been reported.[84]

Rationally based combinations of novel agents

Novel agents such as bortezomib and lenalidomide have demonstrated significant activity, either alone or in combination with Dex or conventional agents, in MM patients with relapsed/refractory MM. However, our increasing knowledge about the cellular and molecular mechanisms of action of these novel agents has facilitated preclinical studies to identify promising, synergistic combinations for evaluation in rationally designed clinical trials.

Bortezomib together with lenalidomide

Mechanistically, bortezomib binds to and reversibly inhibits the chymotryptic-like activity of the 20S proteasome core, thereby leading to the accumulation of proteins that are regulated via proteasomal degradation. This, in turn, results in cellular stress, cell cycle arrest, disruption of MM cell adhesion to bone marrow stroma, inhibition of cytokine signaling, antiangiogenic effects, and modification of bone remodeling by inhibition of osteoclasts and stimulation of osteoblast differentiation. Specifically, bortezomib indirectly blocks the activity of nuclear factor-κB (NF-κB), thereby inhibiting downstream elements important for MM cell survival, such as IL-6 production and caspase inhibitors. In addition, bortezomib leads to upregulation of death receptors and ligand (e.g. Fas and FasL), triggering caspase 8–mediated apoptotic signaling. Moreover, the accumulation of proapoptotic molecules such as Bax, Noxa, and others trigger mitochondrial cytochrome c release and activation of caspase 9–dependent apoptosis. Another important mechanism of action of bortezomib in MM cells involves the unfolded protein response, which takes advantage of the high intracellular protein turnover of MM cells (e.g. production of immunoglobulins), and renders them especially sensitive to the accumulation of misfolded proteins [reviewed in Ref. (69)].

Lenalidomide displays multiple mechanisms of anti-MM activity, including direct induction of cell cycle arrest and apoptosis, as well as inhibition of MM cell adherence to bone marrow stroma, cytokine production, angiogenesis, and osteoclastogenesis [reviewed in Ref. (32)]. Importantly, lenalidomide has been shown to induce its apoptotic effects in MM cells mainly via a caspase 8–mediated pathway. In addition, lenalidomide stimulates T-cell proliferation, as well as NK-cell toxicity by enhancing IL-2 production from T cells, leading to NK-cell proliferation and ADCC activity.

Therefore, the complementary activation of the two major caspase-dependent apoptotic pathways by bortezomib (mainly caspase 9 and caspase 8) and lenalidomide (caspase 8) suggested that combinations of proteasome inhibitors and IMiDs may have synergistic anti-MM activity. Preclinical in vitro studies confirmed enhanced anti-MM effect with combinations of immunomodulatory Thal derivatives, such as lenalidomide, with bortezomib (Figure 5.1).

Since lenalidomide is not associated with PN, its combination with bortezomib was expected to have more favorable safety profile than the bortezomib-Thal combinations. However, both lenalidomide and bortezomib can lead to hematologic toxicity, suggesting the need for careful clinical development of this combination to avoid pronounced myelosuppression. In a phase 1 study combining lenalidomide and bortezomib in refractory MM patients with prior exposure to lenalidomide, bortezomib, Thal, or transplant, the maximum tolerated doses were identified as 15 mg/day of lenalidomide for 14 days and 1.0 mg/m^2 of bortezomib on days 1, 4, 8, and 11 of each 21-day cycle. Consistent with the initial clinical rationale behind this trial, no significant PN was reported. Furthermore, no anticoagulant prophylaxis was required, although aspirin was used in some patients, and DVT was uncommon (5%).[90] After a median of six cycles (range: 4-17) in 36 evaluable patients, a 58% overall response rate to the combination of lenalidomide and bortezomib was observed, including 6% CR/nCR. Responses were durable (median 6 months, range: 1-26), and 11 out of 36 evaluable patients remained on therapy beyond 1 year. Dex was subsequently added in 14 patients who had PD, with 71% of these patients achieving stable disease or response (Table 5.2). The combination of lenalidomide at 15 mg and bortezomib at 1.0 mg/m^2 with Dex at 20-40 mg/day on the day of bortezomib and the day after has been selected for ongoing

phase 2 studies in relapsed/refractory MM, with an overall response rate of 79%, including 33% with VGPR or better, reported at an interim analysis of an ongoing phase 2 study in relapsed and relapsed/refractory MM.[91]

Bortezomib with tanespimycin

One conceptual framework behind the design of new combination regimens involves the pairing of bortezomib with drug classes that may neutralize molecular pathway(s) that can confer resistance to proteasome inhibition. An example is the combination of bortezomib with hsp90 inhibitors: exposure of MM cells to bortezomib triggers upregulation of heat shock proteins, including hsp90.[92] This is likely a stress response, mounted by tumor cells in their effort to counteract the intracellular accumulation of misfolded proteins. This response may be insufficient, at least in vitro, to prevent the induction of cell death by bortezomib; however, it led to the hypothesis that small-molecule hsp90 inhibitors, such as 17-allylamino-17-demethoxy-geldanamcyin (17-AAG), may be able to enhance proapoptotic effects of bortezomib in MM cells. This hypothesis was confirmed in preclinical MM models[92,93] and provided the basis for ongoing clinical trials of tanespimycin (17-AAG in the KOS-953 cremophor-based formulation) as a single agent[94] or combined with bortezomib[95] in patients with relapsed or refractory MM (Table 5.2). To date, tanespimycin has exhibited a manageable profile of adverse events, without significant cardiotoxicity, PN, or DVT. Importantly, tanespimycin has been associated with durable disease stabilization and minor responses with single-agent treatment in relapsed and refractory MM patients. When combined with bortezomib, it has induced responses both in patients who had previously received bortezomib and in patients who were refractory to bortezomib. Early data show an overall response of 44%, with 27% of patients refractory to bortezomib responding to the combination.[96] These results, together with the lack of major additive toxicity or pharmacokinetic interactions with bortezomib as well as remarkably low rates of PN, have provided a platform for future phase 3 trials of tanespimycin in combination with bortezomib.

Bortezomib with perifosine

Similar to the combination with hsp90 inhibitors based on targeting a compensatory upregulation of a chaperone protein by bortezomib, the rationale to clinically investigate the Akt-inhibitor perifosine was based on the preclinical observation that activation of the Akt pathway represents another mechanism by which MM cells try to escape cell death after treatment with bortezomib.[97] Preclinical data showed synergistic activity of bortezomib combined with perifosine, which translated into the initiation of clinical trials. A preliminary report of a phase 1/2 study showed promising clinical activity with overall response rates of approximately 60%, even in patients refractory to bortezomib alone.[98]

Bortezomib with HDAC inhibitors

Previous studies have identified the aggresome as an alternative system for the degradation of proteins if the proteasomal pathway is blocked, thereby providing a salvage mechanism whereby MM cells escape apoptosis induced by proteasome inhibitors.[99] Histone deacetylases (HDACs), specifically HDAC6, seem to play a pivotal role within this aggresome pathway.[100] Importantly, dual inhibition of proteasomal (bortezomib) and aggresomal (HDAC inhibitors) degradation pathways in preclinical studies[101,102] demonstrates synergistic MM cytotoxicity. Ongoing clinical trials of HDAC inhibitors are evaluating the hydroxamic acid analog LBH589 in combination with bortezomib, based on these studies, and two other HDAC inhibitors, the suberoylanalide hydroxamid acid (SAHA) and romidepsin, are already in clinical evaluation in combination with bortezomib. Preliminary results of these latter two phase 1 trials already show promising clinical results, including patients achieving MR+PR+CR in the setting of relapsed/refractory MM in about half of patients, with manageable toxicity.[103-105]

Bortezomib with other investigational agents

The list of novel agents that are theoretically or already proven to be synergistic with bortezomib is rapidly increasing. Examples of those agents include p38 MAP kinase inhibitors (e.g. SC-469, VX-745), targeting another compensatory pathway of MM cells treated with bortezomib[106]; Bcl-2 inhibitors (e.g. ABT-737), enhancing bortezomib efficacy in vitro[107]; Smac peptides, overcoming antiapoptotic mechanisms in MM cells[108]; monoclonal antibodies targeting the new surface antigen on MM cells CS-1 (HuLuc63) or IGF-1R (AVE1642), thereby combining

proteasome inhibition and immunotherapy[109,110]; targeting protein kinase C (by enzastaurin), since low doses of bortezomib and enzastaurin induce synergistic cytotoxicity in vitro[111]; or even combining two proteasome inhibitors that have distinct effects on proteasome activity and mechanisms of action, recently shown for bortezomib and the novel proteasome inhibitor NPI-0052.[112]

These new regimens will be evaluated in clinical trials and offer great promise for more effective treatment of relapsed/refractory MM. Furthermore, the list of novel agents is rapidly increasing as new targets are identified, and further investigation of these novel strategies, both alone and in combination, for the treatment of MM is warranted as part of a continued effort to improve patient outcome. Participation in clinical trials (e.g. with the new proteasome inhibitor PR-171 or novel monoclonal antibodies) is thus critical and a cornerstone of patient management in the relapsed and refractory setting.

TREATMENT CONSIDERATIONS FOR SPECIFIC PATIENT POPULATIONS

Novel agents now offer not only further treatment options for relapsed and refractory MM, but recent data suggest that tailoring therapy according to individual patient features (such as older age, renal disease, and adverse cytogenetics, including chromosome 13 deletion, elevated β_2-microglobulin, low serum albumin, advanced bone disease, and extramedullary disease) may now be possible.

In patients without specific adverse characteristics, bortezomib in combination with liposomal Dox showed a superior TTP over bortezomib alone, regardless of prior therapy including anthracyclin exposure or Thal treatment.[80,113] In contrast, lenalidomide/Dex resulted in a significantly shorter TTP in patients with previous Thal-containing regimens compared to IMiD-naive patients.[63,64]

Bortezomib and lenalidomide have each been shown to be safe and effective in older patients with relapsed/refractory MM.[114,115] Thal is reported to be safe and effective in elderly patients in the frontline setting, but caution is needed and lower doses are required.[116]

Both bortezomib[117] and Thal[118] have been shown to be safe and effective in patients with renal impairment, and to reverse

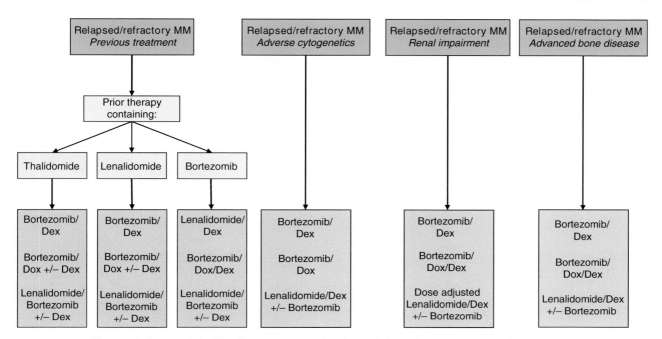

Figure 5.2. Suggested algorithm for treatment considerations and choices in the management of relapsed and refractory multiple myeloma.

renal dysfunction in some patients with relapsed/refractory MM.[119] Lenalidomide has yet to be carefully studied comprehensively in patients with significant renal dysfunction, as it is actively excreted through the kidneys; and patients with serum creatinine >2.5 mg/dL were excluded from the prior trials. However, increased toxicity has been reported in patients with high creatinine levels.[120] Currently, a dose-reduction schedule for lenalidomide in this setting is required.[121]

The poor prognosis conferred by the deletion of chromosome 13 has been shown to be overcome by bortezomib[122] and lenalidomide,[123] while Thal appears to be less effective.[36] Bortezomib has also been shown to overcome the poor prognostic factors of elevated β_2-microglobulin and low serum albumin, as well as being active in patients with bone disease, plasmacytoma, and extramedullary involvement.[115,124,125]

Given that combinations such as bortezomib/Dex, bortezomib/Dox $\pm$ Dex, lenalidomide/Dex, and lenalidomide, bortezomib $\pm$ Dex are currently the most active regimens in patients with relapsed and refractory MM, a treatment algorithm for the management of this group of patients could be proposed as outlined in Figure 5.2.

FUTURE DIRECTIONS

Only a few years ago, effective treatments for relapsed/refractory patients were few and results were disappointing, with options limited to conventional chemotherapy and transplantation. This was especially challenging as patients with relapsed and refractory disease are typically more symptomatic, older, resistant to treatment, and more symptomatic than newly diagnosed patients or patients in first relapse, but the introduction of targeted agents such as Thal, lenalidomide, and bortezomib dramatically improved response rates and prolonged survival, predicated upon targeting MM cells as well as the bone marrow microenvironment. An increasing understanding of these mechanisms in gene regulation, signaling pathways, and microenvironmental interactions has altered the rational design of combination regimens to enhance cytotoxicity, overcome drug resistance, and improve patient outcome in MM (Figure 5.3). With the advent of yet more new drugs, the therapeutic armamentarium continues to expand, the need for more clinical research has grown, and the outlook for this still very challenging group of MM patients has improved.

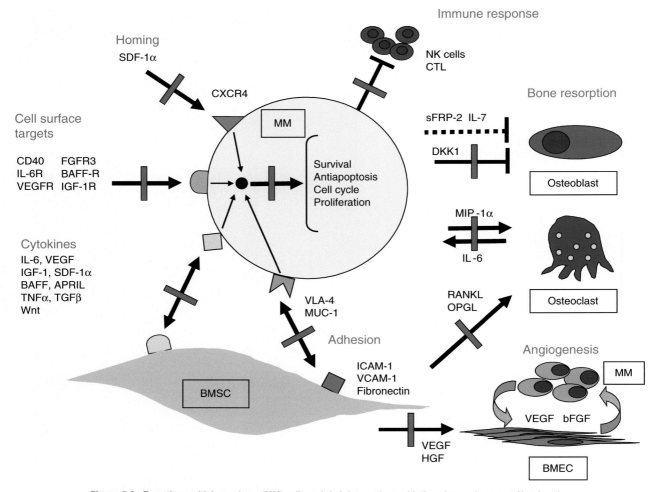

Figure 5.3. Targeting multiple myeloma (MM) cells and their interactions with the microenvironment. Novel, rationally based combination regimens aim to target directly MM cell growth and inhibit their homing to the bone marrow, prevent angiogenesis, disrupt MM cell adhesion to BMSC, decrease cytokine production in the microenvironment, stop bone destruction, and enhance anti-MM immunity.

REFERENCES

1. Anderson KC, Kyle RA, Rajkumar SV, Stewart AK, Weber D, Richardson P. Clinically relevant end points and new drug approvals for myeloma. *Leukemia* 2008;22(2):231-9.
2. Alexanian R, Barlogie B, Dixon D. High-dose glucocorticoid treatment of resistant myeloma. *Ann Intern Med* 1986;105(1):8-11.
3. Barlogie B, Smith L, Alexanian R. Effective treatment of advanced multiple myeloma refractory to alkylating agents. *N Engl J Med* 1984;310(21):1353-6.
4. Anderson H, Scarffe JH, Ranson M, et al. VAD chemotherapy as remission induction for multiple myeloma. *Br J Cancer* 1995;71(2):326-30.
5. Gertz MA, Kalish LA, Kyle RA, Hahn RG, Tormey DC, Oken MM. Phase III study comparing vincristine, doxorubicin (Adriamycin), and dexamethasone (VAD) chemotherapy with VAD plus recombinant interferon alfa-2 in refractory or relapsed multiple myeloma. An Eastern Cooperative Oncology Group study. *Am J Clin Oncol* 1995;18(6):475-80.
6. Lokhorst HM, Meuwissen OJ, Bast EJ, Dekker AW. VAD chemotherapy for refractory multiple myeloma. *Br J Haematol* 1989;71(1):25-30.
7. Phillips JK, Sherlaw-Johnson C, Pearce R, et al. A randomized study of MOD versus VAD in the treatment of relapsed and resistant multiple myeloma. *Leuk Lymphoma* 1995;17 (5-6):465-72.
8. Durie BG, Dixon DO, Carter S, et al. Improved survival duration with combination chemotherapy induction for multiple myeloma: a Southwest Oncology Group Study. *J Clin Oncol* 1986;4(8):1227-37.

9. Giles FJ, Wickham NR, Rapoport BL, et al. Cyclophosphamide, etoposide, vincristine, adriamycin, and dexamethasone (CEVAD) regimen in refractory multiple myeloma: an International Oncology Study Group (IOSG) phase II protocol. *Am J Hematol* 2000;63(3):125-30.

10. Lee CK, Barlogie B, Munshi N, et al. DTPACE: an effective, novel combination chemotherapy with thalidomide for previously treated patients with myeloma. *J Clin Oncol* 2003;21(14):2732-9.

11. MacLennan IC, Chapman C, Dunn J, Kelly K. Combined chemotherapy with ABCM versus melphalan for treatment of myelomatosis. The Medical Research Council Working Party for Leukaemia in Adults. *Lancet* 1992;339(8787):200-5.

12. Berenson JR, Yang HH, Sadler K, et al. Phase I/II trial assessing bortezomib and melphalan combination therapy for the treatment of patients with relapsed or refractory multiple myeloma. *J Clin Oncol* 2006;24(6):937-44.

13. Orlowski RZ, Voorhees PM, Garcia RA, et al. Phase 1 trial of the proteasome inhibitor bortezomib and pegylated liposomal doxorubicin in patients with advanced hematologic malignancies. *Blood* 2005;105(8):3058-65.

14. Orlowski RZ, Nagler A, Sonneveld P, et al. Randomized phase III study of pegylated liposomal doxorubicin plus bortezomib compared with bortezomib alone in relapsed or refractory multiple myeloma: combination therapy improves time to progression. *J Clin Oncol* 2007;25(25):3892-901.

15. Barlogie B, Alexanian R, Dicke KA, et al. High-dose chemoradiotherapy and autologous bone marrow transplantation for resistant multiple myeloma. *Blood* 1987;70(3):869-72.

16. Barlogie B, Hall R, Zander A, Dicke K, Alexanian R. High-dose melphalan with autologous bone marrow transplantation for multiple myeloma. *Blood* 1986;67(5):1298-301.

17. McElwain TJ, Powles RL. High-dose intravenous melphalan for plasma-cell leukaemia and myeloma. *Lancet* 1983;2(8354):822-4.

18. Alexanian R, Dimopoulos MA, Hester J, Delasalle K, Champlin R. Early myeloablative therapy for multiple myeloma. *Blood* 1994;84(12):4278-82.

19. Kumar S, Lacy MQ, Dispenzieri A, et al. High-dose therapy and autologous stem cell transplantation for multiple myeloma poorly responsive to initial therapy. *Bone Marrow Transplant* 2004;34(2):161-7.

20. Vesole DH, Tricot G, Jagannath S, et al. Autotransplants in multiple myeloma: what have we learned? *Blood* 1996;88(3):838-47.

21. Vesole DH, Crowley JJ, Catchatourian R, et al. High-dose melphalan with autotransplantation for refractory multiple myeloma: results of a Southwest Oncology Group phase II trial. *J Clin Oncol* 1999;17(7):2173-9.

22. Lee CK, Barlogie B, Zangari M, et al. Transplantation as salvage therapy for high-risk patients with myeloma in relapse. *Bone Marrow Transplant* 2002;30(12):873-8.

23. Fermand JP, Ravaud P, Chevret S, et al. High-dose therapy and autologous peripheral blood stem cell transplantation in multiple myeloma: up-front or rescue treatment? Results of a multicenter sequential randomized clinical trial. *Blood* 1998;92(9):3131-6.

24. Corradini P, Cavo M, Lokhorst H, et al. Molecular remission after myeloablative allogeneic stem cell transplantation predicts a better relapse-free survival in patients with multiple myeloma. *Blood* 2003;102(5):1927-9.

25. Gahrton G, Svensson H, Cavo M, et al. Progress in allogenic bone marrow and peripheral blood stem cell transplantation for multiple myeloma: a comparison between transplants performed 1983-93 and 1994-8 at European Group for Blood and Marrow Transplantation centres. *Br J Haematol* 2001;113(1):209-16.

26. Maloney DG, Molina AJ, Sahebi F, et al. Allografting with nonmyeloablative conditioning following cytoreductive autografts for the treatment of patients with multiple myeloma. *Blood* 2003;102(9):3447-54.

27. Kroger N, Perez-Simon JA, Myint H, et al. Relapse to prior autograft and chronic graft-versus-host disease are the strongest prognostic factors for outcome of melphalan/fludarabine-based dose-reduced allogeneic stem cell transplantation in patients with multiple myeloma. *Biol Blood Marrow Transplant* 2004;10(10):698-708.

28. Georges GE, Maris MB, Maloney DG, et al. Nonmyeloablative unrelated donor hematopoietic cell transplantation to treat patients with poor-risk, relapsed, or refractory multiple myeloma. *Biol Blood Marrow Transplant* 2007;13(4):423-2.

29. Gerull S, Goerner M, Benner A, et al. Long-term outcome of nonmyeloablative allogeneic transplantation in patients with high-risk multiple myeloma. *Bone Marrow Transplant* 2005;36(11):963-9.

30. D'Amato RJ, Loughnan MS, Flynn E, Folkman J. Thalidomide is an inhibitor of angiogenesis. *Proc Natl Acad Sci USA* 1994;91(9):4082-5.

31. Vacca A, Ribatti D, Roncali L, et al. Bone marrow angiogenesis and progression in multiple myeloma. *Br J Haematol* 1994;87(3):503-8.

32. Anderson KC. Lenalidomide and thalidomide: mechanisms of action—similarities and differences. *Semin Hematol* 2005;42 (4 suppl 4):S3-S8.

33. Hideshima T, Chauhan D, Shima Y, et al. Thalidomide and its analogs overcome drug resistance of human multiple myeloma cells to conventional therapy. *Blood* 2000;96(9):2943-50.

34. Mitsiades N, Mitsiades CS, Poulaki V, et al. Apoptotic signaling induced by immunomodulatory thalidomide analogs in human multiple myeloma cells: therapeutic implications. *Blood* 2002;99(12):4525-30.

35. Singhal S, Mehta J, Desikan R, et al. Antitumor activity of thalidomide in refractory multiple myeloma. *N Engl J Med* 1999;341(21):1565-71.

36. Barlogie B, Desikan R, Eddlemon P, et al. Extended survival in advanced and refractory multiple myeloma after single-agent thalidomide: identification of prognostic factors in a phase 2 study of 169 patients. *Blood* 2001;98(2):492-4.

37. Richardson PG, Mitsiades C, Schlossman R, Munshi N, Anderson K. New drugs for myeloma. *Oncologist* 2007;12(6):664-89.

38. Glasmacher A, Hahn C, Hoffmann F, et al. A systematic review of phase-II trials of thalidomide monotherapy in patients with relapsed or refractory multiple myeloma. *Br J Haematol* 2006;132(5):584-93.

39. Neben K, Moehler T, Benner A, et al. Dose-dependent effect of thalidomide on overall survival in relapsed multiple myeloma. *Clin Cancer Res* 2002;8(11):3377-82.

40. Schey SA, Cavenagh J, Johnson R, Child JA, Oakervee H, Jones RW. An UK myeloma forum phase II study of thalidomide; long term follow-up and recommendations for treatment. *Leuk Res* 2003;27(10):909-14.

41. Richardson P, Schlossman R, Jagannath S, et al. Thalidomide for patients with relapsed multiple myeloma after high-dose chemotherapy and stem cell transplantation: results of an open-label multicenter phase 2 study of efficacy, toxicity, and biological activity. *Mayo Clin Proc* 2004;79(7):875-82.

42. Naina HVK, Lacy MQ, Dispenzieri A, et al. Incidence and clinical course of peripheral neuropathy in patients receiving thalidomide for the treatment of multiple myeloma. *Blood (ASH Annual Meeting Abstracts)* 2005;106(11):3475.

43. Mileshkin L, Stark R, Day B, Seymour JF, Zeldis JB, Prince HM. Development of neuropathy in patients with myeloma treated with thalidomide: patterns of occurrence and the role of electrophysiologic monitoring. *J Clin Oncol* 2006;24(27):4507-14.

44. Rajkumar SV, Blood E, Vesole D, Fonseca R, Greipp PR. Phase III clinical trial of thalidomide plus dexamethasone compared with dexamethasone alone in newly diagnosed multiple myeloma: a clinical trial coordinated by the Eastern Cooperative Oncology Group. *J Clin Oncol* 2006;24(3):431-6.

45. Weber D, Rankin K, Gavino M, Delasalle K, Alexanian R. Thalidomide alone or with dexamethasone for previously untreated multiple myeloma. *J Clin Oncol* 2003;21(1):16-19.

46. Glasmacher A, Hahn C, Hoffmann F, et al. Thalidomide in relapsed or refractory patients with multiple myeloma: monotherapy or combination therapy? A report from systematic reviews. *Blood (ASH Annual Meeting Abstracts)* 2005;106(11):5125.

47. Alexanian R, Weber D, Anagnostopoulos A, Delasalle K, Wang M, Rankin K. Thalidomide with or without dexamethasone for refractory or relapsing multiple myeloma. *Semin Hematol* 2003;40(4 suppl 4):3-7.

48. Dimopoulos MA, Zervas K, Kouvatseas G, et al. Thalidomide and dexamethasone combination for refractory multiple myeloma. *Ann Oncol* 2001;12(7):991-5.

49. Palumbo A, Falco P, Ambrosini MT, et al. Thalidomide plus dexamethasone is an effective salvage regimen for myeloma patients relapsing after autologous transplant. *Eur J Haematol* 2005;75(5):391-5.

50. Palumbo A, Bertola A, Falco P, et al. Efficacy of low-dose thalidomide and dexamethasone as first salvage regimen in multiple myeloma. *Hematol J* 2004;5(4):318-24.

51. Hussein MA. Thromboembolism risk reduction in multiple myeloma patients treated with immunomodulatory drug combinations. *Thromb Haemost* 2006;95(6):924-30.

52. Palumbo A, Rajkumar SV, Dimopoulos MA, et al. Prevention of thalidomide- and lenalidomide-associated thrombosis in myeloma. *Leukemia* 2008;22:414-23.

53. Moehler TM, Neben K, Benner A, et al. Salvage therapy for multiple myeloma with thalidomide and CED chemotherapy. *Blood* 2001;98(13):3846-8.

54. Offidani M, Corvatta L, Marconi M, et al. Low-dose thalidomide with pegylated liposomal doxorubicin and high-dose dexamethasone for relapsed/refractory multiple myeloma: a prospective, multicenter, phase II study. *Haematologica* 2006;91(1):133-6.

55. Dimopoulos MA, Hamilos G, Zomas A, et al. Pulsed cyclophosphamide, thalidomide and dexamethasone: an oral regimen for previously treated patients with multiple myeloma. *Hematol J* 2004;5(2):112-17.

56. Kyriakou C, Thomson K, D'Sa S, et al. Low-dose thalidomide in combination with oral weekly cyclophosphamide and pulsed dexamethasone is a well tolerated and effective regimen in patients with relapsed and refractory multiple myeloma. *Br J Haematol* 2005;129(6):763-70.

57. Glasmacher A, Moehler T, Goldschmidt H, et al. Multicenter phase II trial of patients with refractory or recurrent multiple myeloma with oral treatment of thalidomide combined with oral cyclophosphamide, idarubicin and dexamethasone. *ASH Annual Meeting Abstracts* 2007;110(11):4825.

58. Bartlett JB, Dredge K, Dalgleish AG. The evolution of thalidomide and its IMiD derivatives as anticancer agents. *Nat Rev Cancer* 2004;4(4):314-22.

59. Richardson PG, Schlossman RL, Weller E, et al. Immunomodulatory drug CC-5013 overcomes drug resistance and is well tolerated in patients with relapsed multiple myeloma. *Blood* 2002;100(9):3063-7.

60. Zangari M, Tricot G, Zeldis J, Eddlemon P, Saghafifar F, Barlogie B. Results of Phase I study of CC-5013 for the treatment of multiple myeloma (MM) patients who relapse after high dose chemotherapy (HDCT). *Blood (ASH Annual Meeting Abstracts)* 2001;98(11),775a.

61. Zangari M, Barlogie B, Jacobson J. Revlimid 25mg (REV 25) × 20 versus 50mg (REV 50) × 10 q28 days with bridging of 5mg × 10 versus 10mg × 5 as post-transplant salvage therapy for multiple myeloma. *Blood (ASH Annual Meeting Abstracts)* 2003;102(11).

62. Richardson PG, Blood E, Mitsiades CS, et al. A randomized phase 2 study of lenalidomide therapy for patients with relapsed or relapsed and refractory multiple myeloma. *Blood* 2006;108(10):3458-64.

63. Weber DM, Chen C, Niesvizky R, et al. Lenalidomide plus dexamethasone for relapsed multiple myeloma in North America. *N Engl J Med* 2007;357(21):2133-42.

64. Dimopoulos M, Spencer A, Attal M, et al. Lenalidomide plus dexamethasone for relapsed or refractory multiple myeloma. *N Engl J Med* 2007;357(21):2123-32.

65. Weber D, Knight R, Chen C, et al. Prolonged overall survival with lenalidomide plus dexamethasone compared with dexamethasone alone in patients with relapsed or refractory multiple myeloma. *ASH Annual Meeting Abstracts* 2007;110(11):412.

66. Baz R, Walker E, Karam MA, et al. Lenalidomide and pegylated liposomal doxorubicin-based chemotherapy for relapsed or refractory multiple myeloma: safety and efficacy. *Ann Oncol* 2006;17(12):1766-71.

67. Knop S, Gerecke C, Liebisch P, et al. The efficacy and toxicity of the RAD regimen (Revlimid®, Adriamycin®, dexamethasone) in

relapsed and refractory multiple myeloma—a phase I/II trial of "Deutsche Studiengruppe multiples myelom". *Blood (ASH Annual Meeting Abstracts)* 2007;110(11):2716.

68. Morgan GJ, Schey SA, Wu P, et al. Lenalidomide (Revlimid), in combination with cyclophosphamide and dexamethasone (RCD), is an effective and tolerated regimen for myeloma patients. *Br J Haematol* 2007;137(3):268-9.

69. Hideshima T, Anderson KC. Preclinical studies of novel targeted therapies. *Hematol Oncol Clin North Am* 2007;21(6):1071-91.

70. Richardson PG, Barlogie B, Berenson J, et al. A phase 2 study of bortezomib in relapsed, refractory myeloma. *N Engl J Med* 2003;348(26):2609-17.

71. Jagannath S, Barlogie B, Berenson J, et al. A phase 2 study of two doses of bortezomib in relapsed or refractory myeloma. *Br J Haematol* 2004;127(2):165-72.

72. Jagannath S, Barlogie B, Berenson JR, et al. Updated survival analyses after prolonged follow-up of the phase 2, multicenter CREST study of bortezomib in relapsed or refractory multiple myeloma. *Blood (ASH Annual Meeting Abstracts)* 2007;110(11):2717.

73. Richardson PG, Sonneveld P, Schuster MW, et al. Bortezomib or high-dose dexamethasone for relapsed multiple myeloma. *N Engl J Med* 2005;352(24):2487-98.

74. Richardson PG, Sonneveld P, Schuster M. Extended follow-up of a phase 3 trial in relapsed multiple myeloma: final time-to-event results of the APEX trial. *Blood* 2007;110(10):3557-60.

75. Richardson PG, Briemberg H, Jagannath S, et al. Frequency, characteristics, and reversibility of peripheral neuropathy during treatment of advanced multiple myeloma with bortezomib. *J Clin Oncol* 2006;24(19):3113-20.

76. Miguel JFS, Richardson P, Sonneveld P, et al. Frequency, characteristics, and reversibility of peripheral neuropathy (PN) in the APEX trial. *Blood (ASH Annual Meeting Abstracts)* 2005;106(11):366.

77. Lonial S, Waller EK, Richardson PG, et al. Risk factors and kinetics of thrombocytopenia associated with bortezomib for relapsed, refractory multiple myeloma. *Blood* 2005;106(12):3777-84.

78. Lonial S, Richardson P, Sonneveld P, et al. Hematologic profiles in the phase 3 APEX trial. *ASH Annual Meeting Abstracts* 2005;106(11):3474.

79. Mitsiades N, Mitsiades CS, Richardson PG, et al. The proteasome inhibitor PS-341 potentiates sensitivity of multiple myeloma cells to conventional chemotherapeutic agents: therapeutic applications. *Blood* 2003;101(6):2377-80.

80. Blad E J, Miguel JS, Nagler A, et al. The prolonged time to progression with pegylated liposomal doxorubicin + bortezomib versus bortezomib alone in relapsed or refractory multiple myeloma is unaffected by extent of prior therapy or previous anthracycline exposure. *ASH Annual Meeting Abstracts* 2007;110(11):410.

81. Popat R, Oakervee HE, Foot N, et al. A phase I/II study of bortezomib and low dose intravenous melphalan (BM) for relapsed multiple myeloma. *ASH Annual Meeting Abstracts* 2005;106(11):2555.

82. Davies FE, Wu P, Jenner M, Srikanth M, Saso R, Morgan GJ. The combination of cyclophosphamide, velcade and dexamethasone induces high response rates with comparable toxicity to velcade alone and velcade plus dexamethasone. *Haematologica* 2007;92(8):1149-50.

83. Kropff M, Bisping G, Schuck E, et al. Bortezomib in combination with intermediate-dose dexamethasone and continuous low-dose oral cyclophosphamide for relapsed multiple myeloma. *Br J Haematol* 2007;138(3):330-7.

84. Zangari M, Barlogie B, Burns MJ, et al. Velcade (V)-thalidomide (T)-dexamethasone (D) for advanced and refractory multiple myeloma (MM): long-term follow-up of phase I-II trial UARK 2001-37: superior outcome in patients with normal cytogenetics and no prior T. *ASH Annual Meeting Abstracts* 2005;106(11):2552.

85. Padmanabhan S, Miller K, Musiel L, et al. Bortezomib (Velcade) in combination with liposomal doxorubicin (Doxil) and thalidomide is an active salvage regimen in patients with relapse or refractory multiple myeloma: final results of a phase II study. *Haematologica* 2006;91(suppl 1):277.

86. Hollmig K, Stover J, Talamo G, et al. Bortezomib (Velcade™) + Adriamycin™ + Thalidomide + Dexamethasone (VATD) as an effective regimen in patients with refractory or relapsed multiple myeloma (MM). *ASH Annual Meeting Abstracts* 2004;104(11):2399.

87. Ciolli S, Leoni F, Casini C, Breschi C, Bosi A. Liposomal doxorubicin (Myocet®) enhance the efficacy of bortezomib, dexamethasone plus thalidomide in refractory myeloma. *ASH Annual Meeting Abstracts* 2006;108(11):5087.

88. Palumbo A, Ambrosini MT, Benevolo G, et al. Bortezomib, melphalan, prednisone, and thalidomide for relapsed multiple myeloma. *Blood* 2007;109(7):2767-72.

89. Terpos E, Anagnostopoulos A, Heath D, et al. The combination of bortezomib, melphalan, dexamethasone and intermittent thalidomide (VMDT) is an effective regimen for relapsed/refractory myeloma and reduces serum levels of Dickkopf-1, RANKL, MIP-1{alpha} and angiogenic cytokines. *ASH Annual Meeting Abstracts* 2006;108(11):3541.

90. Richardson PG, Jagannath S, Avigan DE, et al. Lenalidomide plus bortezomib (Rev-Vel) in relapsed and/or refractory multiple myeloma (MM): final results of a multicenter phase 1 trial. *ASH Annual Meeting Abstracts* 2006;108(11):405.

91. Richardson P, Jagannath S, Raje N, et al. Lenalidomide, bortezomib, and dexamethasone (Rev/Vel/Dex) in patients with relapsed or relapsed/refractory multiple myeloma (MM): preliminary results of a phase II study. *Blood (ASH Annual Meeting Abstracts)* 2007;110(11):2714.

92. Mitsiades CS, Mitsiades NS, McMullan CJ, et al. Antimyeloma activity of heat shock protein-90 inhibition. *Blood* 2006;107(3):1092-100.

93. Mitsiades N, Mitsiades CS, Poulaki V, et al. Molecular sequelae of proteasome inhibition in human multiple myeloma cells. *Proc Natl Acad Sci USA* 2002;99(22):14374-9.

94. Richardson PG, Chanan-Khan AA, Alsina M, et al. Safety and activity of KOS-953 in patients with relapsed refractory multiple myeloma (MM): interim results of a phase 1 trial. *ASH Annual Meeting Abstracts* 2005;106(11):361.

95. Richardson P, Chanan-Khan AA, Lonial S, et al. A multicenter phase 1 clinical trial of tanespimycin (KOS-953) + bortezomib

(BZ): encouraging activity and manageable toxicity in heavily pre-treated patients with relapsed refractory multiple myeloma (MM). *Blood (ASH Annual Meeting Abstracts)* 2006;108(11):406.

96. Richardson P, Chanan-Khan AA, Lonial S, et al. Tanespimycin (T) + bortezomib (BZ) in multiple myeloma (MM): Pharmacology, safety and activity in relapsed/refractory (rel/ref) patients (Pts). *J Clin Oncol* 2007;25:3532.

97. Hideshima T, Catley L, Yasui H, et al. Perifosine, an oral bioactive novel alkylphospholipid, inhibits Akt and induces in vitro and in vivo cytotoxicity in human multiple myeloma cells. *Blood* 2006;107(10):4053-62.

98. Richardson P, Jakubowiak A, Wolf J, et al. Phase I/II report from a multicenter trial of perifosine (KRX-0401) + bortezomib in patients with relapsed or relapsed/refractory multiple myeloma previously treated with bortezomib. *ASH Annual Meeting Abstracts* 2007;110(11):1170.

99. Garcia-Mata R, Gao YS, Sztul E. Hassles with taking out the garbage: aggravating aggresomes. *Traffic* 2002;3(6):388-96.

100. Kawaguchi Y, Kovacs JJ, McLaurin A, Vance JM, Ito A, Yao TP. The deacetylase HDAC6 regulates aggresome formation and cell viability in response to misfolded protein stress. *Cell* 2003;115(6):727-38.

101. Hideshima T, Bradner JE, Wong J, et al. Small-molecule inhibition of proteasome and aggresome function induces synergistic antitumor activity in multiple myeloma. *Proc Natl Acad Sci USA* 2005;102(24):8567-72.

102. Mitsiades CS, Mitsiades NS, McMullan CJ, et al. Transcriptional signature of histone deacetylase inhibition in multiple myeloma: biological and clinical implications. *Proc Natl Acad Sci USA* 2004;101(2):540-5.

103. Weber DM, Jagannath S, Mazumder A, et al. Phase I trial of oral vorinostat (Suberoylanilide Hydroxamic Acid, SAHA) in combination with bortezomib in patients with advanced multiple myeloma. *Blood (ASH Annual Meeting Abstracts)* 2007;110(11):1172.

104. Badros A, Philip S, Niesvizky R, et al. Phase I trial of suberoylanilide hydroxamic acid (SAHA) + bortezomib (Bort) in relapsed multiple myeloma (MM) patients (pts). *ASH Annual Meeting Abstracts* 2007;110(11):1168.

105. Prince M, Quach H, Neeson P, et al. Safety and efficacy of the combination of bortezomib with the deacetylase inhibitor romidepsin in patients with relapsed or refractory multiple myeloma: preliminary results of a phase I trial. *ASH Annual Meeting Abstracts* 2007;110(11):1167.

106. Hideshima T, Akiyama M, Hayashi T, et al. Targeting p38 MAPK inhibits multiple myeloma cell growth in the bone marrow milieu. *Blood* 2003;101(2):703-5.

107. Chauhan D, Velankar M, Brahmandam M, et al. A novel Bcl-2/Bcl-X(L)/Bcl-w inhibitor ABT-737 as therapy in multiple myeloma. *Oncogene* 2007;26(16):2374-80.

108. Chauhan D, Neri P, Velankar M, et al. Targeting mitochondrial factor Smac/DIABLO as therapy for multiple myeloma (MM). *Blood* 2007;109(3):1220-7.

109. Tai YT, Dillon M, Song W, et al. Anti-CS1 humanized monoclonal antibody HuLuc63 inhibits myeloma cell adhesion and induces antibody-dependent cellular cytotoxicity in the bone marrow milieu. *Blood* 2007 Oct 9. [Epub ahead of print].

110. Moreau P, Hulin C, Facon T, et al. Phase I study of AVE1642 anti IGF-1R monoclonal antibody in patients with advanced multiple myeloma. *ASH Annual Meeting Abstracts* 2007; 110(11):1166.

111. Podar K, Raab MS, Zhang J, et al. Targeting PKC in multiple myeloma: in vitro and in vivo effects of the novel, orally available small-molecule inhibitor enzastaurin (LY317615.HCl). *Blood* 2007;109(4):1669-77.

112. Chauhan D, Singh A, Brahmandam M, et al. Combination of proteasome inhibitors bortezomib and NPI-0052 trigger in vivo synergistic cytotoxicity in multiple myeloma. *Blood* 2008;111(3):1654-64.

113. Sonneveld P, Hajek R, Nagler A, et al. Impact of prior thalidomide (T) therapy on the efficacy of pegylated liposomal doxorubicin (PLD) and bortezomib (B) in relapsed/refractory multiple myeloma (RRMM). *J Clin Oncol (Meeting Abstracts)* 2007;25(18 suppl):8023.

114. Chanan-Khan AA, Weber D, Dimopoulos M, et al. Lenalidomide (L) in combination with dexamethasone (D) improves survival and time to progression in elderly patients (pts) with relapsed or refractory (rel/ref) multiple myeloma (MM). *ASH Annual Meeting Abstracts* 2006;108(11):3551.

115. Richardson PG, Sonneveld P, Schuster MW, et al. Safety and efficacy of bortezomib in high-risk and elderly patients with relapsed multiple myeloma. *Br J Haematol* 2007;137(5): 429-35.

116. Celegene Corporation. THALOMID (thalidomide) product information. Summit, NJ, USA 2006; Available at: www.celgene.com/PDF/ThalomidPI.pdf.

117. Chanan-Khan AA, Kaufman JL, Mehta J, et al. Activity and safety of bortezomib in multiple myeloma patients with advanced renal failure: a multicenter retrospective study. *Blood* 2007;109(6):2604-6.

118. Tosi P, Zamagni E, Cellini C, et al. Thalidomide alone or in combination with dexamethasone in patients with advanced, relapsed or refractory multiple myeloma and renal failure. *Eur J Haematol* 2004;73(2):98-103.

119. Ludwig H, Adam Z, Hajek R, et al. Recovery of renal impairment by bortezomib-doxorubicin-dexamethasone (BDD) in multiple myeloma (MM) patients with acute renal failure. Results from an ongoing phase II study. *ASH Annual Meeting Abstracts* 2007;110(11):3603.

120. Reece DE, Masih-Khan E, Chen C, et al. Use of lenalidomide (Revlimid(R) ± corticosteroids in relapsed/refractory multiple myeloma patients with elevated baseline serum creatinine levels. *ASH Annual Meeting Abstracts* 2006;108(11):3548.

121. Chen N, Lau H, Kong L, et al. Pharmacokinetics of lenalidomide in subjects with various degrees of renal impairment and in subjects on hemodialysis. *J Clin Pharmacol* 2007;47(12):1466-75.

122. Jagannath S, Richardson PG, Sonneveld P, et al. Bortezomib appears to overcome the poor prognosis conferred by

chromosome 13 deletion in phase 2 and 3 trials. *Leukemia* 2007;21(1):151-7.

123. Bahlis NJ, Mansoor A, Lategan JC, et al. Lenalidomide overcomes poor prognosis conferred by deletion of chromosome 13 and t(4;14) in multiple myeloma: MM016 Trial. *ASH Annual Meeting Abstracts* 2006;108(11):3557.

124. von Metzler, Krebbel H, Hecht M, et al. Bortezomib inhibits human osteoclastogenesis. *Leukemia* 2007;21(9):2025-34.

125. Breitkreutz I, Raab MS, Vallet S, et al. Lenalidomide and bortezomib: targeting osteoclastogenesis, osteoclast survival factors, and bone remodeling markers in multiple myeloma. *ASH Annual Meeting Abstracts* 2007;110(11):1184.

6 Diagnosis and Treatment of Myeloma Bone Disease

G. David Roodman

INTRODUCTION

Multiple myeloma (MM) is the most common cancer to metastasize to bone, with up to 90% of patients developing bone lesions.[1] The bone lesions are purely osteolytic in nature and do not heal in the vast majority of patients. Up to 60% of patients develop pathological fractures over the course of their disease.[2] Bone disease is a hallmark of MM, and myeloma bone disease differs from bone metastasis caused by other tumors. Although myeloma and other osteolytic metastases induce increased osteoclastic bone destruction, in contrast to other tumors, once myeloma tumor burden exceeds 50% in a local area, osteoblast activity is either severely depressed or absent.[3] The basis for this severe imbalance between increased osteoclastic bone resorption and decreased bone formation has been the topic of intensive investigation over the past several years. These studies have helped to identify novel targets for treating myeloma bone disease and are discussed subsequently in this chapter.

The clinical and economic impact of myeloma bone disease in patients with myeloma can be catastrophic. Saad and coworkers[4] retrospectively evaluated data from patients on the control arms of randomized trials of zoledronic acid to assess the impact of pathological fractures on survival of patients with malignant disease. A total of 3049 patients with metastatic bone disease were included in this study, of which 513 had myeloma. Patients with myeloma had the highest incidence of fracture (43%) over the 21 months of the study compared to patients with breast cancer, prostate cancer, and lung cancer. Myeloma patients who experienced pathological fractures had at least a 20% increased risk of death compared to myeloma patients without pathological fractures. Further, patients who had a prior skeletal-related event, which included pathological fracture, spinal cord compression syndrome, surgery to bone, or radiation therapy to bone, were more likely to develop new pathological fractures as compared to patients who did not have a prior skeletal-related event. Patients with a skeletal-related event before entering the studies had a much poorer outcome, including a 40% increase in the risk of sustaining a skeletal-related event compared to patients without a prior history of skeletal-related events.

In addition to the severe clinical consequences of myeloma bone disease, metastatic bone disease has a tremendous economic burden as well. In a recent analysis of the economic burden of metastatic bone disease in the United States, Schulman and Kohles[5] compared patients with metastatic bone disease to patients without metastatic bone disease as controls. In their analysis, they found that the rate of metastatic bone disease in patients with myeloma was the highest of any cancer during the study period (2000-2004). The incremental cost of having bone disease in patients with myeloma was $57 720 per patient compared to that in patients without metastatic bone disease. Furthermore, the total cost in 2004 dollars for patients with myeloma bone disease was estimated at $950 113 852. Thus, myeloma bone disease places a tremendous burden, both economically and clinically, on patients with myeloma.

CLINICAL MANIFESTATIONS OF MYELOMA BONE DISEASE

Bone destruction in MM can involve any bone. In a study of over 250 myeloma patients, bones most likely to be involved included the spine (49%), skull (35%), pelvis (34%), ribs (33%), humeri (22%), femora (13%), and mandible (10%).[6] The most common radiographic findings of bone involvement included osteolysis, osteopenia, pathological fractures, or a combination of the above. Eighty percent of the patients experienced bone pain. Bone pain typically presented in the back or chest and was exacerbated by movement and was less intense at nighttime.

Hypercalcemia occurs in approximately 15% of myeloma patients.[7] The causes of hypercalcemia in myeloma include increased bone resorption, decreased bone formation, impaired renal function, and in a minority of patients, increased production of the hormone parathyroid-related protein (PTHrP) by the myeloma cells. PTHrP is the major mediator of the humoral hypercalcemia of malignancy.[8] In contrast to the humoral hypercalcemia of malignancy, hypercalcemia in myeloma patients is more often secondary to widespread bone involvement and renal impairment as opposed to elevated levels of PTHrP. The level of hypercalcemia in myeloma correlates with tumor burden and not with serum PTHrP levels.[7] The uncoupling of normal bone resorption/formation in myeloma results in markedly increased bone resorption, with an overall net efflux of calcium into the extracellular fluid. Signs and symptoms of hypercalcemia include dry mouth, anorexia, constipation, renal stones, confusion, depression, nausea, vomiting, polydypsia, and polyuria. Renal impairment in myeloma is thought to cause hypercalcemia not only by an inability to clear the excessive calcium released into the serum from increased bone resorption but also from increased renal tubular calcium reabsorption. The etiology of the increased renal tubular calcium reabsorption remains unclear, as elevation of PTHrP is not a consistent finding among myeloma patients.[9]

Myeloma bone disease can also cause neurological complication. Radiculopathy, usually of the thoracic or lumbosacral regions, is the most frequent neurological complication. The radiculopathy is due to expansion of the primary tumor in the vertebrae or collapse of the bone leading to compression of the nerve. Spinal cord compression, which is an oncological emergency, is seen in 2%-3% of patients.[10] Peripheral neuropathy occurs but is typically associated with amyloidosis or more commonly as a side effect of therapy and not bone disease.

EVALUATION OF BONE INVOLVEMENT IN MYELOMA

Metastatic bone surveys using plain radiography have been used as the gold standard to determine the extent of bone involvement in myeloma and monitor progression of bone disease in patients with myeloma. An adequate survey includes imaging X-rays of the skull, vertebral column, pelvis, and extremities. Almost 80% of patients with myeloma will have radiological evidence of skeletal involvement on metastatic bone surveys, with the vertebra, ribs, skull, shoulders and pelvis, and long bones being the most frequently involved.[11] Involvement of lesions in smaller bones is relatively uncommon but can be seen even in the digits (Figure 6.1). However, plain radiography has relatively low sensitivity and can demonstrate lytic bone disease only when at least 30% of trabecular bone has been lost.[12] Furthermore, the skeletal survey is not sensitive enough to be used to assess responses to therapy. If conventional radiography is inconclusive or negative in the setting of high clinical suspicion for bone disease, computerized tomography (CT) without contrast, positron emission tomography (PET)/CT, or magnetic resonance imaging (MRI) may be used. These modalities are more sensitive than conventional radiography for detecting occult bone disease.

Technetium-99m bone scanning is not appropriate for evaluating myeloma bone disease. Bone scans reflect osteoblastic activity and thus underestimate the osteolytic lesions characteristic of myeloma bone disease.[10] Technetium-99-sestamibi scanning has been investigated in myeloma patients because it is concentrated in myeloma tissues. In a multicenter study of 397 whole-body scans compared to standard radiography, sestamibi scanning was found to be more sensitive (77% vs. 45%) than radiographs and was highly specific for staging myeloma patients.[13] These results suggest that sestamibi scanning should be useful for staging myeloma.

The limited reproducibility of bone surveys has led to the use of newer modalities such as CT scan without contrast, MRI scan, and PET scan to evaluate the extent of myeloma bone disease. MRI allows assessment of bone marrow involvement with hematological malignancies and has been used to determine myeloma involvement in the marrow.[14] Myeloma lesions on MRI have a low signal intensity on T1-weighted images and a high signal intensity on T2-weighted images.[15] In contrast to inflammatory lesions, myelomatous lesions do not affect the intravertebral disc space or articular surfaces. The major issue with MRI is a lack of specificity of the findings.[16] MRI findings can be prognostic. Patients found to have more than 10 lesions on MRI imaging of vertebral bodies have a 6- to

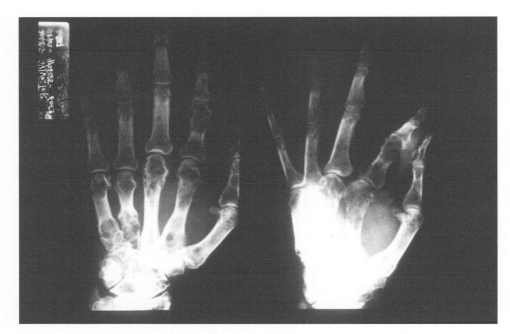

Figure 6.1. Lytic bone lesions in the hands of a patient with myeloma
Source: Courtesy Dr. H. Mankin, Massachusetts General Hospital, Boston, MA.

10-fold higher risk for fracture than patients with less than 10 lesions or a normal appearance on MRI.[17] Walker and coworkers[18] compared MRI with skeletal surveys in 611 patients treated at the University of Arkansas. They found that patients with more than seven focal lesions detected by using MRI had a worse prognosis. In this study, the number of lesions on plain radiography did not contribute to prognosis. In comparison trials, MRI has been shown to have greater sensitivity than plain radiographs in detecting asymptomatic bone disease[19] and provides both anatomical and physiological information about marrow involvement. In one study of 53 patients with MM, 55% of patients with presumed normal plain radiographs had evidence of diffuse or nodular bone involvement on MRI. MRI is also superior to plain radiography for staging patients with MM. One study evaluated 12 patients with presumed solitary plasmacytomas, and on bone survey found four patients to have additional evidence of marrow involvement on MRI evaluation, thus changing their diagnosis to MM.[20] MRI imaging of the head, spine, and pelvis is recommended in all patients with a suspected diagnosis of solitary plasmacytoma to rule out any other bone lesions. MRI is the diagnostic procedure of choice for assessing spinal cord compression.[16]

CT is not used routinely for screening patients with myeloma because of the high levels of radiation exposure. CT has a higher sensitivity than plain radiographs for detecting small lytic lesions and can detect extra-osseous extension of myeloma.[16] CT can be used to determine the presence or absence of bone destruction in cases where the MRI is negative.

More recently, PET has been used to detect metastatic bone lesions in patients with myeloma. Whole-body PET scans using 18F deoxyglucose (FDG-PET) have shown that FDG-PET can identify marrow disease earlier than X-rays or other imaging systems because of its increased sensitivity. Bredella and coworkers[21] examined the ability of whole-body PET to detect bone marrow involvement in patients with myeloma. FDG-PET images were evaluated for the distribution and uptake patterns, and the results were verified using MRI, CT, and radiography. In this study of 13 patients, FDG-PET resulted in upstaging of disease in four patients and was able to detect myelomatous involvement in 85% of patients with a specificity of 92%. Nanni and coworkers[22] compared FDG-PET and FDG-PET combined with CT to whole-body X-rays and MRI in 28 newly diagnosed patients with myeloma. In 57% (16 out of 28 patients) PET-CT detected more bone

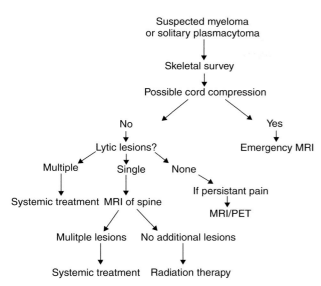

Figure 6.2. Flow diagram for evaluating and treating myeloma bone disease.
Source: Adapted from D'Sa S, Abildgaard N, Tighe J, Shaw P, Hall-Craggs M. Guidelines for the use of imaging in the management of myeloma. *Br J Haematol* 2007;137:49-63. Wiley-Blackwell Publishing, Oxford, UK.

lesions than whole-body X-rays, while in 12 patients the two methods yielded equivalent results. All the lesions that were detected by using PET-CT but were not detected by using whole-body X-rays were small and below the contrast resolution of standard radiographs. In 9 of these 16 patients, whole-body X-rays were completely negative, while PET-CT detected one or more bone lesions. PET-CT also detected more lesions than MRI in 25% of patients studied, and all these lesions were outside the field of view of MRI. Interestingly, MRI detected an osteoporotic pattern in three vertebral pathological fractures that were negative according to PET. Thus, PET-CT appears to be more sensitive than whole-body X-rays for detection of small lytic bone lesions, but has the same sensitivity as MRI for detecting bone disease in the spine and pelvis. These authors recommended using both MRI and PET-CT for evaluating patients with myeloma bone disease. However, the major limitation of PET-CT scanning is that small lesions may not be detected and false-positives can arise from inflammatory lesions from infection or recent chemotherapy or fracture.[23] In the recent guidelines for the use of imaging and management of myeloma by the British Committee for Standards in Hematology, skeletal

surveys, routine MRI, CT, or PET scanning was not recommended for routine follow-up of treated myeloma patients, although these imaging techniques might be useful in selected patients who have persistent unexplained symptoms or in whom there is a concern for increase fracture risk or lack of response to therapy. Figure 6.2 shows a flow diagram for imaging of patients with myeloma or solitary plasmacytoma, which is adapted from the guidelines for imaging by the British Committee for Standards of Hematology.[16]

TREATMENT OF MYELOMA BONE DISEASE

Treatment of myeloma bone disease involves treatment of the underlying malignancy and its manifestations. Current treatments include use of chemotherapy and autologous stem cell transplantation for myeloma; localized radiation therapy to control pain or impending fracture or treat solitary plasmacytoma, kyphoplasty, or vertebraplasty; surgery to bone; and inhibiting bone resorption and osteoclast formation using bisphosphonate therapy.

Bisphosphonate therapy is currently the mainstay of treating myeloma bone disease. Bisphosphonate therapy is used in patients to decrease bone pain, progression of lytic lesions, prevent development of new pathological fractures, and may improve survival. Bisphosphonates are synthetic analogues of pyrophosphate that act to inhibit osteoclast activity.[24] The improvement of bone pain is thought to be due to the inhibition of osteoclast activity mediated by the induction of osteoclast apoptosis through inhibition of protein prenylation by nitrogen-containing bisphosphonates[24] or the generation of toxic ATP derivatives by non-nitrogen–containing bisphosphonates. Of the many different bisphosphonates available in the market, not all have proved to be effective for the treatment of myeloma bone disease. Intravenous pamidronate, 90 mg once monthly, or zoledronate, 4 mg once monthly, is the mainstay of bisphosphonate therapy in myeloma. In the original randomized trial evaluating intravenous pamidronate therapy in myeloma, a significant reduction in the number of skeletal events per patient year was found when compared to placebo (1.3 vs. 2.2) when patients were treated for 21 months.[25] Zoledronate is the most potent bisphosphonate used in the management of myeloma bone disease. When compared with pamidronate in phase 3 trials, zoledronate was found to be as effective as pamidronate in decreasing the number of skeletal complications and need for radiation therapy.[26] The major benefit of zoledronate over pamidronate was that it can be given over a shorter period of time (15 min vs. 2 h).[26] Intravenous and oral ibandronate are used in Europe for the treatment of myeloma bone disease and are being evaluated for use in the United States.[27] Clodronate, an oral bisphosphonate, has also been used for the treatment of myeloma bone disease in Europe at 1600 mg/day.[28] The bioavailability of oral bisphosphonates is less than 4%, so the dose of oral forms of bisphosphonates is much higher when compared to the available intravenous forms.

Current recommendations suggest starting bisphosphonate therapy in myeloma when there is evidence of bone involvement.[29] The optimal duration and frequency of bisphosphonate therapy in myeloma are not well understood and are currently being studied. Current consensus statements recommend treating patients for 2 years and then considering to discontinue therapy at that time if the patient is in remission or a plateau phase of their disease.[29,30] ASCO guidelines currently recommend using either pamidronate or zoledronate in patients with lytic destruction of bone or spinal cord compression on imaging.[29] Patients with renal impairment should receive pamidronate over a longer infusion time.

Zoledronic acid and other bisphosphonates have been reported to have antitumor activity against myeloma cell lines as well as in animal models of myeloma.[31-33] However, it is unclear if zoledronic acid or other bisphosphonates have antitumor activity in patients. In a recent abstract at the American Society of Hematology, Musto et al.[34] reported the final analysis of a multicenter randomized study comparing zoledronic acid versus observation in patients with myeloma. In this study, the effects of zoledronic acid versus placebo were compared in 160 patients with early-stage or smoldering myeloma, who did not require treatment of their myeloma at diagnosis. The end point was the need for chemoradiotherapy. These authors previously reported that pamidronate did not prevent or delay the need for treatment in patients with smoldering myeloma.[35] No significant reduction in the M-component was detected in both groups throughout the study with a medium follow-up of 55 months. Medium time to progression to symptomatic myeloma was not significantly different, although the numbers of bone lesions

and hypercalcemia at the time of progression were significantly lower in the zoledronic acid–treated patients (48.5% vs. 81%; p < 0.05). These data suggest that early treatment with bisphosphonates does not provide any antitumor effect but may reduce the development of skeletal-related events at progression. However, current ASCO guidelines do not recommend treating myeloma patients with bisphosphonate therapy unless they have identifiable bone lesions or osteopenia.[29]

An emerging complication associated with bisphosphonate therapy is osteonecrosis of the jaw (ONJ). In September 2003, Wang et al.[36] and Marx[37] reported the initial cases of ONJ associated with the use of bisphosphonate therapy. An increasing number of reports have pointed out an association between ONJ and the use of bisphosphonate therapy in patients with metastatic bone disease or benign osteoporosis, although a cause-and-effect relationship has not been clearly demonstrated. Patients with myeloma have been reported to have the highest incidence of ONJ [1.6%-11%; reviewed in Ref. (38)] while patients with postmenopausal osteoporosis treated with oral bisphosphonates have an incidence of ONJ of 1/10 000 to 1/100 000 patient treatment years.[39] Bisphosphonate-associated ONJ has been defined as the presence of the exposed bone in the mandible or maxilla in patients receiving bisphosphonate therapy that does not heal within 8 weeks of appropriate dental management in the absence of local metastatic disease or previous radiation therapy.[38] Clinical examination usually shows an exposed alveolar ridge with sequestra of necrotic bone, often with a purulent discharge. The surrounding gums and mucosal tissue are usually inflamed and can be painful to the touch.[38] Patients can have single or multiple lesions, with the mandible more frequently involved than the maxilla. Most patients have only exposed bone, although fistula to the maxillary sinus or the skin can occur and pathological fractures of the mandible have been reported.[38] The overwhelming majority of cases reported have been either case reports or retrospective studies of patients on bisphosphonate therapy. Recently, one long-term follow-up study of myeloma patients with ONJ was reported at the American Society of Hematology meeting.[40] Risk factors for ONJ that were identified included dental extraction, older age, and longer survival. Badros and coworkers[41] have also reported that patients with ONJ have an increased risk of skeletal-related events. In the study reported at the American Society of Hematology, 97 patients (60 from Greece and 37 from the United States) were followed for at least 3.2 years.[40] ONJ resolved in 60 of the 97 patients, resolved and recurred in 12 of the patients, and did not heal over a 9-month period in 26% of the patients. Dental extraction preceded the development of ONJ in 47% of the patients and was more common in patients with a single episode of ONJ than in patients with recurrent or nonhealing ONJ. The recurrence of ONJ in these 12 patients was precipitated by reinitiation of bisphosphonate therapy or by dental procedures. Interestingly, 21 of the ONJ patients developed new skeletal-related events, including fractures of the ribs and long bones and avascular necrosis of the femur. The rate of myeloma relapse was higher in patients with recurrent nonhealing ONJ (84%) compared to patients with a single episode of ONJ. In this series, patients with ONJ following dental procedures were less likely to have a recurrence or nonhealing, although, infrequently, recurrence was linked to retreatment with bisphosphonates in patients with relapsed myeloma. Thus, the risk factors associated with the development of ONJ for patients on bisphosphonate therapy appear to be the duration of bisphosphonate therapy, presence of active myeloma, and a previous dental extraction or dental surgery. The true prevalence of ONJ in myeloma patients on bisphosphonate therapy is unclear but has been reported to range from 3.1% to 11%.[38] Clarke and coworkers,[42] who performed a retrospective chart review of patients who were treated by the Myeloma Institute at the University of Arkansas and were referred to the Head and Neck Surgery Clinic, found that approximately 5% of their patients developed ONJ after an average of 4.4 years of bisphosphonate treatment. Current treatment of ONJ associated with bisphosphonate therapy is conservative management with oral rinses and antibiotic therapy for weeks to months.

The pathophysiology underlying ONJ is still unclear. The jaws are the only bones that have frequent contact with the outside environment and are subject to repeated microtrauma because of chewing. Decreased bone remodeling induced by bisphosphonates has been implicated as a potential mechanism for ONJ but has not been confirmed.[42] Possibly, inhibition of osteoclast function using bisphosphonate therapy is responsible for ONJ. This could interfere with healing of microfractures and trauma that occur especially after tooth extraction and may in part

explain why tooth extraction and surgery to bone are associated with an increased risk of ONJ. No particular myeloma treatments have been clearly implicated in the pathogenesis of ONJ, although the use of dexamethasone and thalidomide has been suggested as additional risk factors.[41] In addition, although bisphosphonates can have effects on new blood vessel formation, biopsies of patients with ONJ show no reduction in capillaries.[38] Interestingly, patients with ONJ more frequently are diabetic or have impaired glucose tolerance than would be expected in an age-matched population.[43] Diabetes is associated with impaired wound healing, and this could play a role in the development of ONJ in patients with myeloma. Infections may also play a role in ONJ, since the oral cavity has an abundance of microorganisms and actinomycetes have been cultured from these lesions.[38]

Stopping or continuing bisphosphonate therapy in myeloma patients who develop ONJ remains a major question. There are no prospective randomized data available to determine the duration or the frequency of treatment with bisphosphonates in patients with myeloma. A retrospective analysis of patients with myeloma treated for 1 year with bisphosphonates and then treated either monthly or every three months thereafter reported an eightfold decrease in the incidence of ONJ in the patients on the reduced schedule.[44] Stopping bisphosphonate therapy has not been shown to accelerate healing in patients with ONJ, and patients can heal with continued bisphosphonate therapy. Furthermore, bisphosphonates have an extremely long half-life in bone, which has been estimated to be greater than 10 years, so stopping bisphosphonates may or may not have any effect on ONJ. However, several consensus statements have suggested stopping or considering stopping bisphosphonate therapy in patients who have received 2 years of bisphosphonate therapy and are in plateau phase or are in complete remission.[29,30] In patients who have progressive bone disease, reinstitution or continuation of bisphosphonate therapy should be considered after the risks and benefits have been discussed with the patient. Several ongoing prospective randomized trials are examining different frequencies of administration of bisphosphonates or treating patients only with bisphosphonates on the basis of their levels of bone resorption markers. However, bone resorption markers are relatively insensitive for determining when to start or stop bisphosphonate therapy in patients with myeloma. Therefore, new therapies for treating myeloma bone disease are currently being explored.

NOVEL THERAPIES FOR MYELOMA BONE DISEASE

Recent studies have identified several important factors produced or induced by myeloma cells that play an important role in the osteolytic bone destruction characteristic of myeloma. These include factors that stimulate osteoclast formation as well as factors that suppress osteoblast activity. These include receptor activator of nuclear factor-κB (NF-κB) ligand (RANKL), macrophage inflammatory peptide-1α (MIP-1α), interleukin-3 (IL-3), IL-6, Dickkopf-1 (DKK1), soluble frizzle-related protein-2, and IL-7 [reviewed in Ref. (45)] (Figure 6.3).

The RANKL signaling pathway plays a critical role in normal bone remodeling. RANK is a transmembrane receptor, which is a member of the tumor necrosis factor (TNF) superfamily and is present on osteoclast precursors. RANKL is a membrane-bound protein expressed on marrow stromal cells and immature osteoblasts and is secreted by activated T cells. RANKL plays an important role in normal osteoclast formation and survival, which has been clearly shown in mice lacking RANKL and RANK. These mice develop severe osteopetrosis.[46] Normally, there is a decoy receptor for RANKL, osteoprotegrin (OPG), which is a member of TNF receptor superfamily.[47] It is produced by osteoblasts and many other cell types and acts as a soluble decoy receptor to block the activity in RANKL. In myeloma, RANKL expression is markedly increased while OPG is decreased.[48] Multiple studies have shown that the circulating levels of RANKL and OPG correlate with both clinical activity of myeloma and the severity of bone disease, and portend a poor prognosis.[49-51] Studies in animal models

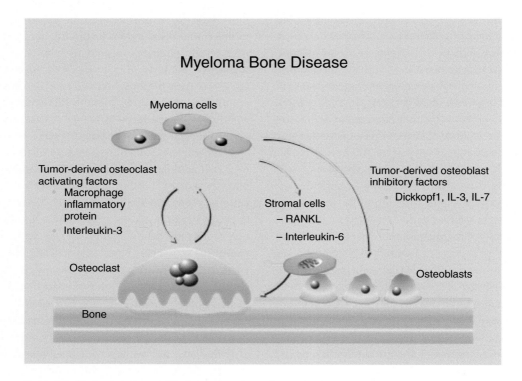

Figure 6.3. Mechanisms responsible for myeloma bone disease. Myeloma cells produce factors that directly or indirectly activate osteoclasts such as MIP-1α and IL-3. In addition, they induce RANK ligand and IL-6 production by marrow stromal cells to enhance osteoclast formation. The bone destructive process releases growth factors that increase the growth of myeloma cells, further exacerbating the osteolytic process. Myeloma cells also produce DKK1, IL-3, soluble frizzle-related protein-2, and IL-7, which suppress osteoblast differentiation and new bone formation.
Source: Derived from Roodman G.D., N Engl J Med. 2004;32:290-2.

have shown that blocking RANKL activity decreases both bone destruction and myeloma tumor burden.[52-54]

Recently, a fully humanized monoclonal antibody to RANKL (Denosumab, Amgen) has been developed. This antibody induces rapid reduction of bone resorption markers in patients, which persisted for up to 90 days after a single dose.[55] This antibody is highly specific for RANKL and does not bind to other members of the TNF-α superfamily. Denosumab is currently in clinical trial for myeloma as well as in other diseases associated with osteoclastic bone destruction. Administration of a single dose of recombinant OPG, which targets the same pathway, also significantly decreases bone resorption markers in myeloma patients for more than a month.[56] However, this drug has not been brought further into clinical development because of concerns about anti-OPG antibodies.

MIP-1α is a chemokine that is a powerful inducer of human osteoclast formation and is produced by myeloma cells in 70% of MM patients.[57] Several groups have shown that osteoclasts also produce MIP-1α and that blocking MIP-1α activity in animal models of myeloma significantly decreased bone destruction and tumor burden.[58] Further, Masih-Khan et al.[59] have reported that myeloma patients with the t(4,14) translocation, which is associated with constitutive expression of fibroblast growth factor receptor 3 (FGFR3) and a very poor prognosis, have very high levels of MIP-1α. Several pharmaceutical companies are evaluating receptor antagonists for MIP-1α in preclinical trials to determine whether they will be active in patients with myeloma bone disease.

In the past few years, signaling pathways involved in osteoblast dysfunction in myeloma have been identified and have also provided potential new targets for treating myeloma bone disease.[60] One of the first to be identified is the Wnt signaling pathway, which plays an important role in normal osteoblast differentiation. Tian and coworkers[61] reported that the Wnt signaling inhibitor, DKK1, was increased in patients with myeloma bone disease and that gene expression profiling showed that it correlated with the extent of bone disease with myeloma. These investigators further showed that DKK1 inhibited osteoblast differentiation of a murine preosteoblast cell line. In addition, other inhibitors of the Wnt signaling pathway such as soluble fizzle-related protein-2 have been identified in marrow samples from patients with myeloma.[62]

Enhancing Wnt signaling either by blocking the activity of Wnt antagonist or increasing Wnt signaling is being explored in animal models of myeloma bone disease and may provide new treatments for patients with myeloma bone disease. Recently, Edwards and coworkers[63] reported that increasing Wnt signaling within the bone marrow microenvironment in myeloma blocks the development of osteolytic lesions. In this study, lithium chloride treatment was used to activate Wnt signaling in osteoblasts. This treatment inhibited myeloma bone disease and decreased tumor burden in bone in a murine model of myeloma. Interestingly, lithium chloride increased tumor growth when the murine myeloma cells were inoculated subcutaneously. These results suggest that increasing Wnt signaling in the bone marrow microenvironment can inhibit myeloma growth and prevent the development of myeloma bone disease but increases myeloma growth in soft tissue. Antibodies to DKK1, a Wnt antagonist, are also being explored in animal models of myeloma. Yaccoby and coworkers[64] have shown that treating mice bearing primary human myeloma cells in a xenograft of rabbit bone with an anti-DKK1 antibody increased both bone formation and blocked tumor growth in the xenograft.

Novel agents recently approved for treating myeloma such as immunomodulatory drugs (IMiDs) and bortezomib can also have effects on myeloma bone disease. Anderson and coworkers[65] reported that immunomodulatory agents such as CC-4047 and thalidomide can inhibit osteoclast formation and activity in vitro, and Terpos and coworkers[66] have reported that thalidomide in combination with dexamethasone reduced bone resorption in 35 patients with relapsed refractory myeloma. The combination of thalidomide (200 mg/day) with dexamethasone (40 mg for 4 days given every 15 days) significantly reduced bone resorption markers, CTX and TRACP-5b, 3 months after initiation of therapy. The reduction in resorption markers persisted for the 6 months of the study. This combination treatment also reduced serum RANKL/OPG ratios at 6 months. Tosi et al.[67] also showed that thalidomide can also reduce bone resorption in newly diagnosed patients with myeloma. They reported a significant reduction in the bone resorption markers urinary NTX and serum CTX, but this was only observed in patients whose myeloma responded to the therapy. Therefore, it is unclear from these studies whether the reduction in bone resorption

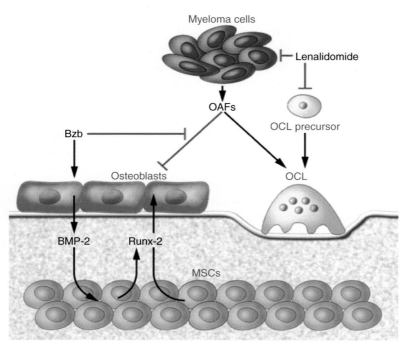

Figure 6.4. Novel therapies for myeloma and myeloma bone disease. Myeloma cells produce or induce osteoclast-activating factors (OAFs), which increase osteoclast formation as well as produce osteoblast-inhibiting factors, which block bone formation. The proteasome inhibitor bortezomib can induce bone formation by increasing BMP-2 production by osteoblasts, which in turn increases the levels of the critical osteoblast transcription factor, Runx-2 levels, to induce mesenchymal stem cells (MSCs) to differentiate into osteoblasts and enhance bone regeneration. In addition, other studies have shown that bortezomib and lenalidomide can inhibit osteoclast (OCL) formation in addition to blocking the growth of myeloma cells. These results suggest that combination therapy that includes bortezomib with lenalidomide or thalidomide may both enhance the antineoplastic effects of either agent and increase bone formation by stimulating osteoblast activity and inhibiting osteoclastic bone destruction, respectively.

markers reflected the antimyeloma effects of the drugs or direct effects on osteoclastic bone resorption.

Bortezomib can also have bone effects in addition to its antimyeloma effects. Zangari and coworkers[68] have reported that a 25% increase from baseline at 6 weeks in the bone formation marker alkaline phosphatase was the most powerful predictor of response to bortezomib in patients with myeloma. Giuliani and coworkers[69] found that bortezomib significantly increased the activity of the critical osteoblast transcription factor RUNX2 in human osteoblast precursors and stimulated bone nodule formation in vitro. Importantly, they found a significant increase in the number of osteoblasts/mm² of bone tissue and the number of RUNX2-positive osteoblastic cells in marrow biopsies

from myeloma patients that responded to bortezomib. Again, the effect on osteoblasts was only seen in patients whose myeloma responded to bortezomib, making it difficult to distinguish if the increase in osteoblast activity was due to the antimyeloma effects of bortezomib or direct effects on osteoblasts or both. In this study, there was no statistically significant effect of bortezomib on bone resorption markers. In a recent abstract at the American Society of Hematology meeting, Zangari et al.[70] reported a prospective evaluation of the bone anabolic effects of bortezomib in patients with relapsed myeloma. In this study, patients received bortezomib as a single agent on days 1, 4, 8, and 11 of a 21-day cycle and were studied prospectively for three cycles. The patients were not receiving bisphosphonates or glucocorticoids during the study. As expected, bone formation markers were initially below normal in 10 out of 11 patients studied, but they increased in 9 out of 11 patients at the end of the third cycle. In addition, bone turnover was increased in 63% of the patients and bone formation rates were increased in two patients. However, it is unclear whether the increase in bone formation will be maintained in patients treated with bortezomib, since Terpos and colleagues[71] in a long-term study did not detect healing of lytic lesions in patients on bortezomib. Bortezomib can also inhibit osteoclast formation.[72] Thus, novel agents for treating myeloma may also directly affect myeloma bone disease (Figure 6.4).

VERTEBROPLASTY AND KYPHOPLASTY FOR MYELOMA BONE DISEASE

Percutaneous vertebroplasty is a technique that involves fluoroscopic percutaneous injection of polymethylmethacrylate, a component of bone cement, into vertebral bodies for stabilization or relief of pain. The diseased vertebral body is injected bilaterally or unilaterally, and the technique provides immediate relief in a significant number of patients. Kyphoplasty is a vertebroplasty technique that involves placement of inflatable bone tamps into the vertebral body. This technique tries to expand the vertebral body back to its original height and provides a compartment into which bone cement can be injected. Both result in decreased myeloma-induced bone pain and improvement in functional activity in patients with vertebral compression fractures secondary to bone involvement.[73] Complications of the procedures are rare and include leakage of cement into surrounding tissues, causing radiculopathy, spinal cord compression, and pulmonary embolism, but most leakage is asymptomatic.[73] Other surgical modalities are also used in managing myeloma bone disease including intramedullary nails and total hip replacement. However, the ability for surgical intervention to succeed depends on the extent of bone disease and inversely correlates with time after development of pathological fracture.

RADIATION THERAPY

Radiation therapy is useful in treating painful bone lesions in patients with myeloma. Approximately 70% of patients with myeloma bone disease receive radiation therapy during the course of their illness.[74] Bone pain is treated typically with 30 Gy of radiation to relieve pain. Higher doses of radiotherapy are avoided because of their ability to reduce or compromise further chemotherapy or prevent subsequent autologous stem cell transplantation.

SUMMARY

Bone disease is responsible for some of the most severe complications and morbidity associated with myeloma. New insights into the pathophysiology underlying myeloma bone disease have provided novel therapeutic targets for treating this devastating complication of myeloma. Denosumab is now in clinical trial, and the potential for anabolic agents that block inhibitors of the Wnt signaling pathway or stimulate bone formation directly are being evaluated in animal models and can be expected to be in clinical trial in the next several years. As treatment for myeloma improve and patients survive longer, therapies to prevent the complications and progression of myeloma bone disease become more important and are vitally needed to improve the quality of life for these patients.

REFERENCES

1. Roodman GD. Pathogenesis of myeloma bone disease. *Blood Cells Mol Dis* 2004;32:290-2.
2. Melton LJ III, Kyle RA, Achenbach SJ, Oberg AL, Rajkumar SV. Fracture risk with multiple myeloma: a population-based study. *J Bone Miner Res* 2005;20:487-93.
3. Taube T, Beneton MN, McCloskey EV, Rogers S, Greaves M, Kanis JA. Abnormal bone remodelling in patients with myelomatosis and normal biochemical indices of bone resorption. *Eur J Haematol* 1992;49:192-8.
4. Saad F, Lipton A, Cook R, Chen YM, Smith M, Coleman R. Pathologic fractures correlate with reduced survival in patients with malignant bone disease. *Cancer* 2007;110:1860-7.
5. Schulman KL, Kohles J. Economic burden of metastatic bone disease in the U.S. *Cancer* 2007;109:2334-42.
6. Kyle RA, Therneau TM, Rajkumar SV, Larson DR, Plevak MF, Melton LJ III. Incidence of multiple myeloma in Olmsted County, Minnesota: trend over 6 decades. *Cancer* 2004;101:2667-74.
7. Oyajobi BO. Multiple myeloma/hypercalcemia [review]. *Arthritis Res Ther* 2007;9(suppl 1):S4.
8. Sourbier C, Massfelder T. Parathyroid hormone-related protein in human renal cell carcinoma. *Cancer Lett* 2006;240:170-82.
9. Horiuchi T, Miyachi T, Arai T, Nakamura T, Mori M, Ito H. Raised plasma concentrations of parathyroid hormone related peptide in hypercalcemic multiple myeloma. *Horm Metab Res* 1997;29:469-71.
10. Wang K, Allen L, Fung E, Chan CC, Chan JC, Griffith JF. Bone scintigraphy in common tumors with osteolytic components [review]. *Clin Nucl Med* 2005;30:655-71.
11. Collins CD. Multiple Myeloma. In: Imaging in Oncology. Ed. by J.E. Husband & R.H. Resnick. Publisher: London; Boca Raton: Taylor & Francis. 2nd Edition, Vol. 2; Chapter 33, pp. 875-89, 2004.
12. Snapper I, Khan A. Myelomatosis: fundamentals and clinical features. University Park Press, Baltimore; 1971.
13. Mele A, Offidani M, Visani G, et al. Technetium-99m sestamibi scintigraphy is sensitive and specific for the staging and the follow-up of patients with multiple myeloma: a multicentre study on 397 scans. *Br J Haematol* 2007;136:729-35.
14. Moulopoulos LA, Dimopoulos MA, Smith TL, et al. Prognostic significance of magnetic resonance imaging in patients with asymptomatic multiple myeloma. *J Clin Oncol* 1995;13:251-6.
15. Lecouvet FE, Vande Berg BC, Malghem J, Maldague BE. Magnetic resonance and computed tomography imaging in multiple myeloma. *Semin Musculoskelet Radiol* 2001;5:43-55.
16. D'Sa S, Abildgaard N, Tighe J, Shaw P, Hall-Craggs M. Guidelines for the use of imaging in the management of myeloma. *Br J Haematol* 2007;137:49-63.
17. Lecouvet FE, Vande Berg BC, Michaux L, et al. Stage III multiple myeloma: clinical and prognostic value of spinal bone marrow MR imaging. *Radiology* 1998;209:653-60.

18. Walker R, Barlogie B, Haessler J. Magnetic resonance imaging in multiple myeloma: diagnostic and clinical implications. *J Clin Oncol* 2007;25:1121-8.

19. Dimopoulos MA, Moulopoulos LA, Datseris I, et al. Imaging of myeloma bone disease—implications for staging, prognosis and follow-up. *Acta Oncol* 2000;39:823-7.

20. Moulopoulos LA, Dimopoulos MA, Weber D, Fuller L, Libshitz HI, Alexanian R. Magnetic resonance imaging in the staging of solitary plasmacytoma of bone. *J Clin Oncol* 1993;11:1311-15.

21. Bredella MA, Steinbach L, Caputo G, Segall G, Hawkins R. Value of FDG PET in the assessment of patients with multiple myeloma. *Am J Roentgenol* 2005;184:1199-204.

22. Nanni C, Zamagni E, Farsad M, et al. Role of 18F-FDG PET/CT in the assessment of bone involvement in newly diagnosed multiple myeloma: preliminary results. *Eur J Nucl Med Mol Imaging* 2006;33:525-31.

23. Fogelman I, Cook G, Israel O, Van der Wall H. Positron emission tomography and bone metastases [review]. *Semin Nucl Med* 2005;35:135-42.

24. Kimmel DB. Mechanism of action, pharmacokinetic and pharmacodynamic profile, and clinical applications of nitrogen-containing bisphosphonates [review]. *J Dent Res* 2007;86:1022-33.

25. Berenson JR, Lichtenstein A, Porter L, et al. Long-term pamidronate treatment of advanced multiple myeloma patients reduces skeletal events. Myeloma Aredia Study Group. *J Clin Oncol* 1998;16:593-602.

26. Rosen LS, Gordon D, Antonio BS, Kaminski M. Zoledronic acid versus pamidronate in the treatment of skeletal metastases in patients with breast cancer or osteolytic lesions of multiple myeloma: a phase III, double-blind, comparative trial. *Cancer J* 2001;7:377-87.

27. Body JJ, Diel IJ, Lichinitser MR, et al. Intravenous ibandronate reduces the incidence of skeletal complications in patients with breast cancer and bone metastases. *Ann Oncol* 2003;14:1399-405.

28. McCloskey EV, Dunn JA, Kanis JA, et al. Long-term follow-up of a prospective, double-blind, placebo-controlled randomized trial of clodronate in multiple myeloma. *Br J Haematol* 2001;113:1035-43.

29. Kyle RA, Yee GC, Somerfield MR, et al. American Society of Clinical Oncology. American Society of Clinical Oncology 2007 clinical practice guideline update on the role of bisphosphonates in multiple myeloma. *J Clin Oncol* 2007;25:2464-72.

30. Lacy MQ, Dispenzieri A, Gertz MA, et al. Mayo clinic consensus statement for the use of bisphosphonates in multiple myeloma [review]. *Mayo Clin Proc* 2006;81:1047-53.

31. Corso A, Ferretti E, Lazzarino M. Zoledronic acid exerts its antitumor effect in multiple myeloma interfering with the bone marrow microenvironment [review]. *Hematology* 2005;10:215-24.

32. Avcu F, Ural AU, Yilmaz MI. The bisphosphonate zoledronic acid inhibits the development of plasmacytoma induced in BALB/c mice by intraperitoneal injection of pristane. *Eur J Haematol* 2005;74:496-500.

33. Croucher P, Jagdev S, Coleman R. The anti-tumor potential of zoledronic acid [review]. *Breast* 2003;12(suppl 2):S30-6.

34. Musto P, Petrucci MT, Bringhen S, et al. Final analysis of a multicenter, randomized study comparing zoledronate vs. observation in patients with asymptomatic myeloma. *Blood* 2007;110:164a.

35. Musto P, Falcone A, Sanpaolo G, et al. Pamidronate reduces skeletal events but does not improve progression-free survival in early-stage untreated myeloma: results of a randomized trial. *Leuk Lymphoma* 2003;44:1545-8.

36. Wang J, Goodger NM, Pogrel MA. Osteonecrosis of the jaws associated with cancer chemotherapy. *J Oral Maxillofac Surg* 2003;61:1104-7.

37. Marx RE. Pamidronate (Aredia) and zoledronate (Zometa) induced avascular necrosis of the jaws: a growing epidemic. *J Oral Maxillofac Surg* 2003;61:1115-17.

38. Van den Wyngaert T, Huizing MT, Vermorken JB. Osteonecrosis of the jaw related to the use of bisphosphonates. *Curr Opin Oncol* 2007;19:315-22.

39. Khosla S, Burr D, Cauley J, et al. American Society for Bone and Mineral Research. Bisphosphonate-associated osteonecrosis of the jaw: report of a task force of the American Society for Bone and Mineral Research. *J Bone Miner Res* 2007;22:1479-91.

40. Badros A, Evangelos T, Goloubeva T, et al. Long-term follow-up of multiple myeloma (MM) patients (pts) with osteonecrosis of the jaw (ONJ). *Blood* 2007;110:1030a.

41. Badros A, Weikel D, Salama A, et al. Osteonecrosis of the jaw in multiple myeloma patients: clinical features and risk factors. *J Clin Oncol* 2006;24:945-52.

42. Clarke BM, Boyette J, Vural E, Suen JY, Anaissie EJ, Stack BC Jr. Bisphosphonates and jaw osteonecrosis: the UAMS experience. *Otolaryngol Head Neck Surg* 2007;136:396-400.

43. Khamaisi M, Regev E, Yarom N, et al. Possible association between diabetes and bisphosphonate-related jaw osteonecrosis. *J Clin Endocrinol Metab* 2007;92:1172-5.

44. Corso A, Varettoni M, Zappasodi P, et al. A different schedule of zoledronic acid can reduce the risk of the osteonecrosis of the jaw in patients with multiple myeloma. *Leukemia* 2007;21:1545-8.

45. Lentzsch S, Ehrlich LA, Roodman GD. Pathophysiology of multiple myeloma bone disease. *Hematol Oncol Clin North Am* 2007;21:1035-49.

46. Li J, Sarosi I, Yan XQ, et al. RANK is the intrinsic hematopoietic cell surface receptor that controls osteoclastogenesis and regulation of bone mass and calcium metabolism. *Proc Natl Acad Sci USA* 2000;97:1566-71.

47. Lacey DL, Timms E, Tan HL, et al. Osteoprotegerin ligand is a cytokine that regulates osteoclast differentiation and activation. *Cell* 1998;93:165-76.

48. Pearse RN, Sordillo EM, Yaccoby S, et al. Multiple myeloma disrupts the TRANCE/osteoprotegerin cytokine axis to trigger bone destruction and promote tumor progression. *Proc Natl Acad Sci USA* 2001;98:11581-6.

49. Terpos E, Szydlo R, Apperley JF, et al. Soluble receptor activator of nuclear factor kappaB ligand-osteoprotegerin ratio predicts

survival in multiple myeloma: proposal for a novel prognostic index. *Blood* 2003;102:1064-9.

50. Sezer O, Heider U, Zavrski I, Kühne CA, Hofbauer LC. RANK ligand and osteoprotegerin in myeloma bone disease. *Blood* 2003;101(6):2094-8.

51. Giuliani N, Bataille R, Mancini C, Lazzaretti M, Barillé S. Myeloma cells induce imbalance in the osteoprotegerin/osteoprotegerin ligand system in the human bone marrow environment. *Blood* 2001;98:3527-33.

52. Croucher PI, Shipman CM, Lippitt J, et al. Osteoprotegerin inhibits the development of osteolytic bone disease in multiple myeloma. *Blood* 2001;98:3534-40.

53. Vanderkerken K, De Leenheer E, Shipman C, et al. Recombinant osteoprotegerin decreases tumor burden and increases survival in a murine model of multiple myeloma. *Cancer Res* 2003;63:287-9.

54. Sordillo EM, Pearse RN. RANK-Fc: a therapeutic antagonist for RANK-L in myeloma [review]. *Cancer* 2003;97:802-12.

55. Body JJ, Facon T, Coleman RE, et al. A study of the biological receptor activator of nuclear factor-kappaB ligand inhibitor, denosumab, in patients with multiple myeloma or bone metastases from breast cancer. *Clin Cancer Res* 2006;12:1221-8.

56. Body JJ, Greipp P, Coleman RE, et al. A phase I study of AMGN-0007, a recombinant osteoprotegerin construct, in patients with multiple myeloma or breast carcinoma related bone metastases. *Cancer* 2003;97(suppl 3):887-92.

57. Choi SJ, Cruz JC, Craig F, et al. Macrophage inflammatory protein 1-alpha is a potential osteoclast stimulatory factor in multiple myeloma. *Blood* 2000;96:671-5.

58. Choi SJ, Oba Y, Gazitt Y, et al. Antisense inhibition of macrophage inflammatory protein 1-alpha blocks bone destruction in a model of myeloma bone disease. *J Clin Invest* 2001;108:1833-41.

59. Masih-Khan E, Trudel S, Heise C, et al. MIP-1alpha (CCL3) is a downstream target of FGFR3 and RAS-MAPK signaling in multiple myeloma. *Blood* 2006;108:3465-71.

60. Giuliani N, Rizzoli V, Roodman GD. Multiple myeloma bone disease: Pathophysiology of osteoblast inhibition. *Blood* 2006;108:3992-6.

61. Tian E, Zhan F, Walker R, et al. The role of the Wnt-signaling antagonist DKK1 in the development of osteolytic lesions in multiple myeloma. *N Engl J Med* 2003;349:2483-94.

62. Oshima T, Abe M, Asano J, et al. Myeloma cells suppress bone formation by secreting a soluble Wnt inhibitor, sFRP-2. *Blood* 2005;106:3160-5.

63. Edwards CM, Edwards JR, Lwin ST, et al. Increasing Wnt signaling in the bone marrow microenvironment inhibits the development of myeloma bone disease and reduces tumor burden in bone in vivo. *Blood* 2008;111:2833-42.

64. Yaccoby S, Ling W, Zhan F, Walker R, Barlogie B, Shaughnessy JD Jr. Antibody-based inhibition of DKK1 suppresses tumor-induced bone resorption and multiple myeloma growth in vivo. *Blood* 2007;109:2106-11.

65. Anderson G, Gries M, Kurihara N, et al. Thalidomide derivative CC-4047 inhibits osteoclast formation by down-regulation of PU.1. *Blood* 2006;107:3098-105.

66. Terpos E, Mihou D, Szydlo R, et al. The combination of intermediate doses of thalidomide with dexamethasone is an effective treatment for patients with refractory/relapsed multiple myeloma and normalizes abnormal bone remodeling, through the reduction of sRANKL/osteoprotegerin ratio. *Leukemia* 2005;19:1969-76.

67. Tosi P, Zamagni E, Cellini C, et al. First-line therapy with thalidomide, dexamethasone and zoledronic acid decreases bone resorption markers in patients with multiple myeloma. *Eur J Haematol* 2006;76:399-404.

68. Zangari M, Esseltine D, Cavallo F, et al. Predictive value of alkaline phosphatase for response and time to progression in bortezomib-treated multiple myeloma patients. *Am J Hematol* 2007;82:831-3.

69. Giuliani N, Morandi F, Tagliaferri S, et al. The proteasome inhibitor bortezomib affects osteoblast differentiation in vitro and in vivo in multiple myeloma patients. *Blood* 2007;110:334-8.

70. Zangari M, Cavallo F, Suza L, et al. Prospective evaluation of the bone anabolic effect of bortezomib in relapsed multiple myeloma (MM) patients. *Blood* 2007;798a.

71. Terpos E, Heath DJ, Rahemtulla A, et al. Bortezomib reduces serum dickkopf-1 and receptor activator of nuclear factor-kappaB ligand concentrations and normalizes indices of bone remodeling in patients with relapsed multiple myeloma. *Br J Haematol* 2006;135:688-92.

72. Zavrski I, Krebbel H, Wildemann B, et al. Proteasome inhibitors abrogate osteoclast differentiation and osteoclast function. *Biochem Biophys Res Commun* 2005;333:200-5.

73. Deramond H, Depriester C, Galibert P, Le Gars D. Percutaneous vertebroplasty with polymethylmethacrylate. Technique, indications, and results. *Radiol Clin North Am* 1998;36:533-46.

74. Bosch A, Frias Z. Radiotherapy in the treatment of Multiple Myeloma. *Int J Radiat Oncol Biol Phys* 1988;15:1363-9.

7 Treatment of Myeloma-Related Complications

Joan Bladé and Laura Rosiñol

INTRODUCTION

Multiple myeloma (MM) is hampered by a number of complications that can result in a poor quality of life and in many instances are contributory causes of death. In this chapter, the treatment of the most frequent complications such as bone disease, renal function impairment, anemia, infections, nervous system involvement, and extramedullary disease are reviewed.

SKELETAL COMPLICATIONS

Incidence and pathogenesis

Bone involvement is the most frequent clinical complication in patients with MM. In this sense, approximately 70% of patients have lytic bone lesions with or without osteoporosis and other 20% have severe osteoporosis without lytic lesions.[1] The skeletal involvement leads to bone pain and can result in pathological fractures. Bone disease in MM results from an imbalance between increased resorption and decreased bone formation. Thus, both malignant plasma cells and bone marrow stromal cells can produce osteoclast-stimulating cytokines such as interleukin-1β (IL-1β), IL-6, and tumor necrosis factor-α (TNF-α).[2-4] Moreover, the interaction between the receptor activator of nuclear factor-κB (NF-κB) (RANK) and RANK ligand can play an important role in cancer-associated bone disease.[5] It seems that the bone involvement in MM is the consequence of an alteration in the cytokine production by the bone marrow microenvironment, thus resulting in the uniform pattern of skeletal involvement. Thus, it has been observed by these authors that patients without lytic lesions at the time of diagnosis usually do not develop lytic lesions later in the course of the disease. These patients commonly have or develop progressive osteopenia resulting in rib or vertebral fractures. In contrast, there are patients developing only a few large lytic lesions, usually in long bones, with a high risk of pathological fractures. On the other hand, other populations of patients present with a pattern of skeletal involvement characterized by multiple small lytic lesions, particularly in the skull and long bones, with no risk of fracture.[6]

Treatment of specific complications of bone disease

Some patients develop long bone pathological fractures and require orthopedic surgery. In the event of extensive lesions, surgery can be followed by radiation therapy. On the other hand, prophylactic orthopedic intervention must be considered in patients with large lytic lesions at high risk of fracture. It is important to consider that patients with severe back pain due to vertebral compression fractures can benefit from vertebroplasty or kyphoplasty.

Spinal cord compression caused by a vertebral fracture is very rare in patients with MM. This complication is usually caused by a plasmacytoma arising from a vertebral body.

Between 15% and 20% of patients with MM have hypercalcemia at the time of diagnosis.[1,7] The symptoms of hypercalcemia can include polydipsia, polyuria, constipation, dehydration, as well as neurological manifestations such as confusion and coma. A common complication of hypercalcemia is renal function impairment caused by interstitial nephritis. Treatment of hypercalcemia with hydration and bisphosphonates is a medical emergency. Zoledronic acid is the bisphosphonate of choice (more rapid response and significantly longer time to recurrence as compared to pamidronate).[8]

TABLE 7.1. Recommendations of bisphosphonate use

- Use of pamidronate over zoledronic acid
- Discontinuation of bisphosphonate therapy after 1 or 2 years of treatment in patients in response
- Restarting the treatment in patients with active disease while receiving chemotherapy
- No treatment with bisphosphonates in patients with asymptomatic monoclonal gammopathies (smoldering myeloma, monoclonal gammopathy of undetermined significance)
- Dental evaluation and follow-up in patients receiving bisphosphonate therapy

General treatment of bone disease

Oral clodronate[9,10] and the intravenous agents pamidronate and zoledronic acid[11,12] are of clinical benefit in the treatment of bone disease in patients with MM. For different reasons (no availability in the United States, poor treatment compliance), clodronate has not been extensively used in clinical practice. Pamidronate is administered at a monthly dose of 90 mg in 2-h i.v. infusion.[11] Zoledronic acid, at a monthly dose of 4 mg, is at least as effective as pamidronate, and it has the advantage in that it can be administered in a 15-min infusion.[12] In patients with renal function impairment the dose of zoledronic acid must be reduced to a maximum of 3 mg. A panel from the American Society of Clinical Oncology recommended the use of either pamidronate or zoledronic acid in patients with MM with either lytic bone lesions or osteoporosis.[13] The panel suggested an indefinite use of bisphosphonates once initiated.[13] However, the appearance of a severe late complication, osteonecrosis of the jaw, related to the time of bisphosphonates exposure has resulted in a reconsideration of the initial recommendations.[14] A recent study by the Nordic Myeloma Group showed no significant difference between monthly infusions of 30 and 90 mg of pamidronate with respect to quality of life and time to first skeletal event.[15] The osteonecrosis of the jaw is associated with the duration of bisphosphonate exposure, type of bisphosphonate (higher with zoledronic acid than with pamidronate), and with a history of recent dental procedure.[16-18] The current recommendations of treatment of myeloma patients with bisphosphonates based on a Mayo Clinic consensus statement[19] as well as in consensus from both the International Myeloma Working Group[20] and the American Society of Clinical Oncology[14] are summarized

in Table 7.1. Finally, in patients in whom bone disease is a consequence of an excess of RANKL activity, newer molecules such as denosumab might be of benefit.[21]

RENAL COMPLICATIONS

Incidence and pathogenesis of renal failure

About one-fifth of patients with MM have a serum creatinine higher than 2 mg/dL at the time of diagnosis.[22-25] The degree of renal failure is usually moderate with a serum creatinine lower than 4 mg/dL. However, in some series up to 10% of patients with newly diagnosed MM have renal failure severe enough to require dialysis at the time of diagnosis.[24] The main causes of renal failure in MM are (1) light chain excretion resulting in cast nephropathy (myeloma kidney); (2) hypercalcemia; and (3) immunoglobulin glomerular deposition (light-chain amyloidosis or immunoglobulin deposition disease).

The main cause of renal failure in patients with MM results from light-chain tubular damage (myeloma kidney). The light chains are filtered by the glomerulus and are catabolized by the proximal tubular cells. In the myeloma kidney, the typical feature consists of the presence of myeloma casts, mainly composed of light chains, in the distal tubules and collecting ducts.[26] There is a correlation between the degree of cast formation and the severity of renal failure.[26] It is to be noted that when a light chain is nephrotoxic it usually causes renal failure from the beginning, even before other clinical features of myeloma develop.[27] It has been recently shown that excessive urine protein overflow, either heavy light chain excretion or massive glomerular proteinuria from nephrotic syndrome, can induce the production of proinflammatory cytokines by renal tubular cells either through NF-κB-dependent or through NF-κB-independent pathways.[28,29] This can result in apoptosis of tubular cells, further inflammation, and progressive fibrosis, leading to end-stage renal failure.[30] On the other hand, the inhibition of NF-κB has significantly reduced the inflammation and fibrosis in experimental glomerulonephritis.[31,32] With the recent availability of therapy with proteasome inhibitors, this pathophysiological mechanism can have an important therapeutic impact.

Light-chain tissue deposition usually consists of glomerular deposits of immunoglobulins resulting in nephrotic syndrome. The amyloid deposits are fibrillar structures of light chains with positive Congo red staining. The frequency of associated AL amyloidosis in MM varies according to the M-protein type, from 2% in IgA myeloma to 19% in IgD myeloma.[33] In light chain deposition disease, the deposit of light-chain immunoglobulins is nonfibrillar (Congo red negative).[34] In contrast with amyloidosis, the light chain is usually of kappa type. The characteristic clinical feature is a nephrotic syndrome, but renal function can rapidly deteriorate resembling glomerulonephritis.[35]

Prognosis and reversibility of renal failure

The median survival of patients with multiple myeloma and renal insufficiency is less than 1 year.[22,23] However, the prognosis mainly depends on the reversibility of renal function.[25] Thus, the median survival of patients with reversible renal failure is similar to that of those with normal renal function, whereas patients with nonreversible renal failure have a median survival of less than 6 months.[23] The reversibility of renal failure is highly variable, ranging from 20% to 60%.[22,23,36-38] In the authors' experience, the factors associated with renal function recovery are a serum creatinine less than 4 mg/dL, a 24-h urine protein excretion less than 1 g, and a serum calcium level greater than 11.5 mg/dL.[23]

Treatment approach

Conventional chemotherapy

In patients with renal failure the response rate to conventional chemotherapy is lower than in those with normal renal function (40% vs. 60%).[23,27] This lower response is at least partially due to the early mortality rate observed in patients with renal failure (30% vs. 7%).[23] In these patients, a melphalan-containing regimen is not the best treatment approach because of the need for the dose adjustment of melphalan to avoid excessive myelosuppression, thus generally leading to suboptimal treatment.[24,25] In addition, the response to melphalan is slow. Vincristine, adriamycin, and high-dose dexamethasone (VAD), or cyclophosphamide and dexamethasone, or even dexamethasone alone in very fragile patients, appear to be better approaches than melphalan-containing regimens because of both a lower myelosuppression and a quicker action.[24] Of these, the most frequently used has been VAD. However, it seems

that the effect of vincristine and adriamycin is only marginal, the efficacy of VAD mainly coming from high-dose dexamethasone.[24] In addition, a randomized trial from the Nordic Myeloma Study Group has recently shown that the association of dexamethasone and cyclophosphamide was more convenient and as effective as VAD when given as up-front therapy.[39] Thus, the best conventional treatment option for patients with MM and renal failure would be cyclophosphamide/dexamethasone. Finally, a recent study has shown that renal failure is reversible in approximately 70% of newly diagnosed myeloma treated with high-dose dexamethasone-containing regimens.[40]

High-dose therapy/autologous stem cell transplantation

The largest experience on high-dose therapy/autologous stem cell transplantation (HDT/ASCT) in patients with MM and renal failure comes from the Arkansas group. Thus, Badros et al.[41] reported a series of 81 patients treated with melphalan 200 mg/m² (MEL-200) or melphalan 140 mg/m² (MEL-140) with renal failure at the time of transplantation. The morbidity and mortality in these patients were higher than those in patients with normal renal function. The transplant-related mortality (TRM) was 6% and 13% after a single or tandem transplant, respectively. The nonhematologic toxicity, particularly the incidence of bacterial infections, atrial arrhythmias, and encephalopathy was high, especially in dialysis-dependent patients who were treated with MEL-200. Chemoresistant disease, low serum albumin, and older age were associated with a poorer outcome. In a shorter series from the Spanish PETHEMA group, the TRM was 29%. The factors associated with TRM were poor performance status, creatinine level > 5 mg/dL, and hemoglobin (Hb) level < 9 g/dL.[42] It seems that in patients with MM and renal failure, the high-dose regimen should consist of MEL-140 and the procedure should be restricted to patients younger than 60 years with chemosensitive disease and good performance status. Another study from the Arkansas group on 59 patients still on dialysis at the time of transplantation showed that 24% became dialysis independent at a median of 4 months after autologous transplantation.[43] In patients with low plasma cell mass in whom the renal function impairment is due to glomerular light chain deposition (light-chain deposition disease) the likelihood of response is higher than in MM because of the low plasma cell mass at the time of transplantation.

In this situation there is no need for tumor reduction with induction chemotherapy before stem cell mobilization and high-dose therapy.[6]

Treatment with novel agents

Bortezomib is a proteasome inhibitor with proven activity in patients with relapsed and refractory MM.[44] Its efficacy as part of frontline therapy is being studied in a number of prospective trials with very encouraging results.[45,46] Taking into account that the action of bortezomib is very rapid it would be an ideal agent to rapidly decrease the light chains in order to prevent the development of irreversible renal failure by avoiding further tubular light chain damage.

A subanalysis of patients with relapsed/refractory myeloma with renal insufficiency in whom bortezomib was administered at the usual dose showed that renal function impairment did not have a negative impact on response rate or on the safety profile.[47] Furthermore, in a retrospective series of 24 patients with relapsed/refractory MM and dialysis-dependent renal failure the overall response rate was 75% with 30% CR or near-CR.[48] Three patients became dialysis-independent following bortezomib therapy. Importantly, the toxicity profile was similar to that reported in patients with normal renal function treated with bortezomib. Ludwig et al.[49] reported the reversal of acute paraprotein-induced renal failure with bortezomib-based therapy in five of eight patients with MM. Improvement of renal function was preceded by a significant reduction in the paraprotein concentration in all patients. These authors suggested that bortezomib may accelerate the kidney response, not only through the rapid decrease in the monoclonal protein concentration but also through its NF-κB inhibitory effect, directly reducing the inflammation in myeloma kidney.[28-30] Hopefully, future studies will more formally evaluate the impact of bortezomib-based therapies in patients with newly diagnosed myeloma and renal failure.

Supportive measures

Plasma exchange

Theoretically, the removal of nephrotoxic light chains with plasma exchange could avoid further renal failure and hopefully prevent irreversible renal failure. The Mayo Clinic group, in a small controlled trial, compared chemotherapy with chemotherapy plus plasma exchange and found only a trend in favor of the group including plasma exchange.[50] Similarly, in a large randomized trial there was no conclusive evidence that plasma exchange improved the outcome of patients with MM and acute renal failure.[51] In our experience, patients with renal failure severe enough to require dialysis do not benefit from plasma exchange.[27] In fact, Johnson et al.[50] reported that the degree of myeloma cast formation is the major factor associated with nonreversible renal failure, even in patients undergoing plasma exchange. However, it is our belief that in nonoliguric patients an early plasma exchange program along with forced diuresis and chemotherapy could be of benefit.

Renal replacement with dialysis

The response rate to conventional chemotherapy in patients on long-term dialysis programs is approximately 50%.[27,52,53] It seems that the presence of renal failure does not have per se a negative impact on the response to chemotherapy. However, the mortality rate in patients with severe renal failure within the first 2 months from diagnosis can be as high as 30%.[27] When excluding patients who die in this early period, the median survival of patients with MM and nonreversible renal failure needing chronic dialysis is almost 2 years, and 30% of them survive for more than 3 years.[27] Thus, long-term dialysis is a worthwhile supportive measure for patients with MM and end-stage renal failure. The removal of free light chains with dialysis is another alternative approach.[54] A new hemodialysis membrane has been recently introduced in order to remove more efficiently the circulating light chains,[55] but the possible benefit of this procedure requires further investigation.

A summary on the treatment approaches for patients with MM and renal failure is shown in Table 7.2.

TABLE 7.2. Treatment of patients with multiple myeloma and renal failure

- Melphalan-containing regimens: should be avoided
- Intermittent pulse cyclophosphamide/dexamethasone: conventional treatment of choice
- HDT/ASCT with MEL-140: feasible in patients younger than 60 years with good PS and chemosensitive disease
- Bortezomib/dexamethasone: highly promising but still investigational in first line
- Plasma exchange: not useful in advanced myeloma kidney
- Dialysis: worthwhile palliative measure

TABLE 7.3. Recommendations for rHuEPO therapy in patients with cancer
• Hb level < 10 g/dL
• Restricted to certain clinical circumstances if Hb is between 10 g/dL and 12 g/dL
• Discontinue therapy if there is no response in 8 weeks (Hb ⇑: 1-2g/dL)
• Dose titration to maintain Hb up to 12 g/dL
• If Hb > 12 g/dL: reduce dose by 50%
• If Hb > 14 g/dL: discontinue EPO and restart at reduced dose if it falls <12 g/dL
• Iron repletion

ANEMIA AND BONE MARROW FAILURE

Incidence and pathogenesis

Approximately, 10% and 35% of patients with newly diagnosed MM have a Hb level lower than 8 and 9 g/dL, respectively.[1,7] In addition to these patients, severe anemia is a frequent complication later in the course of the disease. Anemia is associated with a significant loss in quality of life and poor prognosis. The main causes of anemia in MM are bone marrow replacement by plasma cells, relative erythropoietin (EPO) deficiency, renal insufficiency, chemotherapy with cytotoxic agents, disregulated cell apoptosis, or vitamin B12 or folate deficiencies.[24] Although the main cause of anemia is the bone marrow replacement by plasma cells, some patients with severe anemia have only a moderate increase in bone marrow plasma cells.

Severe granulocytopenia and thrombocytopenia at the time of diagnosis are unusual.[1,7] The authors have seen cases of severe neutropenia in patients with discrete bone marrow plasma cell involvement. In these patients, granulocytopenia characteristically improves when myeloma responds to cytotoxic therapy and recurs at myeloma relapse. This neutropenia responds to granulocyte colony–stimulating factor (G-CSF) and does not preclude peripheral blood stem cell collection. Approximately 10% of patients have a platelet count of less than 100 × 10^9/L, but platelet counts lower than 20 × 10^9/L with risk of severe bleeding are very unusual.[1] The development of an unexplained pancytopenia in patients previously treated with alkylating agents, particularly melphalan, is suspicious of myelodysplasia.[56,57]

Treatment

A number of trials have shown the beneficial effect of recombinant human erythropoietin (rHuEPO) and darbepoetin alfa in the treatment of myeloma-associated anemia.[58] The response to EPO is associated with a significant improvement in quality of life. An important aspect is that the most significant improvement in quality of life is reached when the Hb level increases from 11 to 12 g/dL. There is little further improvement by achieving higher Hb levels. Thus, the goal should be aimed at maintaining a Hb level around 12 g/dL with a careful dose tritiation in order to achieve a good quality of life while minimizing severe complications such as thrombotic events. In fact, the American Societies of Hematology and Clinical Oncology have provided important guidelines to ensure the correct use of rHuEPO in patients with cancer[59,60] (Table 7.3). The most common causes of failure to respond or loss of response to erythropoietin/darbepoetin are functional iron deficiency, infection, surgery, and advanced disease with massive bone marrow plasma cell involvement. The major cause of EPO failure is iron deficiency. Iron repletion should be indicated when there is evidence of functional iron deficiency measured by an increased soluble transferrin receptor. The efficacy of oral iron is limited. It seems that the best iron supplemental therapy is the administration of iron saccharate. When EPO is not effective, packed red cell transfusions are necessary. Treatment with G-CSF may be required to treat chemotherapy-induced severe granulocytopenia. Patients treated with lenalidomide may occasionally require G-CSF therapy.

INFECTION

Incidence and pathogenesis

Infectious complications are the major cause of morbidity and mortality in patients with MM.[24,61] The highest risk of infection is observed during the first 2 months of initiation of therapy, in patients with severe chemotherapy-induced granulocytopenia and in those with relapsed and refractory disease.[6] Patients who have responded to chemotherapy are at a low risk.[62,63] The main cause of infection in MM is the impaired antibody production leading to a decrease in uninvolved immunoglobulins. The remaining more important causes are chemotherapy-induced granulocytopenia, renal function impairment, and glucocorticoid treatment, particularly high-dose dexamethasone.

Most infections in newly diagnosed patients and during the first cycles of chemotherapy are caused by *Streptococcus pneumoniae*, *Staphylococcus aureus*, and *Haemophilus influenzae*, while in patients with renal failure as well as in those with relapsed and/or refractory advanced disease more than 90% of the infectious episodes are caused by gram-negative bacilli or *Staph. Aureus*.[64-66] As already mentioned, active disease is the critical risk factor for infection in MM.[67,68]

Treatment and prophylaxis of infection

An infectious episode in a patient with MM should be managed as a potential serious complication requiring immediate therapy. The frequency of fever from myeloma resembling an active infection is approximately 1%. In case of suspected severe infection and before the identification of the causal microorganism, treatment against encapsulated bacteria and gram-negative microorganisms should be initiated. Of course, the antimicrobial therapy should be selected according to the local flora and the pattern of antibiotic resistance should be observed at each institution.

Although prophylaxis of infection in patients with MM is a controversial issue, some general guidelines can be of interest (Table 7.4).[6] Intravenous immunoglobulin prophylaxis is not recommended.[69] Pneumococcal vaccination is recommended, particularly in patients with IgG myeloma with high-serum M-protein levels, that are usually associated with very low levels of uninvolved immunoglobulins. Although there are patients who develop recurrent pneumococcal infections, the use of prophylactic penicillin is of uncertain efficacy because of the increasing

TABLE 7.4. Infection prophylaxis in multiple myeloma

- Immunoglobulin: not recommended
- Pneumococcal vaccination: recommended, particularly in IgG myeloma with high-serum M-protein levels
- Antibiotic
  - Possible benefit: first 2 months of therapy
  - Recommended in patients at high risk (initiation of therapy in patients with previous serious infections, particularly recurrent pneumonia, renal insufficiency)

emergency of resistant strains. In selected patients at high risk, antibiotic prophylaxis with new macrolides such as telitromicine or new fluoquinolones such as levofloxacin, before a response to chemotherapy is achieved, is worthy of consideration. Antibiotic prophylaxis is likely of benefit within the first 2 months of initiation of therapy, especially in patients at high risk of infection (recent past history of serious infections, such as recurrent pneumonia, or renal failure).[68]

NERVOUS SYSTEM

Incidence

The more frequent neurological complications in patients with MM are spinal cord compression, nerve root compression, peripheral neuropathy, intracranial plasmacytomas, and leptomeningeal involvement.

Spinal cord compression

Spinal cord compression from a plasmacytoma, which occurs in 10%-20% of the patients, is the most frequent and serious neurological complication in MM.[70,71] The dorsal spine is the most common site of involvement, followed by the lumbar region. The clinical picture of spinal cord compression consists of back pain and paraparesis. Although it can evolve for several days or even a few weeks, the onset can be abrupt, resulting in severe paraparesis or paraplegia in a few hours. Lumbar involvement can cause a cauda equina syndrome (low back pain with radicular distribution and leg weakness).[70]

Spinal cord compression is an emergency requiring immediate medical action. When suspected, an urgent magnetic resonance imaging (MRI) should be performed. If it is confirmed, treatment with high-dose dexamethasone must be started immediately at a loading dose of 100 mg followed by 25 mg every 6 h followed by a progressive tapering. Local radiation therapy should be started as soon as possible, simultaneously with high-dose dexamethasone. If the spinal cord compression is caused by a vertebral collapse or by spinal instability rather than from a plasmacytoma (a situation very rare), urgent surgical decompression followed by fixation of a prostheses of bone graft or methacrylate is required.[70]

Nerve root compression

Patients with nerve root compression complain of back pain that follows a radicular distribution. Treatment with radiation therapy is helpful, allowing time to the action of systemic chemotherapy.

Peripheral neuropathy

Clinically significant peripheral neuropathy is very uncommon in newly diagnosed patients with MM. Peripheral neuropathy is more frequent in Waldenström macroglobulinemia (WM) and in monoclonal gammopathy of undetermined significance (MGUS).[70] In the neuropathy associated with IgM antimyelin-associated glycoprotein (anti-MAG) in patients with WM and IgM-MGUS, the M-protein has a definite pathogenetic role. However, in patients with IgG or IgA M-protein it is uncertain whether or not the paraprotein is involved in the pathogenesis. IgM-associated neuropathies are mainly sensory and tend to have a benign course. For this reason, specific treatment for the neuropathy should be restricted to patients with severe disability.[72] Improvement in cases of anti-MAG–associated neuropathy have been reported with plasma exchange, chlorambucil, fludarabine, and rituximab.[61,73,74] Peripheral neuropathies associated with IgG or IgA paraproteins can be either demyelinating or axonal and may resemble chronic inflammatory demyelinating peripheral neuropathy. Patients with IgG- or IgA-associated peripheral neuropathies respond better than the IgM type.[70]

Intracranial plasmacytomas

The presence of an intracranial plasmacytoma involving the brain is extremely rare. However, myeloma involvement of skull base may extend into the orbits and can cause orbital pain, exophthalmos, and diplopia.[70,75] Of interest, diplopia can result either from the direct effect of an orbital plasmacytoma or from ophthalmoplegia due to cranial nerve involvement within the orbits. In rare instances, subdural plasmacytoma, direct leptomeningeal infiltration, or a brain plasmacytoma may occur. Leptomeningeal involvement can result in spastic paraparesis, with the MRI suggesting a parasagittal meningioma.[70,76] Treatment should be based on radiation therapy along with systemic therapy.

Leptomeningeal involvement

Leptomeningeal involvement (CNS) with the detection of plasma cells in the cerebrospinal fluid (CSF) is rare in patients with MM. The largest experience comes from the University of Arkansas. Thus, Fassas et al.[77] reported a series of 25 patients and reviewed the findings of 71 reported cases. The main features are summarized in Table 7.5.

The frequency of CNS involvement is approximately 1%, with paraparesis, symptoms from increased intracranial pressure, cranial nerve palsies, and confusion as the most frequenting presenting features.[77] The CSF exam frequently shows plasma cells of plasmablastic morphology and an increased protein concentration with positive immunofixation for the myeloma protein. The imaging techniques show a diffuse leptomeningeal enhancement, occasionally with prominent masses. Unfortunately, despite active treatment measures such as intrathecal

TABLE 7.5. Leptomeningeal involvement in multiple myeloma

- Frequency: 1%
- Associated features:
  - Unfavorable cytogenetic abnormalities
  - Plasmablastic morphology
  - Other extramedullary locations (65%)
  - Plasma cell leukemia (25%)
  - Increased lactate dehydrogenase (40%)
- MRI: diffuse leptomeningeal enhancement with or without masses
- Median survival: 3 months

therapy (methotrexate, Ara-C, glucocorticoids), cranial, or even craniospinal radiation along with systemic therapy the prognosis is extremely poor with a median survival duration of 3 months from the diagnosis of the CNS involvement.[77]

EXTRAMEDULLARY PLASMACYTOMA IN MULTIPLE MYELOMA

Incidence

Approximately 15% of the patients with newly diagnosed MM have extramedullary plasmacytomas and an additional 20% develop extramedullary plasmacytomas later in the course of the disease.[78] Between 30% and 35% of relapsing patients have soft tissue plasmacytomas either at physical examination or at CT scan or MRI techniques.[79] The incidence seems to be higher in younger patients.[80] In fact, it has been recently described as macrofocal multiple myeloma to indicate a distinct entity with favorable prognosis in young patients.[81]

Treatment

Depending on its location (i.e. causing spinal cord compression) urgent treatment with high-dose dexamethasone and radiation therapy is mandatory. However, the treatment of extramedullary disease generally relies on systemic therapy with or without radiation, depending on the location. It is surprising that the information on both the frequency of plasmacytomas and their specific response to systemic therapy with or without radiation is very scarce, despite the fact that the response of plasmacytomas has been included in all the proposals for myeloma response criteria. As regards the response of extramedullary plasmacytomas to the novel antimyeloma agents, it is the experience of the authors that soft-tissue plasmacytomas respond very poorly to thalidomide.[79] In contrast, bortezomib as single agent is highly effective.[82] There are no data on the possible efficacy of lenalidomide on soft-tissue plasmacytomas. Taking into account the above observations, perhaps thalidomide-containing regimens, such as thalidomide/dexamethasone, would not be an optimal treatment for patients with extramedullary disease because of the lack of efficacy of thalidomide and the transient effect of dexamethasone on soft-tissue plasmacytomas. In these patients, the use of bortezomib-containing regimens is the first treatment option.

REFERENCES

1. Kyle RA, Gertz MA, Witzig TE, et al. Review of 1027 patients with newly diagnosed multiple myeloma. *Mayo Clin Proc* 2003;78:21-33.
2. Lacy MQ, Donovan KA, Heimback JK, Ahmann GJ, Lust JA. Comparison of interleukin-1 beta expression by in situ hybridization in monoclonal gammopathy of undetermined significance and multiple myeloma. *Blood* 1999;93:300-5.
3. Lust JA, Donovan KA. The role of interleukin-1 beta in the pathogenesis of multiple myeloma. *Hematol Oncol Clin North Am* 1999;13:1117-25.
4. Klein B, Zhang XG, Lu ZY, Bataille R. Interleukin-6 in multiple myeloma. *Blood* 1995;85:863-72.
5. Li J, Sarosi I, Yan XQ, et al. RANK is the intrinsic hematopoietic cell surface receptor that controls osteoclastogenesis and regulation of bone mass and calcium metabolism. *Proc Natl Acad Sci USA* 2000;97:1566-71.
6. Bladé J, Rosiñol L. Complications of multiple myeloma. *Hematol Oncol Clin North Am* 2007;21:1231-46.
7. Bladé J, San Miguel JF, Fontanillas M, et al. Initial treatment of multiple myeloma: long-term results in 914 patients. *Hematol J* 2001;2:272-8.
8. Major P, Lortholary A, Hon J, et al. Zoledronic acid is superior to pamidronate in the treatment of hypercalcemia of malignancy: a pooled analysis of two randomized, controlled clinical trials. *J Clin Oncol* 2001;19:558-67.
9. Lathinen R, Laakso M, Palva I, et al. Randomized, placebo-controlled multicentric trial of clodronate in multiple myeloma. *Lancet* 1992;340:1049-52.
10. McCloskey EV, MacLennan IC, Drayson MT, Chapman C, Dunn J, Kanis JA. A randomized trial of the effect of clodronate on skeletal morbidity in multiple myeloma. *Br J Haematol* 1998;100:317-25.
11. Berenson JR, Lichtenstein A, Porter L, et al. Efficacy of pamidronate in reducing skeletal events in patients with advanced multiple myeloma. *N Engl J Med* 1996;334:488-93.
12. Rosen LS, Gordon D, Kaminski M, et al. Zoledronic acid versus pamidronate in the treatment of skeletal metastases in patients with breast cancer or osteolytic lesions of multiple myeloma: a phase III, double blinded, comparative trial. *Cancer J* 2001;7:377-87.
13. Berenson JR, Hillner BE, Kyle RA, et al. American Society of Clinical Oncology practice guidelines: the role of bisphosphonates in multiple myeloma. *J Clin Oncol* 2002;20:3719-36.
14. Kyle RA, Yee GC, Somerfield MR, et al. American Society of Clinical Oncology 2007 clinical practice guideline update on the role of bisphosphonates in multiple myeloma. *J Clin Oncol* 2007;25:2464-72.

15. Gimsing P, Carlson K, Fayers P, Turesson I, Wisloff F. Randomized study on prophylactic pamidronate 30 mg vs. 90 mg in multiple myeloma (Nordic Study Group). *Blood* 2007;110:164a (Abstract 533).

16. Durie BGM, Katz M, Crowley J. Osteonecrosis of the jaw and bisphosphonates (letter). *N Engl J Med* 2005;353:99-100.

17. Badros A, Weikel D, Salama A, et al. Osteonecrosis of the jaw in multiple myeloma patients: clinical features and risk factors. *J Clin Oncol* 2006;24:945-52.

18. Bamias A, Kastritis E, Bamia C, et al. Osteonecrosis of the jaw in cancer after treatment with bisphosphonates: incidence and risk factors. *J Clin Oncol* 2005;23:8580-7.

19. Lacy MQ, Dispenzieri A, Gertz MA, et al. Mayo Clinic consensus statement for the use of bisphosphonates in multiple myeloma. *Mayo Clin Proc* 2006;81:1047-53.

20. Durie BGM, Attal M, Beksac M, et al. Use of bisphosphonates in multiple myeloma: IMWG response to Mayo Clinic consensus statement. *Mayo Clin Proc* 2007; 82:516-22.

21. McClung MR, Lewiecki EM, Cohen SB, et al. Denosumab in postmenopausal women with low bone mineral density. *N Engl J Med* 2006;354:821-31.

22. Alexanian R, Barlogie B, Dixon D. Renal failure in multiple myeloma. Pathogenesis and prognostic implications. *Arch Intern Med* 1990;150:1693-5.

23. Bladé J, Fernández-Lama P, Bosch F, et al. Renal failure in multiple myeloma. Presenting features and predictors of outcome in a series of 94 patients. *Arch Intern Med* 1998;158:1889-93.

24. Bladé J, Rosiñol L. Renal, hematologic and infectious complications in multiple myeloma. *Best Pract Res Clin Haematol* 2005;18:635-52.

25. Papaiakovou VE, Bamias A, Gika D, et al. Renal failure in multiple myeloma: incidence, correlations and prognostic significance. *Leuk Lymphoma* 2007;48:337-41.

26. Sanders PW. Pathogenesis and treatment of myeloma kidney. *J Lab Clin Med* 1994;124:484-8.

27. Torra R, Bladé J, Cases A, et al. Patients with multiple myeloma and renal failure requiring long-term dialysis: presenting features, response to therapy and outcome in a series of 20 cases. *Br J Haematol* 1995;91:854-9.

28. Abbate M, Zoja C, Remuzzi G. How does proteinuria cause progressive renal failure? *J Am Soc Nephrol* 2006;17:2974-84.

29. Mezzano SA, Barria M, Droguett MA, et al. Tubular NF-kappaB and AP-1 activation in human proteinuric renal disease. *Kidney Int* 2001;60:1366-77.

30. Sitia R, Palladini G, Merlini G. Bortezomib in the treatment of AL amyloidosis: targeted therapy? *Haematologica* 2007;92:1302-7.

31. Rangan GK, Wang Y, Tay YC, Harris DC. Inhibition of nuclear factor-κB activation reduces cortical tubulointerstitial injury in proteinuric rats. *Kidney Int* 1999;56:118-34.

32. Takase O, Hirahashi J, Takayanagi A, et al. Gene transfer of truncated IkappaBalpha prevents tubulointerstitial injury. *Kidney Int* 2003;63:501-13.

33. Bladé J, Lust JA, Kyle RA. Immunoglobulin D myeloma: presenting features, response to therapy, and survival in a series of 53 patients. *J Clin Oncol* 1994;12:2398-404.

34. Randall RE, Williamson WC, Mullinax F, Tung MY, Still WJS. Manifestations of systemic light-chain deposition. *Am J Med* 1976;60:293-9.

35. Dhodapkar MV, Merlini G, Solomon A. Biology and therapy of immunoglobulin deposition diseases. *Hematol Oncol Clin North Am* 1997;11:89-110.

36. Bernstein SP, Humes DH. Reversible renal insufficiency in multiple myeloma. *Arch Intern Med* 1982;142:2083-6.

37. Cavo M, Baccarani M, Galieni P, et al. Renal failure in multiple myeloma: a study of the presenting findings, response to treatment, and prognosis in 26 patients. *Nouv Rev Fr Hematol* 1986;28:147-52.

38. Cohen DJ, Sherman W, Osserman EF. Acute renal failure in patients with multiple myeloma. *Am J Med* 1984;76:247-56.

39. Mellquist UH, Lenhoff S, Johnsen HE, et al. Cyclophosphamide plus dexamethasone is an efficient initial treatment before high-dose melphalan and autologous stem cell transplantation in patients with newly diagnosed multiple myeloma: results of a randomized comparison with vincristine, doxorubicin and dexamethasone. *Cancer* 2008;112:129-35.

40. Kastritis E, Anagnostopoulos A, Roussou M, et al. Reversibility of renal failure in newly diagnosed multiple myeloma patients treated with high-dose dexamethasone containing regimens and impact of novel agents. *Haematologica* 2007;92:546-9.

41. Badros A, Barlogie B, Siegel E, et al. Results of autologous stem cell transplantation in multiple myeloma with renal failure. *Br J Haematol* 2001;114:822-9.

42. San Miguel JF, Lahuerta JJ, García-Sanz R, et al. Are myeloma patients with renal failure candidates for autologous stem cell transplantation? *Hematol J* 2000;1:28-36.

43. Lee CK, Zangari M, Barlogie B. Dialysis-dependent renal failure in patients with myeloma can be reversed by high-dose myeloablative therapy and autotransplant. *Bone Marrow Transplant* 2004;33:823-28.

44. Richardson PG, Sonneveld P, Schuster MW, et al. Bortezomib or high-dose dexamethasone for relapsed multiple myeloma. *N Engl J Med* 2005;352:2487-98.

45. Rosiñol L, Oriol A, Mateos MV, et al. Phase II PETHEMA trial of alternating bortezomib and dexamethasone as induction regimen before autologous stem-cell transplantation in younger patients with multiple myeloma: efficacy and clinical implications of tumor response kinetics. *J Clin Oncol* 2007;25:4452-8.

46. Oakervee H, Popat R, Cavenagh J. Use of bortezomib as induction therapy prior to stem cell transplantation in frontline treatment of multiple myeloma: impact on stem cell harvesting and engraftment. *Leuk Lymphoma* 2007;48:1910-21.

47. Jagannath S, Barlogie B, Berenson JR. Bortezomib in recurrent and/or refractory multiple myeloma. Initial clinical experience in patients with impaired renal function. *Cancer* 2005;103:1195-2000.

48. Chanan-Khan AA, Kaufman JL, Metha J, et al. Activity and safety of bortezomib in multiple myeloma patients with advanced renal failure: a multicenter retrospective study. *Blood* 2007;109:2604-6.

49. Ludwig H, Drach J, Graf H, Meran JG. Reversal of acute renal failure by bortezomib-based chemotherapy in patients with multiple myeloma. *Haematologica* 2007;92:1411-14.

50. Johnson WJ, Kyle RA, Pineda AA, O'Brien PC, Holley KE. Treatment of renal failure associated to multiple myeloma. *Arch Intern Med* 1990;150:863-9.

51. Clark WF, Stewart AK, Rock GA, et al. Plasma exchange when myeloma presents as acute renal failure. A randomized, controlled trial. *Ann Intern Med* 2005;143:777-84.

52. Iggo N, Palmer AB, Severn A, et al. Chronic dialysis in patients with multiple myeloma and renal failure: a worthwhile treatment. *Q J Med* 1989;270:903-10.

53. Korzets A, Tam F, Russell G, Freehally J, Walls J. The role of continuous peritoneal dialysis in end-stage renal failure due to multiple myeloma. *Am J Kidney Dis* 1990;6:216-23.

54. Cohen G, Rudnicki M, Schmaldienst S, Horl WH. Effect of dialysis on serum plasma levels of free immunoglobulin light chains in end-stage renal disease patients. *Nephrol Dial Transplant* 2002;17:879-83.

55. Hutchinson CA, Cockwell P, Reid S, et al. Efficient removal of immunoglobulin free-light chains by hemodialysis for multiple myeloma: in vitro and in vivo studies. *J Am Soc Nephrol* 2007; 3:886-95.

56. Bergsagel DE, Bailey AJ, Langley GR, et al. The chemotherapy of plasma cell myeloma and the incidence of acute leukemia. *N Engl J Med* 1979;301:743-8.

57. Finnish Leukemia Group. Acute leukemia and other secondary neoplasms in patients treated with conventional chemotherapy for multiple myeloma: a Finnish Leukemia group study. *Eur J Haematol* 2000;65:123-7.

58. Ludwig H, Rai K, Bladé J, et al. Management of disease-related anemia in patients with multiple myeloma or chronic lymphocytic leukaemia: epoietin treatment recommendations. *Hematol J* 2002;3:121-30.

59. Rizzo JD, Lichtin AE, Woolf SH, et al. Use of epoietin in patients with cancer: evidence-based clinical practice guidelines of the American Society of Clinical Oncology and the American Society of Hematology. *Blood* 2002;100:2303-20.

60. Rizzo JD, Lichtin AE, Woolf SH, et al. Use of epoietin in patients with cancer: evidence-based clinical practice guidelines of the American Society of Clinical Oncology and the American Society of Hematology. *J Clin Oncol* 2002;2:40-63.

61. Kelleher P, Chapel H. Infections: principle of prevention and therapy. In: Metha J, Singhal S, eds. *Myeloma*. London: Martin Dunitz Ldt; 2002:223-39.

62. Hargreaves RM, Lea JR, Griffiths H, et al. Immunological factors and risk of infection in plateau phase myeloma. *J Clin Pathol* 1995;48:260-6.

63. Snowden L, Gibson J, Joshua DE. Frequency of infection in plateau-phase multiple myeloma (letter). *Lancet* 1994;344:262.

64. Savage DG, Lindenbaum J, Garret TJ. Biphasic pattern of bacterial infection in multiple myeloma. *Ann Intern Med* 1982;96:47-50.

65. Meyers BR, Hirschman SZ, Axelrod JA. Current pattern of infection in multiple myeloma. *Am J Med* 1972;52:87-92.

66. Shaikh BS, Lombard RM, Appelbaum PC, Bentz MS. Changing pattern of infection in patients with multiple myeloma. *Oncology* 1982;39:78-82.

67. Perri RT, Hebbel RP, Oken MM. Influence of treatment and response status on infection in multiple myeloma. *Am J Med* 1981;71:935-40.

68. Oken MM, Pomeroy C, Weisdorf D. Prophylactic antibiotics for the prevention of early infection in multiple myeloma. *Am J Med* 1996;100:624-8.

69. Salmon SE, Samal BA, Hayes DM, et al. Role of gammaglobulin for immunoprophylaxis in multiple myeloma. *N Engl J Med* 1967;277:1336-40.

70. Gawler J. Neurological manifestations of myeloma and their management. In: Malpas JS, Bergsagel DE, Kyle RA, Anderson KC, eds. *Myeloma: Biology and Management*, 3rd edn. Philadelphia: Saunders, Elsevier Inc; 2004:269-93.

71. Posner JB. Back pain and epidural spinal cord compression. *Med Clin North Am* 1987;71:185-205.

72. Nobile-Orazio E, Meucci N, Baldini L, Din Troia A, Scarlato G. Long term prognosis of neuropathy associated with antiMAG IgM M-proteins and its relationship to immune therapies. *Brain* 2000;123:710-17.

73. Kilidreas C, Anagnostopoulos A, Karandreas N, et al. Rituximab therapy in monoclonal IgM-related neuropathies. *Leuk Lymphoma* 2006;47:859-64.

74. Levine TD, Pestronk A. IgM antibody related polyneuropathies: B-cell depletion chemotherapy using rituximab. *Neurology* 1999;52:1701-4.

75. Woodruff RK, Ireton HJC. Multiple nerve palsies as the presenting feature of meningeal myelomatosis. *Cancer* 1982;49:1710-12.

76. Spaar FW. Paraproteinemias and multiple myeloma. In: Bryn V, ed. *Handbook of Clinical Neurology*. Amsterdam: Elsevier North Holland Biomedical Press; 1980:131-79.

77. Fassas A, Ward S, Muwalla F, et al. Myeloma of the central nervous system: strong association with unfavourable chromosomal abnormalities and other high-risk disease features. *Leuk Lymphoma* 2004;45:291-300.

78. Bladé J, Kyle RA, Greipp PR. Presenting features and prognosis in 72 patients with multiple myeloma who were younger than 40 years. *Br J Haematol* 1996;93:345-51.

79. Rosiñol L, Cibeira MT, Bladé J, et al. Escape of extramedullary disease to the thalidomide effect in multiple myeloma. *Haematologica* 2004;89:832-6.

80. Bladé J, Kyle RA, Greipp PR. Multiple myeloma in patients younger than 30 years. Report of 10 cases and review of the literature. *Arch Intern Med* 1996;156:1463-8.

81. Dimopoulos MA, Pouli A, Anagnostopoulos A, et al. Macrofocal multiple myeloma in younger patients: a distinct entity with favourable prognosis. *Leuk Lymphoma* 2006;47: 1553-6.

82. Rosiñol L, Cibeira MT, Uriburu C, et al. Bortezomib: an effective agent in extramedullary disease in multiple myeloma. *Eur J Haematol* 2006;76:405-8.

8 Autologous Transplantation for Multiple Myeloma

J.-L. Harousseau

INTRODUCTION

Until now high-dose therapy (HDT) supported by Autologous Stem Cell Transplantation (ASCT) has been considered the standard of care for frontline therapy of multiple myeloma (MM) in younger patients with normal renal function, and MM is currently the first indication of ASCT.[1,2]

However, the introduction of novel agents Thalidomide, bortezomib, and lenalidomide is changing the scenario in two ways. First, these agents can be added to HDT either before or after ASCT, with the objectives of increasing the complete remission (CR) rate and of prolonging first remission duration.

Second, the use of novel agents as frontline therapy in combination with either dexamethasone or alkylating agents yields CR rates and progression-free survival (PFS) rates that are comparable to those achieved with HDT. Therefore the role of ASCT is again a matter of debate: should it be used upfront or only as salvage treatment at progression in patients initially treated with novel agents?

AUTOLOGOUS STEM CELL TRANSPLANTATION IN MM. WHAT HAVE WE LEARNED IN THE PAST 25 YEARS?

The concept of dose intensity in MM

In 1983, Mc Elwain and Powles introduced the concept of HDT in MM. With a single infusion of high-dose intravenous melphalan, they obtained a high response rate including CR in nine patients with high-risk MM, which was in favor of a dose-response effect of melphalan[3]. The results of this pioneer work were confirmed later in a larger study.[4] However, this approach induced severe and prolonged myelosuppression and could be widely developed only when Barlogie showed that infusion of previously collected autologous bone marrow could reduce the risks related to this hematologic toxicity.[5,6]

Autologous bone marrow transplantation was then evaluated in relapsed/refractory MM but also very rapidly in newly diagnosed patients. At that time, the interest for HDT was explained by the absence of significant improvement of conventional chemotherapy. With the combination of melphalan and prednisone (MP), the overall response rate was not superior to 50% and CR were rare (<5%) and the median survival did not exceed 3 years. The addition of other cytotoxic agents did not significantly improve overall survival (OS).[7] Nonrandomized pilot studies showed that with a single course of HDT, 30-50% CR could be achieved in newly diagnosed MM and that this more important tumor burden reduction could be converted into a prolongation of remission and survival[8]. This preliminary experience was in favor of the impact of HDT, but owing to possible selection bias in these trials, comparative studies were needed.

ASCT versus conventional chemotherapy

A first set of three nonrandomized comparative studies confirmed the benefit of HDT compared to conventional chemotherapy.[9,10,11] In these studies, patients treated with HDT were compared with matched controls, and in all the three studies, HDT appeared superior in terms of OS. However, they were partially biased since only patients who actually underwent ASCT were analyzed. A retrospective analysis of survival in potential candidates for HDT who were conventionally treated showed OS similar to that reported in selected series of ASCT.[12] Therefore randomized studies were needed to assess the impact of HDT.

TABLE 8.1. **Conventional chemotherapy versus high-dose therapy: results of randomized studies**

Group/trial (reference)	No. of patients	Age (yr)	Median follow-up	CR rate (%)		Median EFS (mo)		Median OS (mo)	
				CC	HDT	CC	HDT	CC	HDT
IFM 90 (13)	200	<65	7 yr	5	22	18	28	44	57
MAG91 (15)	190	55–65	56 mo	5	19	19	24	50	55
Pethema (17)	164	<65	44 mo	11	30	33	42	66	61
Italian MMSG (16)	195	<70	39 mo	6	25	15.6	28	42	58 +
MRC7 (14)	407	<65	42 mo	8	44	19	31	42	54
MAG95 (18)	190	55–65	10 yr	20*	48*	19	25	48	48
US S9321 (19)	516	≤70	76 mo	15	17	7 yr 14%	7 yr 17%	7 yr 38%	7 yr 38%

The Intergroupe Francophone du Myélome (IFM) was the first to conduct a randomized trial showing the superiority of HDT with ASCT compared to conventional chemotherapy in 200 patients < 65 years of age.[13] In this IFM 90 trial, HDT significantly improved the response rate, event-free survival (EFS), and OS. Similar results were published 7 years later by the British Medical Research Council (MRC).[14] As a consequence of these two studies, ASCT became standard of care for frontline therapy at least in younger patients (up to 65 years of age) with a normal renal function. However, other randomized studies were published in the past 10 years, and not all were that positive.[15-19] Results of seven published randomized studies are in Table 8.1.

In all but one studies, the CR rate was superior in the HDT arm. In five of these seven studies this superior CR rate translated into a significant benefit in terms of PFS. It should be noticed that in the two studies that failed to show an improved PFS with ASCT, randomization was not performed at diagnosis but only after induction treatment, which may have induced a selection bias. In the Spanish study only patients responding to induction chemotherapy were randomized to undergo ASCT or further chemotherapy, and only 75% of the patients entering the study were randomized.[17] In the US Intergroup study the selection bias was even more obvious since only 516 of 813 registered patients (63%) were randomized and only 424 (52%) actually underwent the assigned therapy.[19]

However, as regards OS, the superiority of ASCT was significant in only three out of seven studies. This could be explained by a better salvage treatment in the conventional chemotherapy arms.

WHAT ARE THE CONCLUSIONS OF THESE STUDIES COMPLETED 10 YEARS AGO OR MORE?

1. The benefit of ASCT is more evident when all patients are randomized at diagnosis than when randomization is performed after induction treatment, probably because patients with resistant disease are excluded from late randomization. Patients who do not respond to initial chemotherapy should not be excluded from HDT programs since it has been shown that ASCT is a useful salvage therapy for patients with primary refractory MM.[20,21]

2. Compared to conventional chemotherapy, ASCT almost always increases PFS and time without symptoms or treatment toxicity, as shown in two French studies.[15,18] However, OS is not always significantly improved. A meta-analysis of 2411 patients included into randomized controlled trials comparing HDT and standard dose therapy showed a PFS benefit but no significant OS benefit for HDT.[22] This is partly explained by the impact of ASCT after relapse in patients initially treated with conventional chemotherapy. Therefore, already at that time, delayed ASCT was considered a valuable approach.[15,23]

3. The randomized trials confirmed that ASCT significantly increased not only the response rate but also the CR rate. An important finding from the IFM 90 trial was the strong relationship between quality of response and OS.[13] Patients achieving CR or at least very good partial remission (VGPR) had longer OS than patients who had only partial remission (PR). This finding was confirmed in all subsequent IFM trials[24,25] and by other groups, at least for PFS.[14,26-31] Although the relationship

between quality of response and PFS or OS is not found in all types of myeloma[32,33] and has not been shown by all investigators,[34,35] a recently published meta-analysis confirmed the highly significant association between maximal response and long-term outcome.[36]

This important finding from studies on ASCT induces three consequences.

1. The prognostic impact of CR achievement that has been shown in the great majority of hematological malignancies could not be shown in MM before the introduction of HDT since the CR rate was so low with conventional chemotherapy.[35] However, when large numbers of patients are evaluated[37] or when results are improved by novel agents,[38,39] it is possible to show the benefit of CR achievement, even in studies not involving ASCT and even in relapsed MM. Therefore, CR or at least CR plus VGPR is now considered an objective of any treatment.

2. While the majority of randomized studies show a PFS benefit of ASCT over conventional chemotherapy, this is not the case when there is no difference in the CR rate. Indeed, in the US Intergroup trial, PFS achieved with ASCT and with conventional chemotherapy were similar.[19] This was not explained by lower results of the ASCT arm (as compared to results achieved in the IFM 90 trial, for instance) but by better results with conventional chemotherapy. The CR rate obtained with chemotherapy was much better than in other trials and almost identical to that achieved with ASCT. That means that if results of chemotherapy can be improved specially with novel agents, the difference in PFS may disappear.[40]

3. Response criteria have been redefined in order to introduce the notions of CR (negative immunofixations), near-CR (negative electrophoresis but positive immunofixation) and VGPR.[41,42]

The current ASCT procedure

Studies performed since the early eighties have clearly defined the standard of care for stem cell collection and conditioning regimen.

Stem cell collection

Peripheral blood progenitor cells have completely replaced bone marrow as the source of stem cells in ASCT for MM. The main reasons for this choice are easier accessibility and availability, faster hematopoietic recovery, and possibly lower tumor contamination.[43] There is a significant correlation between the number of CD34+ cells infused and the speed of engraftment, specially of platelet recovery.[44] The dose of CD34+ cells necessary for prompt engraftment is at least 2×10^6/kg. Currently, two different methods are used to mobilize stem cells into the peripheral blood, either chemotherapy (usually cyclophosphamide) plus G-CSF (5 μg/kg) or G-CSF alone (10 μg/kg).[42] High doses of cyclophosphamide are more efficient and increase the number of CD34+ cells harvested but are associated with significant toxicity. In newly diagnosed patients, priming with G-CSF alone is sufficient to allow adequate stem cell collection in most cases.[43]

When stem cells are collected early in the course of the disease, the proportion of poor mobilizers is very low. Prior exposure to chemotherapy, especially to alkylating agents, decreases the hemopoietic quality of the graft. It is recommended to avoid alkylating agents and to prefer dexamethasone-based regimens in the induction chemotherapy when stem cell collection is planned. Although contamination of the graft by tumor cells is associated with poorer outcome,[45] this could just reflect more advanced disease at the time of collection, and the benefit of graft purging or of CD34+ cells selection has never been proven.

Conditioning regimen

The standard conditioning regimen is currently melphalan 200 mg/m² IV. This regimen was introduced by the London group in the early nineties.[46] At that time, following the Arkansas group, total body irradiation was still the most frequently used in preparation for ASCT. The IFM group compared melphalan 200 mg/m² and melphalan 140 mg/m² plus 8-Gy total body irradiation and showed that melphalan 200 mg/m² was at least as effective and better tolerated than the total body irradiation-containing regimen.[48] Moreover, while EFS was identical in both groups, OS was significantly longer with melphalan 200 mg/m² because of a longer OS after first relapse. Then, melphalan 200 mg/m² became the preferred preparative regimen. Higher doses of melphalan (up to 300 mg/m²) have been tested prior to ASCT since extrahematologic toxicity is low.[49] A small phase 2 study showed encouraging results with melphalan 220 mg/m² in relapsed/refractory patients.[50] This regimen was tolerable and induced mostly a high incidence of severe mucositis. It was then used as

TABLE 8.2. Single versus double autologous stem cell transplantation (ASCT): results of published randomized trials

	Number of patients	EFS	OS
IFM 94 (24)	399	7 years = 10% vs 20% (p < 0.03)	7 years, 21% vs 42% (p < 0.01)
Bologna 96 (56)	321	Median 23 months vs 35 months (p < 0.001)	7 years, 46% vs 43% (p = 0.90)
Hovon 24 (31)	304	Median 22 months vs 21 months 6 years, 15% vs 7% (p = 0.013)	Median 50 months vs 55 months (p = 0.51)

preparative regimen for second ASCT for high-risk de novo MM (IFM 99-04 protocol).[51] Again the most frequent adverse event was grade 3-4 mucositis. Overall results with two courses of HDT plus ASCT (melphalan 200 mg/m² followed by melphalan 220 mg/m²) were very encouraging in this subgroup of high-risk patients (30 months EFS). However, in the absence of a randomized trial comparing 200 mg/m² and 220 mg/m² of melphalan, the impact of the highest dose is unknown.

The addition of another cytotoxic agent or of a radioisotope to melphalan has not been convincing. While the antimyeloma activity might be superior, the toxicity was increased. For instance, the addition of Holmium-DOTMP induced delayed thrombotic thrombocytopenic purpura.[52] In a Spanish trial the combination of busulfan plus melphalan was stopped because of a high incidence of veno-occlusive disease.[53]

Currently no randomized trial has shown the superiority of any other conditioning regimen compared to melphalan 200 mg/m².

Single versus double ASCT

While attempts to improve results of ASCT by improving either the quality of the graft or the conditioning regimen were unsuccessful, another strategy based on further intensification was tested. The concept of double intensive therapy was introduced in the late eighties with the objective of further increasing the CR rate.[54] The Arkansas group developed a double ASCT program that yielded encouraging median EFS and OS of 43 months and 68 months, respectively, in newly diagnosed patients.[55]

The IFM was again the first to conduct a randomized trial comparing single and double ASCT in 599 patients up to 60 years of age.[24] On an intent-to-treat basis, the 7-year EFS and OS were significantly improved in the double

ASCT arm. The benefit in EFS but not in OS was confirmed by two other randomized studies.[31,56] Results of these published studies are in Table 8.2. Final results of two other randomized studies from France and Germany are pending. Currently results of randomized trials are in favor of double ASCT. Again all three published studies showed that achievement of CR (or at least a VGPR) had a favorable impact on EFS and/or OS.

The IFM 94 trial confirmed the feasibility of double ASCT, since 75% of patients underwent the second ASCT, and the toxic death rate was less than 5%. However, many investigators considered the benefit of this approach to be marginal and were concerned by cost and morbidity. Therefore, defining which patients benefited more from this aggressive management seemed important. In the IFM 94 trial, the only parameter defining patients who did not benefit from double ASCT was response to the first ASCT.[24] Patients with less than 90% reduction of their M-component after one ASCT had a longer OS in the double ASCT arm, whereas patients experiencing CR of VGPR after the first ASCT had the same OS with or without the second. This finding was confirmed by the Italian group.[56]

Which patients benefit from autologous stem cell transplantation?

Randomized studies showing the superiority of ASCT compared to conventional chemotherapy have been performed in patients aged ≤ 65 years and with a normal renal function. Although ASCT is feasible in selected patients over 65 years of age,[57,58] the usual preparative regimen (melphalan 200 mg/m²) may be too toxic, especially in patients over the age of 70.[59]

Palumbo et al. showed that two or three courses of melphalan 100 mg/m² supported by ASCT were feasible in patients up to 75 years of age[10] and were superior to conventional chemotherapy using the classical regimen melphalan-prednisone (MP) in patients aged 65-70.[16] However, the IFM group failed to confirm this finding. In the three-arm randomized IFM 9906 trial for patients aged 65-75, this regimen gave a higher CR rate than MP, but on an intent-to-treat basis, PFS and OS were not superior. This was due to a poor feasibility of tandem ASCT in elderly patients and to rapid post-ASCT relapses. Moreover, the combination of MP plus thalidomide was significantly superior.[60] Results of this IFM study do not support the use of ASCT in older patients outside a clinical trial.

Although ASCT is feasible in patients with renal failure,[61-63] the preparative regimen is more toxic, and no randomized trial has evaluated the impact of ASCT compared to conventional chemotherapy. Therefore ASCT should not be performed in patients with end-stage renal failure outside a clinical trial.

A number of prognostic factors have been defined in the context of ASCT, including β_2-microglobulin level and cytogenetic abnormalities.[64] While patients with a low β_2-microglobulin level and without deletion 13 have a prolonged EFS[65-67] patients with a high β_2-microglobulin level and unfavorable cytogenetics (deletion 13 or hypodiploidy) have a poor outcome even with double ASCT.[65,67,68]

Prognostic impact of cytogenetic abnormalities in the context of ASCT has been recently re-evaluated. Beside chromosome 13 deletion/monosomy, two other frequent abnormalities are associated with a poor prognosis: t (4;14) and del (17 p), which are found in 14-15% and 10-11% of cases, respectively. Patients with these abnormalities have significantly shorter EFS and OS despite HDT and ASCT.[69-72] Interestingly, t (4;14) and del (17p) are often associated with del (13), and it appears that most of the negative impact of del (13) is related to t (4;14) and del (17p) (73). In multivariate analysis of the IFM 99 trials (with double transplantation for all patients), del (13) was not found to be an independent prognostic factor, and in patients without t (4;14) and del (17p) there was no statistically significant difference between patients with or without del (13).

Finally, the combination of β_2-microglobulin level or International Staging System with assessment of t (4;14) and del (17p) appeared to be the most important prognostic factor.[73] Patients with both a high β_2-microglobulin level and one of these abnormalities had a very poor outcome even with double ASCT. In these patients, novel

approaches are clearly needed, and the role of bortezomib and lenalidomide is currently being evaluated in this subgroup of patients.

ASCT IN THE ERA OF NOVEL AGENTS: NOVEL AGENTS IN COMBINATION WITH ASCT

Novel agents as induction treatment prior to ASCT

The standard induction therapy in patients candidate for ASCT was dexamethasone-based, either dexamethasone alone[74] or VAD-like therapy. The primary objective of novel agents given in this context is to increase the CR rate not only prior to but also after ASCT. The increased CR rate could be converted into longer EFS and OS. Another interest would be to reduce the proportion of patients needing a second ASCT due to a less than VGPR after the first.

Thalidomide-based regimens
Thalidomide was the first novel agent to be used in this setting, either in combination with dexamethasone (TD), or in combination with adriamycin and dexamethasone (TAD). These combinations have been compared with dexamethasone or VAD[75-78] (Table 8.3).

In all studies, TD and TAD were both superior to dexamethasone alone or VAD in terms of response rate or VGPR rate (TAD) (19-35% vs 13-15%). However, the thalidomide-based regimens did not increase the CR rate prior to ASCT, which remained very low ($\leq$10%). Post-ASCT results were analyzed in 2 trials: while VGPR rates with TD and VAD were similar,[77] VGPR rates were superior with TAD compared to VAD.[78] Moreover, these combinations with thalidomide induced a high incidence of deep-vein thrombosis (DVT). Stem cell collection after TD or TAD was sufficient for single ASCT[77] and even for double ASCT in 82% of patients.[79] Therefore the benefit of TD compared to VAD remained modest.

Other combinations with thalidomide have also been evaluated. The TCD regimen (thalidomide, cyclophosphamide, dexamethasone) is currently tested in a large randomized study in the United Kingdom. Preliminary results show high CR rates both before ASCT (20%) and after ASCT (58%). These CR rates are superior to those achieved with CVAD.[80] The addition of cyclophosphamide apparently improves the results compared to those obtained with TD.

TABLE 8.3. Thalidomide-based regimens before ASCT

	Rajkumar (75) N = 207 (%)		Cavo (76) N = 200 (%)		Macro (77) N = 204 (%)		Lokhorst (78) N = 402 (%)	
	TD	D	TD	VAD	TD	VAD	TAD	VAD
Post-Induction	4	0	10	8	NA	NA	4	2
CR	NA	NA	19	14	35*	13*	33*	15*
≥ VGPR CR + PR	63*	41*	76*	52*	NA	NA	72*	54*
Post-ASCT	NA	NA	NA	NA	NA	NA	16	11
CR	NA	NA	NA	NA	44	42	49*	32*
≥ VGPR CR + PR	NA	NA	NA	NA	NA	NA	79	76
DVT	17	3	15	2	23	7.5*	8	4
PN	7	4	4	7	17	13*	12	7

A, Adriamycin; CR, complete remission; D, dexamethasone, DVT, deep vein thrombosis; PN, peripheral neuropathy; PR partial remission; T, thalidomide, V. vincristine; VGPR, very good partial remission. * significant

Bortezomib-based regimens

Bortezomib has more recently been evaluated as induction treatment before ASCT. Several nonrandomized studies have been performed with bortezomib combined with dexamethasone (VD) or included into multiagent combinations (Table 8.4).

Phase 2 studies of VD regimens show very high response rates (66%-88%) and an apparent increase in the CR plus VGPR rate before ASCT (22.5%-31%).[81-83] These CR plus VGPR rates are comparable to those achieved with single ASCT and could be converted to even higher CR plus VGPR rates (approximately 55%) after ASCT. The most frequent adverse event with these regimens was peripheral neuropathy, which was observed in 25 to 30% of cases, but grade 3 was rare. However, only randomized trials could demonstrate the superiority of bortezomib-based regimens compared to classical induction treatment.

In 2005, the IFM initiated a randomized trial (IFM 2005-01) comparing four courses of induction treatment prior to ASCT with either VAD or VD.[84] Compared to VAD, VD regimen increased not only the overall response rate (60% vs 13%; p < 0.0001) but also CR plus n-CR rate (21% vs 8%; p < 0.0001) and the CR plus VGPR rate (47% vs 19%; p < 0.0001). More importantly, this higher pre-ASCT efficacy translated into a higher post-ASCT CR plus n-CR rate (35% vs 24%; p = 0.0056) or CR plus VGPR (62% vs 42%; p < 0.0001) on an intent-to-treat analysis. Moreover, when focusing on patients who actually underwent ASCT, the post-ASCT CR plus VGPR was 72% versus 51% (p < 0.0001) in the VD arms, which is quite comparable to the results achieved after a double ASCT and thalidomide maintenance in the IFM 9902 trial (despite the fact that in this later trial, poor-risk patients were excluded).[85]

The VD regimen was well tolerated with no more adverse events than with the standard VAD except peripheral neuropathy (35% vs 23% but only 6% grade ≥ 3 with VD). Stem cell collection after priming with G-CSF alone was sufficient to allow one ASCT in 97% of patients.

Therefore VD should now be considered a standard induction treatment prior to ASCT, to which other more complex regimens should be compared.

The addition of third agent (doxorubicin or thalidomide) was tested in small phase 2 studies, and the outcome appeared even better (Table 8.4) with response rates around 90% and CR rates up to 24%.[86-88] Again this higher efficacy appeared to translate into very high CR plus n-CR rates (>50%) after ASCT. The Italian group recently confirmed these results in a randomized trial comparing VTD and TD.[89] The CR plus n-CR or CR plus VGPR rates look even better than with VD (Table 8.5).

Lenalidomide-based regimens

Experience with lenalidomide in induction treatment is more limited. A small pilot study of lenalidomide plus dexamethasone (RD) in newly diagnosed patients showed an overall response rate of 91% with 56% CR plus VGPR. In

TABLE 8.4. Bortezomib-based regimens before ASCT

Author	Treatment	Number of cycles	Number of patients	Response before ASCT	Response after ASCT	Peripheral neuropathy
Bortezomib + dexamethasone						
Jagannath (81)	1.3 mg/m² D1, 4, 8, 11 Dex 40 mg D 1–2, 4–5, 8–9 < PR on cycle 2 or < CR or cycle 4	4	32	RR = 88% CR = 6% nCR = 19%	NA	31% Grade ≥ 3 6%
Harousseau (82)	B 1.3 mg/m² D1, 4, 8, 11 Dex 40 mg D1–4, 8–11 On cycle 1–2, D1–4 m cycles 3–4	4	48	RR = 66% CR + nCR = 21% VGPR = 10%	RR = 40% CR + VGPR = 54%	30% Grade ≥ 3 6%
Rosinol (83)	B 1.3 mg/m² D1, 4, 8, 11 Cycles 1–3-5 Dex 40 mg D1–4, 6–12, 17–20 Cycles 2–4-6	6	40	RR = 65% CR = 12.5% VGPR = 10%	RR = 88% CR + VGPR = 55%	25% Grade ≥ 3 0%
Bortezomib + dexemathasone + adriamycin						
Oakervee (86)	B 1.3 mg/m² D1, 4, 8, 11 A escalating doses 0, 4.5, or 9 mg/m² D1–4 Dex 40 mg D1–4, D8–11 and 15–18 cycle 1, D1–4 cycles 2–4	21		RR = 95% CR = 24% nCR = 5% VGPR = 33%	CR = 43% CR + nCR = 57% CR + nCR = VGR = 81%	48% Grade 35%
Popat (87)	B 1 mg/m² D1, 19, 4, 8, 11 A Dex as in 9 mg/m² D1–4	19		RR = 89% CR = 11% nCR = 5% VGPR= 26%	RR = 100% CR + nCR = 54%	16% grade 30%
Bortezomib + dexamethasone + thalidomide						
Wang (88)	B 1.3 mg/m² D 20 mg/m² D1–4, D9–12 D17–20 T100 ->200 mg/D	38		RR = 87 % CR = 16	CR = 37%	

A, Adriamycin ; B, bortezomib; CR, complete remission (immunofixations negative); Dex, dexamethasone; n-CR, near complete remission (immunofixations positive); RR, response rate; VGPR, very good partial remission.

patients proceeding to ASCT, the 2-year PFS and OS were very promising (83% and 92% respectively).[90] Recently a randomized study comparing lenalidomide combined with either high-dose (RD) or low-dose dexamethasone (RD) showed a very high short-term OS rate with low-dose dexamethasone specially in younger patients up to 65 years of age[91]. However, in these two studies, the role of this combination as induction treatment is unclear, since only part of

TABLE 8.5. Randomized trials on bortezomib-based combination as induction treatment prior to ASCT				
	Harousseau (84)		Cavo (89)	
	VAD	VD	VTD	TD
	N = 242	N = 240	N = 129	N = 127
CR + nCR	8	21	36	9
≥VGPR	19	47	60	27
≥PR	63	80	93	80
Response to first ASCT	N = 198	N = 206	N =	N =
CR + nCR	29	41	57	28
≥VGPR	51	72	77	54

the patients were actually candidates for ASCT. Moreover, lenalidomide induces some degree of myelosuppression, and two recent publications addressed the question of the impact of lenalidomide on mobilization of peripheral blood stem cells in previously untreated patients.[92,93] Therefore, although the combination of lenalidomide plus dexamethasone appears to be very active, more studies in the field of ASCT are needed to evaluate the efficacy/toxicity ratio. The same statement applies to the lenalidomide-bortezomib-dexamethasone (RVD) combination, which also induced a very high response rate in a pilot phase 1/2 study.[94]

To summarize, induction regimens including novel agents look very promising since they increase the response rate compared to classical regimens like VAD. Currently, VD appears superior to TD because of higher pre- and post-ASCT CR or CR plus VGPR rates. The addition of a third agent to either TD or VD could further improve results. The impact of this better tumor reduction on PFS and OS is still unknown.

Novel agents in the preparative regimen

On the basis of the synergy of Bortezomib with alkylants, studies of a combination of high-dose melphalan plus bortezomib as preparative regimen prior to ASCT have been performed. They showed the feasibility of this combination, even if bortezomib was administered partly after stem cell infusion. Preliminary results are encouraging and justify further evaluation of this approach.[95,96]

Maintenance therapy after ASCT

While ASCT improves CR rate and PFS, almost all patients ultimately relapse. Therefore attempts to prolong remission duration with a maintenance therapy are logical. The

impact of chemotherapy as maintenance after ASCT has never been demonstrated by a randomized trial.

In the eighties it was hoped that α–interferon, which prolonged remission duration after conventional chemotherapy, could be even more effective in the context of HDT since the tumor burden was lower. Although the preliminary results of a small randomized study were in favor of α–interferon maintenance after ASCT, the differences with longer follow-up were no longer significant.[97] The end of the story came with the results of the US Intergroup study, which failed to show any difference in PFS and OS between α–interferon and no further treatment in 242 patients responding to either conventional chemotherapy or to ASCT.[19]

Thalidomide has been tested in this setting by several groups. Several phase 2 studies have shown the feasibility of thalidomide maintenance and have suggested that it could improve OS.[98,99] At least four randomized studies have been completed and are summarized in Table 8.6. The Arkansas group has performed a large randomized trial testing the impact of thalidomide in the context of a complex protocol including induction treatment, double ASCT, consolidation therapy, and α–interferon plus dexamethasone maintenance (Total Therapy 2).[100] In this trial thalidomide was administered from the onset until disease progression or undue adverse effects, and 70% of patients received more than 2 years of treatment. While CR rate and 5-year EFS were significantly better in the thalidomide arm (respectively 62% and 43%, 56%, and 44%), 5-year OS were exactly the same (65% in both arms). This was explained by a shorter OS after relapse in the thalidomide arm (median OS 1.1 years vs 2.7 years in the control group).

In the IFM 9902 trial, 2 months after double ASCT, 597 patients with standard-risk MM (β_2-microglobulin 3mg/L

Author	N	ASCT	Dose of thalidomide	Duration of treatment	CR rate	PFS	OS	PN	Grade 3–4
Barlogie (100)	668	Double	Start	* Relapse 70% >2 yr	62% vs 43%	5-yr PFS 56% vs 44%	5-yr OS 65% vs 65%		27%
Attal (85)	597	Double	Median 200 mg/D	Until relapse or toxicity (median 1 month)	67% vs 55% or 57%	3-yr PFS 52% vs 36% or 37%	4-yr OS 87% vs 74or77%		7%
Abdelkefi (101)	140	Single	100 mg/D	6 months	67% vs 51%	3-yr PFS 85% vs 57%	3-yr OS 85% vs 65%		4%
Spencer (102)	243	Single	200 mg/D	12 months	24% vs 15%	2-yr PFS 63% vs 36%	2-yr OS 51% vs 80%		

TABLE 8.6. Randomized studies testing thalidomide as maintenance after ASCT

* From the onset until relapse or toxicity.

or less and/or no deletion 13 by FISH) were randomly assigned to receive no further treatment, pamidronate or thalidomide plus pamidronate.[85] Thalidomide increased the CR plus VGPR rate (67% vs 55% and 57% in the other two arms), the 3-year PFS (52% vs 36% and 37%), and the 4-year OS (87% vs 77% and 74%).

The Tunisian study showed that single ASCT plus thalidomide maintenance was superior to double ASCT in terms of CR plus VGPR rate, PFS, and OS.[101]

Finally, the Australian study is also in favor of thalidomide maintenance.[102]

To summarize:

1. All studies showed a significant benefit in terms of CR (or CR + VGPR) rate and PFS, and in three out of four OS was significantly prolonged as well.
2. In the IFM 9902 trial the effect of thalidomide on EFS differed according to the response achieved after double ASCT. Patients who had at least a VGPR did not benefit from thalidomide, while patients who failed to achieve at least VGPR had a significantly longer EFS in the thalidomide arm. This could mean that thalidomide mostly acts by further reducing the tumor mass after HDT, like a consolidation therapy rather than by a pure maintenance effect. It should be noticed that in the other two studies where thalidomide was given only after ASCT, PFS and OS improvement were also associated with an increase of CR rates.

3. Except in the Arkansas study, in which thalidomide was given during induction treatment in combination with dexamethasone and chemotherapy, there is no risk of deep-vein thrombosis since the tumor burden is low.
4. The optimum duration of thalidomide maintenance is not known. However, the incidence of peripheral neuropathy observed with thalidomide is cumulative and is related to the duration of treatment. The incidence of grade ¾ peripheral neuropathy was 27% in the Arkansas study, where treatment was prolonged, and only 4% in the Tunisian study, where thalidomide was given only for 6 months. If thalidomide acts mostly like a consolidation, long-term treatment might not be necessary. Reducing duration of treatment could not only decrease the incidence of adverse events but also decrease the risk of resistant clones selection and improve the therapeutic efficacy at relapse.
5. In the pioneer study on thalidomide[103] and in the IFM 9902 study, patients with chromosome 13 deletions benefit less from this treatment. Preliminary results with bortezomib or lenalidomide suggest that these agents may overcome the poor prognosis associated with this cytogenetic abnormality.[104-106] Therefore, these agents are attractive alternatives for post-ASCT treatment that are currently evaluated in randomized trials.

TABLE 8.7. Combinations including novel agents as primary treatment

Authors	Regimen	Number of patients	Age	CR (%)	CR + VGPR (%)	CR + PR (%)	EFS
Palumbo (107)	MPT	129	60–85	15.5	36	76	54% at 2 years
Facon (60)	MPT	12	65–75	16	50	81	Median 28 months
Mateose (108)	MPV	60	<65	32	43	89	82% at 16 months
San Miguel (109)	MPV	344	Median 71	35	45	82	Median 24 months
Palumbo (110)	MPR	54*	Median 71	24	48	81	87% at 16 months
Lacy (90)	RD	34	Median 34	18	56	91	59% at 2 years †

* At the dose levels of 0.18 mg/kg melphalan and 10 mg Lenalidomide (N = 21) † without SCT

ASCT IN THE ERA OF NOVEL AGENTS: NOVEL AGENTS IN PLACE OF ASCT

Can novel agents replace ASCT in all patients?

Novel agents given in addition to ASCT in frontline therapy already improve the outcome. Their use either in induction or after ASCT will probably reduce the proportion of patients needing a second transplant since more patients will achieve CR or VGPR after one transplant. The next question is "Should regimens including novel agents replace ASCT as frontline treatment even in younger patients?"

Frontline therapy with novel agents is dramatically improving the outcome in patients who are not candidates for ASCT, especially elderly patients. Several groups have evaluated the combination of one novel agent with melphalan-prednisone (Table 8.7).[60,89,107-110]

The IFM and the Italian group have compared MP with the same combination plus thalidomide in patients older than 65 years of age.[106-107] In both studies the response rate (including CR rate) and PFS were superior in the thalidomide arm. The OS was also longer in the thalidomide arm, although the difference was not yet significant at the time of publication in the Italian study. The logical consequence of these studies is that MP should no longer be considered the standard of care for older patients. These results also question the value of early ASCT, because MP-thalidomide used in older patients yielded CR and EFS rates that are comparable to those achieved in younger patients who had HDT plus ASCT.

The Spanish group has evaluated the combination of MP with bortezomib (MPV) in a phase 1/2 trial on patients.[108] This combination yielded 43% CR including

32% CR with negative immunofixation. These results are fully confirmed by the first results of VISTA trial[109]. In this large phase 3 randomized trial, the MPV combination was significantly superior to MP in terms of response rate (82% vs 50%) but, most importantly, yielded an outstanding CR rate of 35%, which appears to be superior to the CR rate achieved with HDT.

Results with lenalidomide also show high CR plus VGPR rates and promising short-term PFS.[90,91,110] These results have been obtained mostly in elderly patients. One can speculate that they could be similar or even better in younger patients. Therefore, some investigators already state that ASCT should no longer be used in frontline therapy but that stem cells could be collected during the first months of therapy with novel agents and used only as a rescue at time of relapse or progression. However, although these results are impressive, they do not necessarily indicate the end of ASCT as primary therapy in MM for a number of reasons.

1. In the past, the arguments against ASCT were morbidity and cost. Since the combinations using novel agents have been given for at least 9 months, they have induced toxicities (peripheral neuropathy, infections, thrombosis) and are expensive as well.
2. Quality of life is an important aspect of modern treatments. While ASCT, as a "single shot" treatment, induces a severe impairment of quality of life during the short period following HDT, prolonged treatment with novel agents could also induce a delayed quality-of-life impairment.
3. More importantly, results of combinations including novel agents are often compared with results achieved

in the 1990s with single ASCT. But the results of ASCT have recently improved, especially with double ASCT and with the introduction of novel agents. For instance, in the IFM 99 trial with double stem cell transplantation, median PFS was 39 months.[25] In the thalidomide arm of Total Therapy 2, the CR rate was 62% and 5-year PFS was 56%. These results compare favorably with those achieved with MPT. Longer follow-up is needed to evaluate the impact of bortezomib and/or lenalidomide on PFS and OS.

4. Results of ASCT could be further improved with the addition of novel agents before and after HDT. Early results of Total Therapy 3 with the addition of bortezomib to the multidrug induction DT-PACE and of VTD as consolidation and TD as maintenance after double ASCT are impressive with 83% n-CR at 2 years, and 84% 2-year EFS.[111] Moreover, results of the VISTA trial confirm that, even in the era of novel therapies, melphalan remains an important agent in the therapy of MM and the best way to administer melphalan is at high dose with stem cell rescue.

5. The combination of novel agents plus ASCT could improve not only the quantity of responses but also the magnitude of response. The Italian group recently showed that consolidation with VTD after ASCT was able to induce molecular remissions in 22% of patients who were in CR or VGPR after HDT.[112] Molecular remission is a very rare event after ASCT and has been observed mostly after allogeneic SCT. Since molecular remission may be associated with long-term disease control and possibly cure, this approach opens a new avenue with ASCT.

Therefore, rather than comparing ASCT and novel agents, it should be more useful to combine ASCT with novel agents in order to further increase the CR rate, to reduce the need for a second ASCT, and to prolong remission duration. Another possibility could be to compare novel agents with ASCT at the time of relapse versus frontline ASCT plus novel agents.

Can novel agents replace ASCT in selected patients?

While HDT even without novel agents can induce long-term remission in patients with good prognosis characteristics,[113] it is now possible to define a subgroup of patients who do poorly even after double ASCT. Gene expression profiling is a powerful method for predicting outcome but is not yet easily available. Combination of biologic markers (β_2-microglobulin, albumin) and cytogenetic abnormalities by conventional karyotype or by FISH are currently used for prognosis assessment. There is some preliminary evidence that the poor prognosis associated with del (13) and t(4;14) could be overcome by novel agents.[104-106]

This finding is the basis of a risk strategy proposed by the Mayo Clinic.[113] With this approach, ASCT is deferred in 25% of patients with poor-risk characteristics who are initially treated with novel agents. This innovative strategy raises two issues.

1. Until now the benefit of bortezomib and lenalidomide in patients with del (13) or t(4;14) has been shown mostly in terms of response achievement. Longer follow-up and more patients are needed to confirm that the good response rate translates into prolonged PFS.
2. But if novel agents are useful in this subgroup of patients, they could be even more active in combination with HDT.[111]

CONCLUSION

ASCT has been the first improvement in MM therapy and has dramatically increased OS in younger patients. The introduction of three active novel agents in the past few years is going to completely change the frontline strategy not only in older patients who could not benefit from ASCT but also in younger patients. We already know that post-ASCT thalidomide prolongs PFS and probably OS and that novel agents prior to ASCT increase the pre- and post-ASCT CR plus VGPR rates. Therefore we can hope that these combinations of novel agents with ASCT will induce very high CR rates, including CR in poor-risk patients, and high-quality response and prolong PFS. However, since combination with novel agents without ASCT induce high CR rates as well, it could be useful in the near future to design randomized studies comparing the best regimen with early ASCT with the best nonintensive regimen with ASCT at relapse. These studies would also have to address the important question of salvage treatment when several active agents have been used upfront.

REFERENCES

1. Gratwohl A, Baldomero H, Frauendorfer K, et al. The EBMT activity survey 2006 on hematopoietic stem cell transplantation: focus on the use of cord blood products. *Bone Marrow Transplant* 2007;online.

2. Harousseau JL, Shaughessy J, Richardson P. Multiple myeloma. *Hematology Am Soc Hematol Educ Program* 2004;237-56.

3. Mc Elwain TJ, Powles RL. High-dose intravenous melphalan for plasma-cell leukaemia and myeloma. *Lancet* 1983;16:822-4.

4. Selby PJ, Mc Elwain TJ, Nandi AC, et al. Multiple myeloma treated with high-dose intravenous melphalan *Br J Haematol* 1987;66:55-62.

5. Barlogie B, Hall R, Zander A, Dicke K, Alexanian R. High-dose melphalan with autologous bone marrow transplantation for multiple myeloma. *Blood* 1986;67:1298-301.

6. Barlogie B, Alexanian R, Dicke KA, et al. High dose chemoradiotherapy and autologous bone marrow transplantation for resistant multiple myeloma. *Blood* 1987;70:869-72.

7. Myeloma Trialists' Collaborative group. Combination chemotherapy versus melphalan plus prednisone as treatment for multiple myeloma: an overview of 6633 patients from 27 randomized trials. *J Clin Oncol* 1998;16:3832-42.

8. Harousseau JL, Attal M. The role of autologous hematopoietic stem cell transplantationin multiple myeloma. *Semin hematol* 1997;34 (suppl 1):61-6.

9. Barlogie B, Jagannath S, Vesole DH, et al. Superiority of tandem autologous transplantation over standard therapy for previously untreated multiple myeloma. *Blood* 1997;89:789-93.

10. Palumbo A, Triolo S, Argentino C, et al. Dose-intensive melphalan with stem cell support is superior to standard treatment in elderly myeloma patients. *Blood* 1999;94:1248-53.

11. Lenhoff S, Hjorth M, Holmberg E, et al. Impact of high-dose therapy with autologous stem cell support in patients younger than 60 years with newly diagnosed multiple myeloma: a population-based study. *Blood* 2000;95:7-11.

12. Blade J, San Miguel JF, Fontanillas M, et al. Survival of multiple myeloma patients who are potential candidates for early high-dose therapy intensification/autotransplantation and who were conventionally treated. *Blood* 1996;14:2167-73.

13. Attal M, Harousseau JL, Stoppa AM, et al. A prospective randomized trial of autologous bone marrow transplantation and chemotherapy in multiple myeloma. *N Engl J Med* 1996;335:91-7.

14. Child JA, Morgan GJ, Davies FE, et al. High-dose chemotherapy with hematopoietic stem-cell rescue for multiple myeloma. *N Engl J Med* 2003;348:1875-83.

15. Fermand JP, Ravaud P, Chevret S, et al. High-dose therapy and autologous peripheral blood stem cell transplantation in multiple myeloma: upfront or rescue treatment? Results of a multicenter sequential randomized trial. *Blood* 1998;92:3131-6.

16. Palumbo A, Bringhen S, Petrucci MT, et al. Intermediate-dose melphalan improves survival of myeloma patients aged 50-70: results of a randomized controlled trial. *Blood* 2004;104:3052-7.

17. Blade J, Rosinol L, Sureda A, et al. High-dose therapy intensification compared with continued standard chemotherapy in multiple myeloma patients responding to the initial chemotherapy: long-term results from a prospective randomized trial from the Spanish Cooperative Group PETHEMA. *Blood* 2005;106:3755-9.

18. Fermand JP, Katsahian S, Divine M, et al. High-dose therapy and autologous blood stem-cell transplantation compared with conventional treatment in myeloma patients aged 55 to 65 years: long-term results of a randomized control trial from the Group Myelome-Autogreffe. *J Clin Oncol* 2005;23:9227-33.

19. Barlogie B, Kyle RA, Anderson KC, et al. Standard chemotherapy compared with high-dose chemoradiotherapy for multiple myeloma: final results of Phase III US Intergroup trial S9321. *J Clin Oncol* 2006;24:929-36.

20. Alexanian R, Dimopoulos MA, Hester J, Delasalle K, Champlin R. Early myeloablative therapy for multiple myeloma. *Blood* 1994;84:4278-82.

21. Rajkumar SV, Fonseca R, Lacy MQ, et al. Autologous stem cell transplantation for relapsed and primary refractory myeloma. *Bone Marrow Transplant* 1999;23:1267-72.

22. Koreth J, Cutler CS, Djulbegovic B, et al. High-dose therapy with single autologous transplantation versus chemotherapy for newly diagnosed multiple myeloma: a systematic review and meta-analysis of randomized controlled trials. *Biol Blood Marrow Transplant* 2007;13:183-96.

23. Gertz M, Lacy MQ, Inwards DJ, et al. Delayed stem cell transplantation for the management of relapsed or refractory multiple myeloma. *Bone Marrow Transplant* 2000;26:45-50.

24. Attal M, Harousseau JL, Facon T, et al. Intergroupe Francophone du Myelome: single versus double autologous stem cell transplantation for multiple myeloma. *N Engl J Med* 2003;349:2495-502.

25. Harousseau JL, Attal M, Moreau P, et al. The prognostic impact of complete remission plus very good partial remission in a double-transplantation program for newly diagnosed multiple myeloma. *Blood* 2006;108:877a (abstract).

26. Vesole DH, Tricot G, Jagannath S, et al. Autotransplants in multiple myeloma: what have we learned? *Blood* 1996;88: 838-47.

27. Fassas A, Shaughnessy J, Barlogie B. Cure of myeloma: hype or reality? *Bone Marrow Transplant* 2005;35:215-24.

28. Lahuerta JJ, Martinez-Lopez J, de la Serna J, et al. Remission status defined by immunofixation vs electrophoresis after autologous transplantation has a major impact on the outcome of multiple myeloma patients. *Br J Haematol* 2000;109:438-46.

29. Wang M, Delasalle K, Thomas S, Giralt S, Alexanian R. Complete remission represents the major surrogate marker of long survival in multiple myeloma. *Blood* 2006;108:123a (abstract).

30. Lenhoff S, Hjorth M, Turesson I, et al. Intensive therapy for multiple myeloma in patients younger than 60 years. Long-term results focusing on the effect of the degree of response on survival and relapse pattern after transplantation. *Haematologica* 2006;01:1228-33.

31. Sonneveld P, van der Holt B, Segeren CM, et al. Intermediate-dose melphalan compared with myeloablative treatment in multiple myeloma: long-term results of the Dutch Cooperative group HOVON 24 trial. *Haematologica* 2007;92:928-35.

32. Pineda-Roman M, Bolejack V, Arzoumian V, et al. Complete response in myeloma extends survival, but not with history of prior monoclonal gammopathy of undetermined significance or smouldering disease. *Br J Haematol* 2007;136:393-9.

33. van Rhee F, Bolejack V, Hollmig K, et al. High serum-free light chain levels and their rapid reduction in response define an aggressive multiple myeloma subtype with poor prognosis. *Blood* 2007;110:827-32.

34. Rajkumar SV, Fonseca R, Dispenzieri A, et al. Effect of complete response on outcome following autologous stem cell transplantation for myeloma. *Bone Marrow Transplant* 2000;26:979-83.

35. Durie BG, Jacobson J, Barlogie B, Crowley J. Magnitude of response with myeloma frontline therapy does not predict outcome: importance of time to progression in SWOG chemotherapy trials. *J Clin Oncol* 2004;22(10):1857-63.

36. van de Velde HJK, Liu X, Chen G, Cakana A, Draedt W, Bayssas M. Complete response correlates with long-term survival and progression-free survival in high-dose therapy in multiple myeloma. *Haematologica* 2007;92:1399-406.

37. Kyle RA, Leong T, Li S, et al. Complete response in multiple myeloma. Clinical trial E9486, an Eastern Cooperative Oncology Group study not involving stem cell transplantation. *Cancer* 2006;106:1958-66.

38. Richardson PG, Sonneveld P, Schuster M, et al. Extended follow-up of a Phase III trial in relapsed multiple myeloma: final time-to-event results of the Apex trial. *Blood* 2007;110:3557-60.

39. Harousseau JL, Weber D, Dimopoulos M, et al. Relapsed/Refractory multiple myeloma patients treated with lenalidomide/dexamethasone who achieve a complete or near complete response have longer overall survival than patients achieving a partial response. *Blood* 2007;110:1052a (abstract).

40. Harousseau JL. Role of stem cell transplantation. Hematol Oncol Clin North Am 2007;21:1157-74.

41. Blade J, Samson D, Reece D, et al. Criteria for evaluating disease response and progression in patients treated with high-dose therapy and haematopoietic stem cell transplantation. *Br J Haematol* 1998;102:1115-23.

42. Durie BG, Harousseau JL, San Miguel JS, et al. International uniform response criteria for multiple myeloma. *Leukemia* 2006;20:1467-73.

43. Harousseau JL. Optimizing peripheral blood progenitor cell autologous transplantation in multiple myeloma. *Haematologica* 1999;84:548-53.

44. Tricot G, Jagannath S, Vesole D, et al. Peripheral blood stem cell transplants for multiple myeloma: identification of favourable variables for rapid engraftment in 225 patients. *Blood* 1996;85:588-96.

45. Gertz MA, Witzig TE, Pineda AA, et al. Monoclonal plasma cells in the blood stem-cell harvest from patients with multiple myeloma are associated with shortened relapse-free survival after transplantation. *Bone marrow Transplant* 1999;19:337-42.

46. Cunningham D, PAZ-Ares L, Milan S, et al. High-dose melphalan and autologous bone marrow transplantation as consolidation in previously untreated myeloma. *J Clin Oncol* 1994;12:759-63.

47. Lopez-Perez R, Garcia-Sanz R, Gonzalez D, et al. The detection of contaminating clonal cells in apheresis products is related to response and outcome in multiple myeloma undergoing autologous peripheral blood stem cell transplantation. *Leukemia* 2000;14:1493-9.

48. Moreau P, Facon T, Attal M, et al. Comparison of 200 mg/m^2 melphalan and 8 Gy total body irradiation plus 140mg/m^2 melphalan as conditioning regimen for peripheral blood stem cell transplantation in patients with newly diagnosed multiple myeloma: final analysis of the Intergroupe Francophone du Myelome 9502 trial. *Blood* 2002;99:731-5.

49. Philips GL, Meisenberg BR, ReeceDE, et al. Activity of single-agent melphalan 220 to 300 mg/m^2 with amifostine cytoprotection and autologous hematopoietic stem cell support in non-Hodgkin and Hodgkin lymphoma. *Bone marrow Transplant* 2004;33:781-7.

50. Moreau P, Milpied N, Mahe B, et al. Melphalan 220 mg/m^2 followed by peripheral stem cell transplantation in 27 patients with advanced multiple myeloma. *Bone Marrow Transplant* 1999;23:1003-6.

51. Moreau P, Hulin C, Garban F, et al. Tandem autologous stem cell transplantation in high risk-de novo multiple myeloma: final results of the prospective and randomized IFM 99-04 protocol. *Blood* 2006;107:397-403.

52. Giralt S, Bensinger W, Goodman M, et al. 166Ho-DOTMP plus melphalan followed by peripheral blod stem cell transplantation in patients with multiple myeloma. *Blood* 2003;102:2684-91.

53. Carreras E, Rosinol L, Terol MF, et al. Veno-occlusive disease of the liver after high-dose cytoreductive therapy with busulfan and melphalan for autologous blood stem cell transplantation in multiple myeloma patients. *Biol Blood Marrow Transplant* 2007;13:1448-54.

54. Harousseau JL, Milpied N, Laporte JP, et al. Double intensive therapy in high-risk multpile myeloma. *Blood* 1992;79:2827-33.

55. Barlogie B, Jagannath S, Desikan KR, et al. Total therapy with tandem autotransplants for newly diagnosed multiple myeloma. *Blood* 1999;93:55-65.

56. Cavo M, Tosi P, Zamagni E, et al. Prospective randomized study of single compared with double autologous stem cell transplantation for multiple myeloma: Bologna 96 clinical study. *J Clin Oncol* 2007;25:2434-41.

57. Siegel DS, Desikan KR, Mehta J, et al. Age is not a prognostic variable with autotransplants for multiple myeloma. *Blood* 1999;93:51-4.

58. Jantunen E, Juittinen T, Penttila K, et al. High-dose melphalan (200 mg/m^2) supported by autologous stem cell transplantation is safe and effective in elderly (>65 years) myeloma patients: comparison with younger patients treated with the same protocol. *Bone marrow Transplant* 2006;37:917-22.

59. Badros A, Barlogie B, Siegel D, et al. Autologous stem cell transplantation in elderly multiple myeloma patients over the age of 70 years. *Br J Haematol* 2001;114:1248-53.

60. FaconT, Mary JY, Hulin C, et al. Melphalan and prednisone plus thalidomide versus melphalan and prednisone or reduced-intensity autologous stem cell transplantation in elderly patients with multiple myeloma (IFM 99-06): a randomized trial. *Lancet* 2007;370:1209-18.

61. Badros A, Barlogie B, Siegel D, et al. Results of autologous stem cell transplant in multiple myeloma patients with renal failure. *Br J Haematol* 2001;114:822-9.

62. Tosi P, Zamagni E, Ronconi S, et al. Safety of autologous hematopoietic stem cell transplantation in patients with multiple myeloma and renal failure. *Leukemia* 2000;14:1310-3.

63. San Miguel J, Lahuerta JJ, Garcia-Sanz R, et al. Are myeloma patients with renal failure candidate for autologous transplantation. *The Hematology Journal* 2000;1:28-36.

64. Desikan R, Barlogie B, Sawyer J, et al. Results of high-dose therapy for 1000 patients with multiple myeloma: durable complete remission and superior survival in the absence of chromosome 13 abnormalities. *Blood* 2000;95:4008-10.

65. Facon T, Avet-Loiseau H, Guillerm G, et al. Chromosome 13 abnormalities identified by Fish analysis and serum β_2 microglobulin produce powerful myeloma staging system for patients receiving high-dose therapy. *Blood* 2001;97:1566-71.

66. Tricot G, Spencer T, Sawyer J, et al. Predicting long-term (>5years) event-free survival in multiple myeloma patients following planned tandem autotransplants. *Br J Haematol* 2002;116:211-7.

67. Shaughnessy J, Jacobson J, Sawyer J, et al. Continuous absence of metaphase-defined cytogenetic abnormalities especially of chromosome 13 and hypodiploidy ensures long-term survival in multiple myeloma treated with Total Therapy 1: interpretation in the context of global gene expression. *Blood* 2003;101:3849-56.

68. Fassas AT, Spencer T, Sawyer J, et al. Both hypodiploidy and deletion of chromosome 13 independently confer poor prognosis in multiple myeloma. *Br J Haematol* 2002;118:1041-7.

69. Chang H, Sloan S, Li D, et al. The t(4;14) is associated with poor prognosis in myeloma patients undergoing autologous stem cell transplant. *Br J Haematol* 2004;125:64-8.

70. Gertz M, Lacy MQ, Dispenzieri A, et al. Clinical implications of t(11;14)(q13;q32), t(4;14)(p16.3;q32) and -17p13 in myeloma patients treated with high-dose therapy. *Blood* 2005;125:2837-40.

71. Jaksic W, Trudel S, Chang H, et al. Clinical outcomes in t(4;14) multiple myeloma: a chemotherapy sensitive disease characterized by rapid relapse and alkylating agent resistance. *J Clin Oncol* 2005;105:7069-73.

72. Chang H, Qi C, Yi QL, et al. P53 gene deletion detected by fluorescence in situ hybridisation is an adverse prognostic factor for patients with multiple myeloma following autologous stem cell transplantation. *Blood* 2005;105:358-60.

73. Avet-Loiseau H, Attal M, Moreau P, et al. Genetic abnormalities and survival in multiple myeloma:the experience of the Intergroupe Francophone du Myeloma. *Blood* 2007;109:3489-95.

74. Kumar S, Lacy MQ, Dispenzieri A, et al. Single agent dexamethasone for prestem cell transplant induction therapy for multiple myeloma. *Bone Marrow Transplant* 2004;34:485-90.

75. Rajkumar SV, Blood E, Vesole D, et al. Phase III clinical trial of Thalidomide plus dexamethasone compared with dexamethasone alone in newly diagnosed multiple myeloma: a clinical trial coordinated by the Eastern Cooperative Oncology Group. *J Clin Oncol* 2006;24:431-6.

76. Cavo M, Zamagni E, Tosi P, et al. Superiority of thalidomide and dexamethsone over vincristine-doxorubicine-dexamethasone (VAD) as primary therapy in preparation for autologous transplantation for multiple myeloma. *Blood* 2005;106:35-9.

77. Macro M, Divine M, Uzunban Y, et al. Dexamethasone + thalidomide compared to VAD as pretransplant treatment in newly diagnosed multiple myeloma: a randomized trial. *Blood* 2006;108:22a (abstract).

78. Lokhorst HM, Schidt-Wolf I, Sonneveld P, et al. Thalidomide in induction treatment increases the very good partial remission rate before and after high-dose therapy in previously untreated multiple myeloma. *Haematologica* 2008;93:124-7.

79. Breitkreutz I, Lokhorst HM, Raab MS, et al. Thalidomide in newly diagnosed multiple myeloma: influence of thalidomide treatment on peripheral blood stem cell collection yield *Leukemia* 2007;21:1294-9.

80. Morgan GJ, Davies FE, Owen RG, et al. Thalidomide combinations improve response rates: results from the MRC IX study. *Blood* 2007;110:1051a (abstract).

81. Jagannath S, Durie B, Wolf J, et al. Bortezomib therapy alone and in combination with dexamethasone for previously untreated symptomatic multiple myeloma. *Br J Haematol* 2005;129:776-83.

82. Harousseau JL, Attal M, Leleu X, et al. Bortezomib plus dexamethasone as induction treatment prior to autologous stem cell transplantation in patients with newly diagnosed multiple myeloma. *Haematologica* 2006;91:1498-505.

83. Rosinol L, Oriol A, Mateos MV, et al. Phase II Pethema trial of alternating bortezomib and dexamethasone as induction regimen before autologous stem-cell transplantation in younger patients with multiple myeloma: efficacy and clinical implications of tumor response kinetics. *J Clin Oncol* 2007;25:4452-8.

84. Harousseau JL, Mathiot C, Attal M, et al. Velcade/dexamethasone versus VAD as induction treatment prior to autologous stem cell transplantation in newly diagnosed multiple myeloma: updated results of the IFM 2005/01 trial. *Blood* 2007;110:139a (abstract).

85. Attal M, Harousseau JL, Leyvraz S, et al. Maintenance therapy with thalidomide improves survival in multiple myeloma patients. *Blood* 2006;15:3289-94.

86. Oakervee R, Pollat R, Curry N, et al. PAD combination (PS341, doxorubicin and dexamethasone for previously untreated symptomatic multiple myeloma. *Br J Haematol* 2005;129:776-83.

87. Popat R, Oakervee HE, Curry N, et al. Reduced dose PAD for previously untreated patients with multiple myeloma. *Blood* 2005;106:717a (abstract).

88. Wang M, Giralt S, Delasale K, Handy B, Alexanian R. Bortezomib in combination with thalidomide-dexamethasone for previously untreated multiple myeloma. *Hematology* 2007;12:235-9.

89. Cavo M, Patriarca F, Tacchetti P, et al. Bortezomib-thalidomide-dexamethasone vs thalidomide-dexamethasone in preparation for autologous stem-cell transplantation in newly diagnosed multiple myeloma. *Blood* 2007;110:30a.

90. Lacy MQ, Gertz MA, Dispenzieri A, et al. Long-term results of response to therapy, time to progression, and survival with lenalidomide plus dexamethasone in newly diagnosed myeloma. *Mayo Clin Proc* 2007;82:1179-84.

91. Rajkumar SV, Jacobus S, Callander N, et al. A randomized trial of lenalidomide plus high-dose dexamethasone versus lenalidomide plus low-dose dexamethasone in newly diagnosed multiple myeloma (E403): a trial coordinated by the Eastern Cooperative Oncology Group. *Blood* 2007;110:31a (abstract).

92. Kumar S, Dispenzieri A, Lacy MQ, et al. Impact of lenalidomide on stem cell mobilization and engraftment post-peripheral blood stem cell transplantation in patients with newly diagnosed multiple myeloma. *Leukemia* 2007;21:2035-42.

93. Mazumder A, Kaufman J, Niesvizky R, Lonial S, Vesole D, Jagannath S. Effect of lenalidomide on mobilization of peripheral blood stem cells in previously untreated multiple myeloma patients. *Leukemia* 2008;22:1280-1.

94. Richardson P, Jagannath S, Raje N, et al. Lenalidomide, bortezomib, and dexamethasone as frontline therapy for patients with multiple myeloma: preliminary results of a Phase ½ study. *Blood* 2007;110:63a (abstract).

95. Hollmig K, Stover J, Talamo G, et al. Addition of bortezomib to high dose melphalan as en effective conditioning regimen with autologous stem cell support in multiple myeloma. *Blood* 2004;103:266a (abstract).

96. Attal M, Harousseau JL. Role of autologous stem-cell transplantation in multiple myeloma. Best Practice & Research. *Clin Haematol* 2007;20:747-59.

97. Cunningham D, Powles R, Malpas JS, et al. A randomized trial of maintenance therapy with intron A following high dose melphalan and ABMT in myeloma. *Br J Haematol* 1998;102:195-202.

98. Stewart AK, Chen CI, Howson-Jan K, et al. Results of a multicenter randomized trial of thalidomide and prednisone maintenance therapy for multiple myeloma after autologous stem cell transplant. *Clin Cancer Res* 2004;10:8170-6.

99. Brinker BT, Walker EK, Leong T, et al. Maintenance therapy with thalidomide improves overall survival after autologous hematopoietic progenitor cell transplantation for multiple myeloma. *Cancer* 2006;106:2171-80.

100. Barlogie B, Tricot G, Anaissie E, et al. Thalidomide and hematopoietic stem cell transplantation for multiple myeloma. *N Engl J Med* 2006;354:1021-30.

101. Abdelkefi A, Ladeb S, Torjman L, et al. Single autologous stem cell transplantation followed by maintenance therapy with thalidomide is superior to double autologous transplantation in multiple myeloma: results of a multicenter randomized clinical trial. *Blood* 2008;111:1805-1810.

102. Spencer A, Prince HM, Roberts A, et al. Thalidomide improves survival when used following ASCT. *Haematologica* 2007;92:41-2 (abstract).

103. Singhal S, Mehta J, Desikan R, et al. Antitumor activity of thalidomide in refractory multiple myeloma. *N Engl J Med* 1999;341:1565-71.

104. Jagannath S, Richardson PG, Sonneveld P, et al. Bortezomib appears to overcome the poor prognosis conferred by chromosome 13 deletion in phase 2.3 trials. *Leukemia* 2007;21:151-7.

105. Sagaster V, Ludwig H, Kaufmann H, et al. Bortezomib is relapsed multiple myeloma: response rates and duration are independent of a chromosome 13q- deletion. *Leukemia* 2007;21:164-8.

106. Bahlis NJ, Mansoor B, Lategan JC, et al. Lenalidomide overcomes poor prognosis conferred by deletion of chromosome 13 and t(4;14) : MM016 trial. *Blood* 2006;108:1016a (abstract).

107. Palumbo A, Bringhen S, Caravita T, et al. Oral melphalan and prednisone chemotherapy plus thalidomide compared with melphalan and prednisone alone in elderly patients with multiple myeloma: randomized controlled trial. *Lancet* 2006;367:825-31.

108. Mateos MV, Hernandez JM, Hernandez MT, et al. Bortezomib plus melphalan and prednisone in elderly untreated patients with multiple myeloma: results of a multicenter phase ½ study. *Blood* 2006;108:2165-72.

109. San Miguel JF, Schlag R, Khuageva N, et al. MMY-3002: a Phase III study comparing bortezomib-melphalan-prednisone with melphalan-prednisone in newly diagnosed multiple myeloma. *Blood* 2207;110:31a (abstract).

110. Palumbo A, Falco P, Corradini P, et al. Melphalan, prednisone and lenalidomide treatment for newly diagnosed myeloma: a report from the GIMEMA-Italian Multiple Myeloma Network. *J Clin Oncol* 2007;25:4459-65.

111. Barlogie B, Anaissie E, van Rhee F, et al. Incorporating bortezomib into upfront treatment for multiple myeloma: early results of total therapy 3. *Br J Haematol* 2007;138:176-85.

112. Ladetto M, Pagliano G, Avonto I, et al. Consolidation with bortezomib, thalidomide and dexamethasone induces molecular remissions in autografted multiple myeloma patients. *Blood* 2007;110:163a (abstract).

113. Barlogie B, Tricot GJ, van Rhee F, et al. Long-term outcome results of the first tandem autotransplant trial for multiple myeloma. *Br J Haematol* 2006;135:158-64.

114. Bergsagel PL. Individualizing therapy using molecular markers in multiple myeloma. *Clin Lymphoma Myeloma* 2007;(suppl 4):S170-4.

9   Allogeneic Stem Cell Transplantation for Multiple Myeloma

William I. Bensinger

INTRODUCTION

The outlook for patients with multiple myeloma (MM) has greatly improved in the past decade. Before 1995, melphalan and prednisone were considered the standards of treatment since newer regimens such as vincristine, adriamycin, and dexamethasone (VAD) or vincristine, melphalan, cyclophosphamide, and prednisone (VMCP) produced faster responses but did not improve overall survival. Progress in the treatment of MM occurred when it was shown that high-dose therapy followed by autologous stem cell transplantation (ASCT) when compared to VAD could increase complete remission rates (CR), improve disease-free survival and increase overall survival. As such, ASCT has become the standard of care for many patients with MM. ASCT is, unfortunately, not curative for the vast majority of patients with MM. Furthermore, it has been shown that autologous transplants can produce survival benefits when used as part of initial therapy or later in the disease course, which means more recent studies of the timing of ASCT, when compared to conventional therapy, have shown equivalent survival since patients failing conventional therapy can eventually receive a transplant.

New insights into the biology and genetics of myeloma cells have resulted in the rapid introduction of new drugs with unique mechanisms of action. These drugs, which include thalidomide, lenalidomide, and bortezomib, have shown significant activity in MM, and when these new agents are combined with more traditional drugs, the response and complete remission rates are as high as responses achieved with ASCT.[1,2] Despite these advances, long-term survival after treatment with ASCT or the newly developed drugs is rare and virtually all patients recur.

Stem cell transplantation from allogeneic donors can cure 10% to 20% of patients with chemotherapy-resistant hematologic malignancies and up to 80% of patients who are transplanted in remission. A large part of the high response and curative potential of allografts is attributed to a "graft-versus-tumor" effect. In patients with MM this graft-versus-myeloma (GVM) effect has been well documented.[3-5] In contrast, stem cell transplantation from autologous or syngeneic donors provides little or no immunologic effect against the myeloma cell. Thus autologous or syngeneic stem cell transplants are essentially a form of supportive care after intensive chemotherapy +/− radiation designed to accomplish eradication of disease. Long-term follow-up of recipients of ASCT indicate a continuing risk of disease recurrence after 5 years and arguably few, if any, patients are cured. In contrast, allogeneic stem cell transplants, with long-term follow-up appear to result in durable remissions and a lower risk of recurrence after 5 years presumably due to the continuous immune surveillance of the donor graft.

Although treatment with high-dose chemoradiotherapy followed by allogeneic SCT is capable of producing remissions and long-term survival for patients with MM, the high transplant-related mortality of 25% to 50% limits the wide application of this approach. Patients who have failed a prior autologous transplant or who have advanced, refractory disease are generally poor candidates for a full-dose allogeneic SCT owing to treatment-related mortality that exceeds 50%. Furthermore, since more than 80% of patients who develop MM are greater than age 55 years and need closely HLA-matched family member or unrelated

Supported in part by grants: CA-18029, CA-47748, CA-18221, CA-15704, from the National Cancer Institute, and HL 36444 from the National Heart, Lung and Blood Institute, National Institutes of Health, Bethesda, MD., The Jose Carreras Foundation against Leukemia, Barcelona, Spain.

individuals to serve as stem cell donors, less than 10% of patients are even eligible to receive an allogeneic stem cell transplant.

IMMUNOLOGIC EFFECT OF THE ALLOGRAFT

The principal advantage of an allograft is derived from the immunocompetent cells in the donor graft, which are potent enough to eradicate residual MM in the recipient. The therapeutic benefit of GVM is frequently associated with graft-versus-host-disease (GVHD), a result of the immunocompetent donor T cells attacking normal host recipient tissues in the skin, liver, gastrointestinal tract, and lungs. Because of small patient numbers and heterogeneity of risk factors in registry data, few conventional transplant studies to date have been able to identify a graft-versus-myeloma effect. A small retrospective report of 37 patients who received conventional allografts for MM found that among 15 patients who achieved complete response, 11 had chronic GVHD while 4 did not.[6] Individual case reports have documented a graft-versus-myeloma effect in association with GVHD when immunosuppression was withdrawn.[7] Small series of patients with MM who developed postallograft relapses and who subsequently were infused with allogeneic leukocytes from their original stem cell donors have clearly demonstrated a graft-versus-myeloma effect that was associated with GVHD.[3-5,8,9] In initial studies, 50% to 70% of patients receiving donor lymphocyte infusions for relapsed MM have been reported to achieve complete responses.[5,10,11] A more recent survey of 25 patients at 15 centers reported complete responses in only 7 (28%) patients who received 1 or more infusions of donor lymphocytes.[9] In a review of donor lymphocyte infusions for relapsed MM, a graft-versus-myeloma effect was noted in 18 of 22 patients who developed GVHD compared to only 2 of 7 patients who did not develop GVHD ($p = 0.02$).[12] These studies suggest that clinical GHVD is not essential for a graft-versus-myeloma effect, but the relationship between the two is very strong. Unfortunately, despite obtaining a CR after DLI, few of these remissions are durable.

In an attempt to reduce transplant-related complications, some groups have utilized partially T-depleted allografts after ablative or reduced-intensity conditioning, followed by pre-emptive donor lymphocyte infusions.[13] Retrospective studies of reduced-intensity transplants have shown a strong linkage between the development of chronic GVHD and a diminished risk of relapse (HR, 0.37, $p = 0.02$).[14,15] Furthermore, when one compares response rates to donor lymphocyte infusions among different diseases, it appears that the graft-versus-tumor effects in patients with MM are less potent than other diseases such as chronic myeloid leukemia, chronic lymphocytic leukemia, mantle cell or follicular lymphoma.[16-18] This suggests that reduced-intensity allografting for MM is less likely to be successful unless patients can first be treated to a state of minimal disease. The majority of studies analyzing outcomes after nonablative allografting have confirmed this prediction.

ABLATIVE ALLOGRAFTS

The US intergroup trial of early versus late autologous transplant suggested that autologous transplant produced equivalent survival to standard chemotherapy when transplant could be given as salvage treatment for patients failing conventional therapy.[19] The trial was started in 1993 and had a third option that allowed patients with matched siblings to undergo allogeneic transplant using an ablative regimen of melphalan and total body irradiation. That arm of the study was closed after 36 patients were treated, owing to excessively high transplant-related mortality (TRM) of 53%. After 7 years of follow-up, however, the overall survivals are identical at 39% for both autologous and allogeneic recipients, while the progression-free survivals are 15% for autologous recipients compared to 22% for allogeneic recipients. In addition, while the risk of relapse and death continues in the groups that received autologous transplants, the overall survival curve for the allogeneic group has reached a plateau with follow-up extending to 10 years. Thus, at the present time only allogeneic stem cell transplantation is capable of producing long-term, durable remissions with the potential for cure. This would argue that allogeneic transplants should continue to have a role in the management of MM, even if only as a continuing investigational field.

Although early studies of myeloablative allogeneic transplants were plagued by prohibitively high TRM, improved supportive care and patient selection has led to a reduction of complications in more recently reported studies. One of the largest series of patients comes from the EBMT Registry where data on 690 patients with MM have been reported.[20] The EBMT registry analysis examined transplants performed on 334 patients from 1983 to 1993 and 356 patients from 1994 to 1998. Of the patients transplanted during the latter period 133 (37%) received peripheral blood stem cells (PBSC) rather than marrow. The most important observation was a marked reduction in TRM from 46% to 30% between the two time periods. The reduction in mortality was a result of fewer deaths from opportunistic infections and interstitial pneumonias. This was due, in part, to better patient selection with less prior treatment as well as improvements in supportive care. The superior results did not appear to be a result of the introduction of PBSC. The overall survival after 3 years improved from 35% during the 1983-93 periods to 56% during the 1994-98 period.

A phase 2 study utilizing high-dose busulfan and mephalan followed by allogeneic peripheral blood stem cells from matched sibling donors in 30 patients with MM has reported a TRM of 16% at 100 days, 30% overall with an 81% CR rate.[21] Survival and progression-free survivals at 6 years were 65% and 70%. A single center study reviewed the 10-year results of myeloablative allografts (n = 72) and compared them with patients who received autologous transplants (n = 86).[22] One-year mortality was 22% for allogeneic recipients; the 5- and 10-year survivals were not significantly different at 48% and 40% for allograft recipients compared to 46% and 31% for autologous patients. The 10-year progression-free survivals were 33% for the allogeneic group and 15% for the autologous group, although these differences were not statistically significant.

Thus improvements in patient selection and supportive care have narrowed the differences in TRM between ablative (25%-30%) and reduced-intensity (15%-20%) allogeneic stem cell transplants. This suggests that there may be strategies to make ablative regimens more tolerable that would still preserve the cytoreductive benefits of an allograft. One such strategy would be to substitute novel drugs into the ablative conditioning regimen such as treosulfan, which in preliminary reports can reduce TRM to 10% at 100 days and 25% at 1 year.[23]

NONABLATIVE ALLOGENEIC TRANSPLANTS

The high-intensity conditioning regimens customarily used before allogeneic transplants are designed to produce cytoreduction, which is primarily designed to reduce the myeloma disease burden, and immunosuppression designed to allow establishment of the donor graft. These high-dose therapies result in myeloablation, which requires transplant using the donor graft. The demonstrated efficacy of donor lymphocyte infusions in relapsed allograft patients suggests that the allogeneic graft-versus-myeloma effect is an important component for cure. This has led to the exploration of reduced-intensity conditioning regimens, designed more for immunosuppression rather than tumor cytoreduction, with the aim of establishing consistent donor engraftment while minimizing toxicity and damage to normal host tissues. The approach using reduced-intensity immunosuppression minimizes or eliminates the period of severe pancytopenia that always occurs after myeloablative conditioning. In theory, once donor engraftment is achieved, this approach will allow the GVM effects to operate while reducing the high TRM.

The most widely used reduced-intensity regimen was developed in Seattle on the basis of canine transplant studies where it was shown that reliable allogeneic donor peripheral blood stem cell engraftment could be achieved with a very low dose of total body irradiation of 200 cGy and a combination of two potent immunosuppressive drugs, including mycophenolic acid and cyclosporine.[24] This strategy was applied to 18 patients undergoing allogeneic transplant for MM. Seven patients had refractory disease and six had failed a prior autograft. Two patients of the first four rejected the donor graft, leading to the addition of fludarabine, which provided additional immunosuppression.[25] There were no further occurrences of rejection following the addition of fludarabine to the regimen. Although only 1 of 18 died of transplant-related toxicities, complete responses occurred in only 2 patients and only 3 others achieved partial responses. None of the responses were durable. These results confirmed that in MM the GVM effects are relatively modest and that additional therapy would be needed prior to a reduced-intensity allograft in order to improve the results.

In order to accomplish the goal of treating patients to a state of minimal disease, an autologous stem cell transplant was performed first followed by a reduced-intensity allograft in patients with MM who had not received a prior high-dose regimen. Patients first have autologous peripheral blood stem cells collected, followed by melphalan 200 mg/m^2 and reinfusion of autologous stem cells to provide cytoreduction and some immunosuppression. In this way the high-dose therapy is separated in time from the introduction of the allograft. Two to four months later, after recovery from the autologous stem cell transplant, patients received a regimen of 200 cGy total body irradiation, mycophenolic acid, and cyclosporine with allogeneic peripheral blood stem cells. Fifty-four patients aged 29-71 years, with median age of 52 years, received this tandem autologous, allogeneic transplant strategy. All 52 except 1 achieved full donor chimerism, with a single patient requiring donor lymphocyte infusions on day 84 for partial chimerism. The overall transplant mortality was 22% and the complete remission rate was 57%. Four patients developed severe acute GVHD (grades 3-4), and chronic GVHD developed in 60%.[26] These results were recently updated to include 102 patients with a median follow-up of 5 years.[27] Sixty-three percent of patients achieved CR, and the progression-free and overall survivals at 5 years were 35% and 63%, respectively. Unfortunately, patients treated with the tandem-auto allogeneic approach continue to experience relapse beyond 3 years.

More than 400 patients who have received allogeneic stem cell transplants after reduced-intensity regimens for MM with results reported in full manuscript or abstract form in 13 phase 2 studies (Table 9.1). The types of regimens used varied widely and include melphalan 100-180 mg/m^2 often with added fludarabine, TBI 200 cGy, with fludarabine, or sometimes with added cyclophosphamide or low-dose busulfan. Antithymocyte globulin (ATG) or the anti-CD52 antibody alemtuzumab have been included with some regimens in order to facilitate engraftment and reduce GVHD. GVHD prophylaxis regimens have included cyclosporine or tacrolimus and mycophenolic acid or methotrexate. There is currently no consensus on which of these regimens is superior in terms of toxicity or efficacy. G-CSF-mobilized PBSC have been used for the majority of studies owing to fewer graft failure/rejections and putatively greater graft-versus-myeloma effects when compared to bone marrow. Unrelated donors were utilized in 121 transplants. Approximately 120 of these patients had the reduced-intensity allograft performed as part of a tandem strategy following an ablative autologous transplant.

Acute GVHD grades 2-4 occurred in 25-58% of patients. Chronic GVHD was reported in 7% to 70% of patients. Overall TRM has ranged from a low of 0% to a high of 41%.

Survival has ranged from 50% to 100% at 1 year, 26% to 74% at 2 years, 36% to 70% at 3 years and as high as 69% at 4 years. Complete response rates have ranged from a low of 10% to as high as 73%.

The Arkansas group utilized melphalan 100 mg/m^2 to prepare 45 patients before RIC allografting. These patients had either failed two or three prior autologous transplants or received the allograft as part of a tandem autologous-allogeneic transplant strategy (n = 12). The patients had a median age of 56 years and donors were all HLA matched; 12 were unrelated volunteer donors. TBI and fludarabine were added to the regimens of patients receiving transplants from unrelated donors. The day 100 TRM was 15%, overall transplant mortality was 38%, and 64% achieved CR or near CR. Overall survival at 3 years was poor, only 36%. There was a significantly better 3-year survival for patients transplanted as part of the planned tandem strategy versus failed autografts, 86% versus 31%, p = 0.01.[28]

Several other studies of reduced-intensity allografts from family members or unrelated donors have confirmed that results are poor when patients have failed a prior autologous transplant or have chemotherapy-resistant disease.[29-31] A study combining data from several centers including approximately 120 patients found that relapse from a prior autologous transplant was the most significant risk factor for transplant mortality (HR 2.80; p = 0.02), relapse (HR 4.14; p < 0.001), and death (HR 2.69; p = 0.005).[14] At least one trial comparing autologous with reduced-intensity allografts following relapse from a prior autologous transplant found no differences in progression-free and overall survival.[32] A more recent study has demonstrated that a second autologous transplant performed only after relapse or progression can result in major responses with prolonged survival.[33] Thus it remains to be determined whether a reduced-intensity allograft or a second autograft is the best choice once patients have failed a prior autograft. Conversely, complete response rates and early survivals were very good when a planned tandem, reduced-intensity allograft approach was utilized as part of the initial treatment.[26,34-36] In a retrospective review of 834 patients undergoing reduced-intensity allograft for a variety of hematologic malignancies of which 165 patients had MM, relapse rates per year of follow-up were lower at 0.19 if patients were in CR prior to allograft compared to a yearly relapse rate of 0.27 per year if patients with MM were not in CR.[37]

TABLE 9.1. Phase 2 trials of reduced-intensity allogeneic transplantation from related and unrelated donors for the treatment of MM

Reference	No.	Regimen	# Tandem Auto	Proph GVHD	%Graft Chim	AGVHD %, 2–4	CGVH %	TRM %	CR %	%Survival at (yr)
Maloney[26]	54 (0)	TB!2Gy, Flu	54	CSA Mmf	100	45	60	22	57	69 (5)
Lee[28]	45* (12)	HDM100 (TBI2Gy, Flu)	12	CSA	89	58	13	38	64	36 (3)
Kroger[34]	17 (8)	HDM100, Flu, ATG	17	CSA, Mtx	100	38	7	18	73	74 (2)
Kroger[35]	21 (21)	HDM100–140, Flu, ATG	9	CSA, Mtx	100	38	12	24	40	74 (2)
Gerull[60]	52 (20)	TBI2Gy, Flu	0	CSA Mmf	90	37	70	17	27	41 (1.5)
Mohty[41]	41	Bu, Flu, ATG	0	CSA Mtx (13)	98	36	41	17	24	62 (2)
Peggs[40]	20 (8)	TBI, Flu, alemtuzumab	0	CSA Mmf	nr	25*	nr	15	10	71 (2)
Einsele[31]	22 (15)	TBI2Gy, Flu, Cyclo	0	ATG, CSA Mmf	nr	38	32	23	27	26 (2)
Giralt[30]	22 (9)	Flu, HDM 140–180	0	FK506 Mtx	100	46	27	41	32	30 (2)
Qazilbash[38]	22 (0)	Flu, HDM 100–140	Nr	FK506 Mtx	Nr	32	47	nr	18	48 (2)
Hoepfner[29]	19 (6)	TBI2Gy, Flu	0	CSA Mmf	nr	37	nr	32	nr	50 (2)
Galimberti[36]	20 (0)	TBI2Gy, Flu (10) Cy, Flu (10)	20	CSA Mmf	nr	25	30	20	35	58 (2)
Ma[61]	10 (0)	TBI3Gy, FLU	0	CSA Mmf	80	60	40	0	30	100 (1)
Perez-Simon[62]	29 (nr)	Mel, Flu	10	CSA Mtx		41	51	21	28	60 (2)
Sorasio[63]	22 (22)	TBI2Gy, Flu	nr	CSA Mmf	91	50	59	18	20	73 (1)
Majolino[64]	53	Thiotepa, Flu, Mel	0	CSA Mtx		45	64	13	62	45 (3)

No., total number of patients (number from matched unrelated donors); regimen HDM, high-dose melphalan; TBI, total body irradiation; Flu, fludarabine; cyclo, cyclophosphamide; # tandem auto-planned prior to autologous transplant; ProphGVHD, graft-versus-host disease prophylaxis; CSA, cyclosporine; ATG, antithymocyte globulin; Mtx, methotrexate; Mmf, mycophenolic acid; FK506, tacrolimus; AGVHD, acute graft-versus-host disease; CGVH, chronic GVHD; TRM, transplant-related mortality rate; CR, complete response rate; nr, not reported; *14 patients given DLI

The MD Anderson group has explored a regimen of fludarabine and melphalan 100-180 mg/m^2 and found significantly greater toxicities associated with melphalan doses >100 mg/m^2.[30,38] Other groups using the fludarabine-melphalan combination have reported less toxicity using the 100 mg/m^2 dose of melphalan.[34,39]

In one study the anti-CD52 antibody, alemtuzumab was added to total body irradiation and fludarabine in 20 patients with MM undergoing reduced-intensity allografting as part of frontline therapy.[40] Fourteen of 20 were given donor lymphocyte infusions post-transplant for residual or progressive disease. Although transplant mortality and survival at 2 years were acceptable at 15% and 71%, respectively, the complete response rate of 10% was disappointing. The low response rate may have been due to the addition of alemtuzumab, which may have interfered with the GVM effect. In another study antithymocyte globulin (ATG) at doses of 2.5 to 12.5 mg/kg were added to a busulfan-fludarabine regimen. The incidences of transplant mortality and GVHD were relatively low at 17% and 27%, respectively, but the complete response rate was also low at 24%.[41] Both these studies suggest that antibodies such as alemtuzumab or ATG to prevent GVHD must be used cautiously and probably at reduced doses since these antibodies can also abrogate the GVM effect. More recently, a European group has examined the influence of ATG in 79 patients undergoing allografting with a melphalan/fludarabine regimen and compared results with 59 patients who did not receive ATG.[13] They reported a higher complete remission rate that was dose dependently associated with the use of ATG. This analysis further found that ATG was associated with trends to better EFS and OS. This beneficial effect could be due in part to the known antimyeloma activity of ATG; however, as noted before, this may be a "double-edged sword" since ATG may negatively impact GVM.

Recently the European Group for Blood and Marrow Transplant (EBMT) has summarized registry data containing 229 patients undergoing reduced-intensity allogeneic stem cell transplants in 33 centers.[42] The regimens varied widely, but almost all utilized fludarabine, with a large majority receiving either low-dose total body irradiation, melphalan, or cyclophosphamide. Approximately 50% of the reduced-intensity regimens also contained antithymocyte globulin or alemtuzumab. Eighty percent of patients were transplanted with peripheral blood stem cells. Acute GVHD grades 2-4 occurred in 31% of patients and extensive chronic GVHD was reported in 25%. Although the TRM was low at 22%, the 3-year overall survivals and progression-free survivals were disappointing at 41% and 22%. Disease status and duration at transplant and the use of alemtuzumab for conditioning were found in multivariate analysis to be adverse risk factors for transplant mortality, progression-free survivals, and overall survivals. The development of limited chronic GVHD was associated with better overall survivals and progression-free survivals, 84% and 46%, while patients with extensive chronic GVHD had overall survivals and progression-free survivals of 58% and 30%. Interestingly, patients without chronic GVHD had the worst outcomes, with overall survivals and progression-free survivals of 29% and 12%, deaths being mainly due to recurrent disease.

More recently, the EBMT has compared reduced-intensity conditioning with standard ablative conditioning for allografting in MM.[43] Between 1998 and 2002, 196 patients conditioned with ablative regimens were compared with 321 patients undergoing reduced-intensity conditioning. TRM was significantly lower for the reduced-intensity group, p = 0.001. There was, however, no statistical difference in overall survivals between the two groups, and progression-free survivals were inferior for patients receiving reduced-intensity regimens, p = 0.009. This was due to a rate of relapse for the reduced-intensity group that was more than double the rate for standard conditioning patients, p = 0.0001.

COMPARATIVE TRIALS

No prospective randomized trials have been published comparing ablative with nonablative conditioning regimens for the transplant of patients with MM. There are, however, a number of studies reported or underway comparing tandem autologous transplants to a tandem autologous, nonablative allograft approach (Table 9.2). The randomization for these studies was "genetic," in that patients with available related donors were typed, and if an HLA-identical donor was identified, they were offered a nonablative transplant as the second transplant. While not truly randomized, they provide some comparative data on the relative risks and benefits of the two techniques.

A French trial using 2 parallel studies compared outcomes in 284 patients with MM who were high risk by virtue of elevated β_2-microglobulin and deletion of chromosome 13 by fluorescence in-situ hybridization.[44] All patients first had an autologous transplant with high-dose melphalan. The 65 patients with HLA-matched donors underwent an allogeneic transplant on one protocol after conditioning with busulfan, fludarabine, and a high dose of antithymocyte globulin 12.5 mg/kg. They were compared with 219 patients without donors who were treated on another protocol with a second autologous transplant with melphalan 220 mg/m². Transplant mortality was 5% for the tandem auto group compared to 11% for the auto-allo group. The complete response and very good PR rates were 51% and 62% respectively for the tandem auto and auto-allo groups. With a relatively short follow-up of a median 2 years, the overall survivals and event-free survivals were not statistically different, 35%

TABLE 9.2 Comparison trials of tandem autologous transplant with autologous + reduced-intensity allografting

Author	Regimens	Number	TRM (%)	Response CR/VGPR	DFS (f/u yr)	OS (f/u yr)
Garban[*44]	Auto mel200/220	219	5	33%/18%	0% 5 yr	44% 5 yr
	Auto mel200	65[†]	11	33%/29%	0% 5 yr	33% 5 yr
	Allo bu, flu, ATG					
Bruno[46]	Auto mel200	80[‡]	4	26%/ nr	20% 4 yr	53% 4 yr
	Auto mel200	82[§]	10	55%/ nr	42% 4 yr**	75% 4 yr**
	Allo 2Gy TBI					
Blade[††65]	Auto BuMel-Mel, CBV	88	5	11%/6%	Med 26 mo	Med 57 mo
	Auto BuMel-Mel	26	16	33%/nr	Med 19 mo	Med "not reached"
	Allo FluMel140					

nr, not reported [*]high-risk patients with elevated B-2M and deletion 13 by FISH.[†]19/65 patients did not receive the reduced-intensity allograft [‡]46/80 patients completed the tandem autograft [§]58/82 patients received the reduced-intensity allograft ** statistically significant [††]only patients not in CR after autograft 1 proceeded to second autograft or RIC allograft

versus 41%, and 25% versus 30% for the tandem auto and auto-allo studies, respectively. Although this study indicates that patients with high-risk features do not benefit from a tandem auto-reduced-intensity allograft approach, the regimen utilized a high dose of ATG 12.5 mg/kg. This resulted in a low incidence of chronic GVHD (7%) but a relatively low complete response rate (33% of evaluable patients). This study agrees with another report analyzing the outcome of RIC allografting in patients with or without del13.[45] This study demonstrated that del13 was an independent, adverse risk factor for overall survivals and progression-free survivals after reduced-intensity allografting primarily due to a greater risk of relapse. Whether any allograft procedure can overcome this adverse risk factor remains to be determined.

Another study followed 162 patients with stage II or III MM to induction with VAD for 2 to 3 cycles, followed by autologous peripheral blood stem cell collection following cyclophosphamide and granulocyte colony stimulating factor.[46] All patients then received high-dose melphalan followed by autologous peripheral blood stem cells. Patients with an HLA-identical sibling (N = 80) were prospectively assigned to receive a reduced-intensity allogeneic transplant using the Seattle regimen, while patients without a matched sibling (N = 82) were assigned to receive a second course of high-dose melphalan and autologous stem cell transplant. Only 58 and 46 patients in the auto-allo and auto-auto groups completed their assigned treatments. The complete response rate was 26%

with the tandem auto and 55% with the auto-allo group (p = 0.004). The transplant mortality was 2% and 10% for the tandem auto and auto-allo groups, respectively, p = ns. Based on intention to treat, and with a 45-month median follow-up, the median overall survivals were 54 months and 80 months, for the tandem auto versus auto-allo groups, respectively, p = 0.01. The progression-free survivals were 29 months versus 35 months for the auto-auto and auto-allo groups, respectively, p = 0.02. An important strength of this trial is the treatment assignment based solely on donor availability and analysis on intention to treat. This study has been criticized, however, because of the relatively large fallout of patients who were assigned to receive tandem autologous transplants yet did not receive the actual treatment and because of the relatively poor outcome of patients assigned to tandem autologous transplant.

Nevertheless, these results suggest a possible advantage for the auto-allo approach, although longer follow-up is needed. Another concern in this study was that high lactate dehydrogenase and low platelet count and diagnosis were both independent predictors of survival and progression-free survival. This would suggest that allogeneic transplant may not be able to overcome high-risk prognostic factors, although a recent update of this trial, with 56 months of follow-up suggested that in subgroup analysis patients with deletion 13 or high β_2-microglobulin retained benefits of improved survival and event-free survival if assigned to the allograft group.[47] The PETHEMA group has reported on a small trial in which patients first received an autologous transplant after conditioning with melphalan +/− busulfan. Only patients not in CR or near-CR proceeded to a second autologous transplant using melphalan or CBV (cyclophosphamide, etoposide, and carmustine) n = 88, or if an HLA-matched donor was available patients were given fludarabine + melphalan followed by an allograft n = 26. There were differences in the rates of CR after second transplant, 11% autologous versus 33% Allogeneic. As expected TRM was different, 5% autologous versus 16% Allogeneic. Owing to small numbers the median EFS and OS were not different; however, the authors noted a "plateau" in the Allogeneic group.

In the United States a large multicenter trial comparing tandem autologous transplants with autologous reduced-intensity allografts for patients with MM was recently closed upon meeting target accrual. This trial also relied on the availability of an HLA-identical sibling for assignment to the Allogeneic group. It is likely that at least two more years of follow-up will be required before the results of this study are reported.

It is clear that reduced-intensity allogeneic transplant regimens can result in reliable donor engraftment with a relatively low mortality compared to high-dose regimens. The immunologic effect of the allograft is, however, relatively modest, resulting in reduced rates of complete response and a higher rate of progression compared to ablative regimens. Therefore, it appears that substantial cytoreduction preallografting is required in order to facilitate the success of a reduced-intensity allograft. Preliminary results suggest the tandem auto/reduced-intensity allogeneic strategy can result in complete responses in over 50% of patients with MM, similar to what can be achieved with a high-dose conditioning regimen. In studies with longer follow-up, however, the risks of disease progression appear to be continuous for at least 5 years. Although reduced-intensity regimens are a promising strategy to ensure reliable engraftment, low mortality and high response rates, as well as the ability to expand this technique to older patients or patients with co-morbid conditions, it will be important to have longer follow-up of patients transplanted with nonablative regimens in order to document the durability of these remissions and to document the rates and severity of chronic GVHD.

HOW DO WE IMPROVE ALLOGENEIC TRANSPLANTS FOR MM?

A possible reason for the high transplant mortality after allografting for patients with MM may be related to the primary immunodeficiency in this disease. Thus improved sources of stem cells such as peripheral blood which result in earlier engraftment and immune reconstitution[48] should reduce infectious complications. The large number of CD34 cells collected from peripheral blood should allow exploration of engineered grafts such as CD4 enrichment to increase the GVM effect without an increase in graft-versus-host disease.[49]

At the present time, allogeneic stem cell transplant remains the only modality with the potential for long-term disease control in more than a handful of patients. Significant progress has been achieved in reducing transplant mortality but the problems of disease recurrence and graft-versus-host disease remain. Future work should focus on novel techniques for cytoreduction and enhancing GVM while reducing or controlling graft-versus-host disease. The reduced-intensity allogeneic transplant technique can serve as a platform from which to build unique conditioning regimens, engineered grafts, or post-transplant therapies in an effort to improve results.

A novel technique for improving the ability to eradiate residual host myeloma utilizes targeted radiation delivered by antibodies or chemically specific uptake. High-energy, short-acting radioisotopes linked to bone-seeking compounds have been utilized in this manner. Holmium-166 (^{166}Ho) a beta-emitting radiometal with a half-life of 26 hours has been linked to a tetra phosphonate chelate (DOTMP) to achieve rapid and specific uptake in bone and bone surfaces. In phase 1-2 trials, increasing doses of ^{166}Ho-DOTMP were given, along with high-dose melphalan, followed by autologous stem cell transplant.[50] A complete response rate of 38% was observed with a median overall survival in excess of 48 months. Sammarium-153, another high-energy isotope was linked to another tetra-phosphonate chelate (EDTMP) and studied in 18 patients with MM, who received melphalan 200 mg/m^2 following the isotope.[51] Five patients achieved complete responses. The samarium isotope has also been given to nine patients in a pilot study along with cyclophophamide as a preparative regimen for allografting in MM.[52] Tolerance was very good, with only one patient dying from transplant complications; responses were disappointing, with only two patients achieving complete response. Nevertheless, this is an attractive way to increase treatment to tumor-bearing areas while sparing nontarget tissues that deserve further study.

CONCLUSIONS AND MANAGEMENT OF POTENTIAL ALLOGRAFT PATIENTS

Future studies of allogeneic marrow transplantation in MM should focus on regimens that are less toxic but able to preserve antitumor effects such as radioisotopes linked to bone-seeking chelates[53,54] or dose-adjusted chemotherapy.[55] It should be relatively easy to combine targeted radiotherapy and dose-adjusted chemotherapy to create a more tolerable regimen.

The studies using nonablative regimens appear to reduce effectively the early complications and mortality of allogeneic transplants, but are relatively ineffective at eradicating residual disease unless accompanied by cytoreduction delivered with a prior autograft. Such treatments could be combined with infusions of allogeneic donor lymphocytes or subsets of lymphocytes in the form of "engineered grafts", for example CD4 lymphocytes, which may have a graft-versus-myeloma effect without increasing graft-versus-host disease.[49] It may also be possible to exploit killer-immunoglobulin-like mismatching between donor and recipient, which has been shown to result in improved progression-free survival due to a reduced rate of relapse.[56] Finally, it may be worthwhile to exploit monoclonal antibodies targeting myeloma cells such as the CD40 antigen[57] or CS-1 antigen,[58] in order to increase the ability of donor allogeneic cells to eliminate residual host disease.[59]

While it is still not possible to recommend allogeneic transplants outside the context of a clinical trial, the results from the recent Italian trial are encouraging.[46] The small number of patients actually transplanted should encourage further studies exploring this approach. Patients who should be considered for allogeneic stem cell transplant are relatively young, that is, age less than 60, those with high-risk cytogenetics such as 17p deletion or 4;14 translocation, high β_2-microglobulin, or lactate dehydrogenase at diagnosis. In addition, patients who have a relatively short duration of response after autologous transplant should be considered for allografting.

REFERENCES

1. Kumar S, Anderson KC. Drug insight: thalidomide as a treatment for multiple myeloma (Review). *Nat Clin Prac Oncol* 2005;2:262-70.
2. Anderson KC, Shaughnessy JD, Jr., Barlogie B, Harousseau J-L, Roodman GD. Multiple myeloma. In: Broudy VC, Abkowitz JL, Vose JM, eds. *Hematology*: American Society of Hematology Education Program Book. Washington, DC: American Society of Hemtology; 2002;214-40.
3. Tricot G, Vesole DH, Jagannath S, Hilton J, Munshi N, Barlogie B. Graft-versus-myeloma effect: Proof of principle. *Blood* 1996;87:1196-8.
4. Verdonck LF, Lokhorst HM, Dekker AW, Nieuwenhuis HK, Petersen EJ. Graft-versus-myeloma effect in two cases. *Lancet* 1996;347:800-1.
5. Aschan J, Lonnqvist B, Ringden O, Kumlien G, Gahrton G. Graft-versus-myeloma effect (Letter). *Lancet* 1996;348:346.
6. Le Blanc R, Montminy-Métivier S, Bélanger R, et al. Allogeneic transplantation for multiple myeloma: further evidence for a GVHD-associated graft-versus-myeloma effect. *Bone Marrow Transplant* 2001;28:841-8.
7. Libura J, Hoffmann T, Passweg J, et al. Graft-versus-myeloma after withdrawal of immunosuppression following allogeneic peripheral stem cell transplantation. *Bone Marrow Transplant* 1999;24:925-7.
8. Bertz H, Burger JA, Kunzmann R, Mertelsmann R, Finke J. Adoptive immunotherapy for relapsed multiple myeloma after allogeniec bone marrow transplantation (BMT): evidence for a graft-versus-myeloma effect. *Leukemia* 1997;11:281-3.
9. Salama M, Nevill T, Marcellus D, et al. Donor leukocyte infusions for multiple myeloma. *Bone Marrow Transplant* 2000;26:1179-84.
10. Collins RH, Jr., Shpilberg O, Drobyski WR, et al. Donor leukocyte infusions in 140 patients with relapsed malignancy after allogeneic bone marrow transplantation. *J Clin Oncol* 1997;15:433-44.
11. Alyea E, Ritz J. Induction of graft versus myeloma by donor lymphocyte infusions following allogeneic bone marrow transplant. In: Anderson KC, ed. *VI International Workshop on Multiple Myeloma* 1997; Harvard Medical School and the Dana Farber Cancer Center, Boxton, MA.
12. Mehta J, Singhal S. Graft-versus-myeloma (Review). *Bone Marrow Transplant* 1998;22:835-43.
13. Ayuk F, Perez-Simon JA, Shimoni A, et al. Anti-thymocyte globulin induces higher response rates and less graft-versus-host disease in multiple myeloma patients undergoing allogeneic stem cell transplantation [abstract]. *Blood* 2007;110 (Part 1):875a, 2980.
14. Kroger N, Perez-Simon JA, Myint H, et al. Relapse to prior autograft and chronic graft-versus-host disease are the strongest prognostic factors for outcome of melphalan/fludarabine-based dose-reduced allogeneic stem cell transplantation in patients with multiple myeloma. *Biol Blood Marrow Transplant* 2004;10:698-708.
15. Einsele H, Schäfer HJ, Bader P, et al. Allografts after reduced intensity conditioning can induce long-term remission in

patients with chemosensitive relapsed multiple myeloma (MM). *Blood* 2002;100 (Part 1):635a, 2499.

16. Cwynarski K, Dazzi F, Cross NCP, et al. Response to donor lymphocyte infusions (DLI) of patients with CML in relapse after allografting: a long-term follow-up study using RT-PCR [abstract]. *Blood* 1999;94 (suppl 1):669a, 2968.

17. Dazzi F, Szydlo RM, Cross NC, et al. Durability of responses following donor lymphocyte infusions for patients who relapse after allogeneic stem cell transplantation for chronic myeloid leukemia. *Blood* 2000;96:2712-6.

18. Helg C, Starobinski M, Jeannet M, Chapuis B. Donor lymphocyte infusion for the treatment of relapse after allogeneic hematopoietic stem cell transplantation (Review). *Leuk Lymphoma* 1998;29:301-13.

19. Barlogie B, Kyle RA, Anderson KC, et al. Standard chemotherapy compared with high-dose chemoradiotherapy for multiple myeloma: final results of phase III US Intergroup Trial S9321. *J Clin Oncol* 2006;24:929-36.

20. Gahrton G, Svensson H, Cavo M, et al. Progress in allogeneic bone marrow and peripheral blood stem cell transplantation for multiple myeloma: a comparison between transplants performed 1983-93 and 1994-98 at European Group for Blood and Marrow Transplantation centres. *Br J Haematol* 2001;113:209-16.

21. Majolino I, Corradini P, Scimè R, et al. Allogeneic transplantation of unmanipulated peripheral blood stem cells in patients with multiple myeloma. *Bone Marrow Transplant* 1998;22:449-55.

22. Kuruvilla J, Shepherd JD, Sutherland HJ, et al. Long-term outcome of myeloablative allogeneic stem cell transplantation for multiple myeloma. *Biol Blood Marrow Transplant* 2007;13:925-31.

23. Schmidt-Hieber M, Blau IW, Trenschel R, et al. Reduced-toxicity conditioning with fludarabine and treosulfan prior to allogeneic stem cell transplantation in multiple myeloma. *Bone Marrow Transplant* 2007;39:389-96.

24. Storb R, Yu C, Sandmaier B, et al. Mixed hematopoietic chimerism after hematopoietic stem cell allografts. *Transplant Proc* 1999;31:677-8.

25. McSweeney PA, Niederwieser D, Shizuru JA, et al. Hematopoietic cell transplantation in older patients with hematologic malignancies: replacing high-dose cytotoxic therapy with graft-versus-tumor effects. *Blood* 2001;97:3390-400.

26. Maloney DG, Molina AJ, Sahebi F, et al. Allografting with non-myeloablative conditioning following cytoreductive autografts for the treatment of patients with multiple myeloma. *Blood* 2003;102:3447-54.

27. Rotta M, Storer B, Sahebi F, et al. Long-term outcome of autologous followed by nonmyeloablative allografting from HLA-identical sibling for multiple myeloma (MM) [abstract]. *Blood* 2007;110 (Part 1): 889a, 3029.

28. Lee C-K, Badros A, Barlogie B, et al. Prognostic factors in allogeneic transplantation for patients with high-risk multiple myeloma after reduced intensity conditioning. *Exp Hematol* 2003;31:73-80.

29. Hoepfner S, Probst SM, Breitkreutz I, et al. Non-myeloablative allogeneic transplantation as part of salvage therapy for relapse of multiple myeloma after autologous transplantation. *Blood* 2002;100 (Part 1):859a, 3387.

30. Giralt S, Aleman A, Anagnostopoulos A, et al. Fludarabine/melphalan conditioning for allogeneic transplantation in patients with multiple myeloma. *Bone Marrow Transplant* 2002;30:367-73.

31. Einsele H, Schafer HJ, Hebart H, et al. Follow-up of patients with progressive multiple myeloma undergoing allografts after reduced-intensity conditioning. *Br J Haematol* 2003;121:411-8.

32. Qazilbash MH, Saliba R, de Lima M, et al. Second autologous or allogeneic transplantation after the failure of first autograft in patients with multiple myeloma. *Cancer* 2006;106:1084-9.

33. Elice F, Raimondi R, Tosetto A, et al. Prolonged overall survival with second on-demand autologous transplant in multiple myeloma. *Am J Hematol* 2006;81:426-31.

34. Kroger N, Schwerdtfeger R, Kiehl M, et al. Autologous stem cell transplantation followed by a dose-reduced allograft induces high complete remission rate in multiple myeloma. *Blood* 2002;100:755-60.

35. Kroger N, Sayer HG, Schwerdtfeger R, et al. Unrelated stem cell transplantation in multiple myeloma after a reduced-intensity conditioning with pretransplantation antithymocyte globulin is highly effective with low transplantation-related mortality. *Blood* 2002;100:3919-24.

36. Galimberti S, Benedetti E, Morabito F, et al. Prognostic role of minimal residual disease in multiple myeloma patients after non-myeloablative allogeneic transplantation. *Leuk Res* 2005;29:961-6.

37. Kahl C, Storer BE, Sandmaier BM, et al. Relapse risk among patients with malignant diseases given allogeneic hematopoietic cell transplantation after nonmyeloablative conditioning. *Blood* 2007;110:2744-8.

38. Qazilbash MH, Saliba RM, Parikh GC, et al. A non-myeloablative regimen of fludarabine and melphalan is safe and well tolerated for allogeneic transplantation in multiple myeloma [abstract]. *Blood* 2007;110 (Part 1):890a, 3032.

39. Desikan R, Barlogie B, Sawyer J, et al. Results of high-dose therapy for 1000 patients with multiple myeloma: durable complete remissions and superior survival in the absence of chromosome 13 abnormalities. *Blood* 2000;95:4008-10.

40. Peggs KS, Mackinnon S, Williams CD, et al. Reduced-intensity transplantation with in vivo T-cell depletion and adjuvant dose-escalating donor lymphocyte infusions for chemotherapy-sensitive myeloma: Limited efficacy of graft-versus-tumor activity. *Biol Blood Marrow Transplant* 2003;9:257-65.

41. Mohty M, Boiron JM, Damaj G, et al. Graft-versus-myeloma effect following antithymocyte globulin-based reduced intensity conditioning allogeneic stem cell transplantation. *Bone Marrow Transplant* 2004;34:77-84.

42. Crawley C, Lalancette M, Szydlo R, et al. Outcomes for reduced-intensity allogeneic transplantation for multiple myeloma: an analysis of prognostic factors from the Chronic Leukemia Working Party of the EBMT. *Blood* 2005;105:4532-9.

43. Crawley C, Iacobelli S, Björkstrand B, Apperley JF, Niederwieser D, Gahrton G. Reduced-intensity conditioning for myeloma: lower nonrelapse mortality but higher relapse

rates compared with myeloablative conditioning. *Blood* 2007;109:3588-94.

44. Garban F, Attal M, Michallet M, et al. Prospective comparison of autologous stem cell transplantation followed by dose-reduced allograft (IFM99-03 trial) with tandem autologous stem cell transplantation (IFM99-04 trial) in high-risk de novo multiple myeloma. *Blood* 2006;107:3474-80.

45. Kroger N, Schilling G, Einsele H, et al. Deletion of chromosome band 13q14 as detected by fluorescence in situ hybridization is a prognostic factor in patients with multiple myeloma who are receiving allogeneic dose-reduced stem cell transplantation. *Blood* 2004;103:4056-61.

46. Bruno B, Rotta M, Patriarca F, et al. A comparison of allografting with autografting for newly diagnosed myeloma. *N Engl J Med* 2007;356:1110-20.

47. Bruno B, Sorasio R, Patriarca F, et al. An update on a comparison of nonmyeloablative allografting with autografting for newly diagnosed myeloma [abstract]. *Blood* 2007;110 (Part 1): 149a, 482.

48. Bensinger WI, Martin PJ, Storer B, et al. Transplantation of bone marrow as compared with peripheral-blood cells from HLA-identical relatives in patients with hematologic cancers. *N Engl J Med* 2001;344:175-81.

49. Champlin R, Giralt S, Gajewski J, Hester J, Körbling M, Deisseroth A. CD8 depleted donor lymphocytes for CML relapsing post BMT. *ISEH* 1995;23:939.

50. Giralt S, Bensinger W, Goodman M, et al. [166]HO-DOTMP plus melphalan followed by peripheral blood stem cell transplantation in patients with multiple myeloma: Results of two phase 1/2 trials. *Blood* 2003;102:2684-91.

51. Dispenzieri A, Wiseman GA, Lacy MQ, et al. A phase I study of 153Sm-EDTMP with fixed high-dose melphalan as a peripheral blood stem cell conditioning regimen in patients with multiple myeloma. *Leukemia* 2005;19:118-25.

52. Kennedy GA, Durrant S, Butler J, et al. Outcome of myeloablative allogeneic stem cell transplantation in multiple myeloma with a 153Sm-EDTMP-based preparative regimen. *Leukemia* 2005;19:879-80.

53. Macfarlane DJ, Durrant S, Bartlett ML, Allison R, Morton AJ. 153Sm EDTMP for bone marrow ablation prior to stem cell transplantation for haematological malignancies. *Nucl Med Commun* 2002;23:1099-106.

54. Giralt S, Bensinger W, Goodman M, et al. Long-term follow-up of 83 patients with multiple myeloma (MM) treated on a phase I-II study of skeletal targeted radiotherapy (STR) using [166]Ho-DOTMP plus melphalan with or without total body irradiation (TBI) and autologous hematopoietic stem cell transplant (AHSCT) [abstract]. *Blood* 2002;100 (Part 1):179a, 670.

55. Deeg HJ, Storer B, Slattery JT, et al. Conditioning with targeted busulfan and cyclophosphamide for hemopoietic stem cell transplantation from related and unrelated donors in patients with myelodysplastic syndrome. *Blood* 2002;100:1201-7.

56. Kroger N, Shaw B, Iacobelli S, et al. Comparison between anti-thymocyte globulin and alemtuzumab and the possible impact of KIR-ligand mismatch after dose-reduced conditioning and unrelated stem cell transplantation in patients with multiple myeloma. *Br J Haematol* 2005;129:631-43.

57. Bensinger W, Jagannath S, Becker PS, et al. A phase 1 dose escalation study of a fully human antagonist anti-CD40 anti-body, HCD122 (formerly CHIR-12.12) in patients with relapsed and refractory multiple myeloma [abstract]. *Blood* 2006;108 (Part 1):1021a, 3575.

58. Hsi ED, Steinle R, Balasa B, et al. CS1: a potential new therapeutic target for the treatment of multiple myeloma [abstract]. *Blood* 2006;108 (Part 1):986a, 3457.

59. Hussein MA, Berenson JR, Niesvizky R, et al. A phase I humanized anti-CD40 monoclonal antibody (SGN-40) in patients with multiple myeloma [abstract]. *Blood* 2005;106 (Part 1):723a, 2572.

60. Gerull S, Goerner M, Benner A, et al. Long-term outcome of nonmyeloablative allogeneic transplantation in patients with high-risk multiple myeloma. *Bone Marrow Transplant* 2005;36:963-9.

61. Ma SY, Lie AK, Au WY, Chim CS, Kwong YL, Liang R. Non-myeloablative allogeneic peripheral stem cell transplantation for multiple myeloma. *Hong Kong Med J* 2004;10:77-83.

62. Couriel D, Carpenter PA, Cutler C, et al. Ancillary therapy and supportive care of chronic graft-versus-host disease: National Institutes of Health consensus development project on criteria for clinical trials in chronic graft-versus-host disease: V. Ancillary Therapy and Supportive Care Working Group report. *Biol Blood Marrow Transplant* 2006;12:375-96.

63. Sorasio R, Giaccone L, Patriarca F, et al. Unrelated donor hematopoietic cell transplantation after nonmyeloablative conditioning for patients with high risk multiple myeloma [abstract]. *Blood* 2006;108 (Part 1):901a, 3158.

64. Majolino I, Davoli M, Carnevalli E, et al. Reduced intensity conditioning with thiotepa, fludarabine, and melphalan is effective in advanced multiple myeloma. *Leuk Lymphoma* 2007;48:759-66.

65. Blade J, Rosinol L, Lahuerta JJ, et al. Tandem autologous transplant versus reduced intensity conditioned allogeneic transplant (allo-RIC) as second intensification in chemosensitive patients with multiple myeloma (MM) not achieving complete remission (CR) or near-CR with a first autologous transplant. Results from a Spanish PETHEMA/GEM study [abstract]. *Blood* 2007;110 (Part 1):224a, 729.

10   Immunoglobulin Light Chain Amyloidosis

Morie A. Gertz and Suzanne R. Hayman

INTRODUCTION

For over 90 years, amyloidosis has been defined by its tinctorial properties. Any histologic tissue section that binds the cotton wool dye Congo red[1] and demonstrates green birefringence when viewed under polarized light is, by definition, an amyloid deposit, and the patient with this deposit has amyloidosis. Refinements of the original Congo red stain include the alkaline Congo red technique[2] of including the use of permanganate and performate pretreatment to enhance the sensitivity of the test. Congo red fluorescence has been introduced to detect small amyloid deposits that would be missed with traditional staining. Phenol Congo red staining has been suggested to enhance the sensitivity of the traditional Congo red study.[3]

All amyloid deposits are amorphous under the light microscope and appear pink with standard hematoxylin and eosin staining. With electron microscopy, amyloid is not amorphous but represents nonbranching fibrils that are composed of protofilaments that are wound into the fibril. The width of the fibril is approximately 10 nm. Amyloid is insoluble in aqueous solution, and repeated homogenizations that discard the supernatant have been used for 40 years to purify amyloid deposits. The resulting pellet, when suspended in distilled water, contains relatively pure amyloid fibrils that can then be separated by high-performance liquid chromatography and sequenced.[4]

CLASSIFICATION

When amyloidosis was first described in the latter half of the 19th century, biochemical composition and ultrastructure of the amyloid deposit was unknown. The disease was, therefore, classified into three categories. It was well recognized that there were patients who had amyloidosis with identical clinical phenotype in a first-degree relative.

These were labeled familial amyloid.[5] Amyloidosis was also recognized to involve the liver, spleen, and kidneys at autopsy in patients with long-standing suppurative infections including deep-seated abscesses, osteomyelitis, and bronchiectasis. In the 19th century, tuberculosis was an exceedingly common cause of secondary amyloidosis as leprosy remains a cause today. Both are related to chronic mycobacterial infection. All other forms were labeled primary, essentially a waste basket for heterogeneous forms of amyloid where a specific cause could not be identified. Primary was subsequently supplanted by idiopathic amyloidosis, which essentially adds no additional information. Today, amyloidosis is classified on the basis of the subunit protein that forms the fibril.[6] An abridged nomenclature for amyloidosis is given in Table 10.1. Briefly, familial amyloidosis is generally composed of a mutant protein that has a high propensity to form the β-pleated sheet configuration. Worldwide, the most common is mutant transthyretin. However, there are patients well recognized who have inheritable amyloidosis due to mutations in fibrinogen-A α chain, apolipoprotein A1, and apolipoprotein A2, as well as lysozyme.[7] All forms of secondary amyloidosis relate to the improper processing of serum amyloid A (SAA) protein, which instead of being broken down to constituent amino acids cannot be broken down beyond an 8.5-kDa fragment labeled AA protein.[8] This is the protein common to all forms of amyloidosis related to long-standing infections, inflammatory bowel disease, Castleman disease, and patients with familial periodic fever syndrome, the most common being familial Mediterranean fever.[9] All forms of amyloidosis, formerly referred to as idiopathic or primary, have subsequently been found to be due to misfolding of intact or a fragment of immunoglobulin light chains or heavy chains leading to the nomenclature of amyloid light chain or AL. All forms of AL are associated with a plasma cell dyscrasia.[10]

TABLE 10.1. Nomenclature of amyloidosis

Protein	Precursor	Clinical
AL or AH	Immunoglobulin light or heavy chain	Primary or localized; myeloma- or macroglobulinemia-associated
AA	SAA	Secondary or familial
		Mediterranean fever, familial periodic fever syndromes
ATTR	Transthyretin	Familial and senile
A Fibrinogen	Fibrinogen	Familial renal amyloidosis (Ostertag)
Aβ₂M	β₂-Microglobulin	Dialysis-associated; carpal tunnel syndrome
Aβ	ABPP	Alzheimer disease
A Apo A-I/A-II	Apolipoprotein A-I	Proteinuria
	Apolipoprotein A-II	Cardiac
		Neuropathy
A Lysozyme	Lysozyme	Gastrointestinal tract
		Liver
		Renal

ABPP, amyloid β protein precursor; AH, amyloid heavy chain; SAA, serum amyloid A.
Source: From Gertz MA, Lacy MQ, Dispenzieri A. Immunoglobulin light chain amyloidosis (primary amyloidosis, AL). In Gertz MA, Greipp PR (eds), *Hematologic Malignancies: Multiple Myeloma and Related Plasma Cell Disorders*. Springer-Verlag, New York, 2004, pp. 157–95. Used with permission of Mayo Foundation for Medical Education and Research.

The inherent amyloidogenicity of immunoglobulin light chains can be demonstrated in vitro under harsh denaturing conditions using guanidine or peptic digestion. When the disulfide bonds, linking immunoglobulin light and heavy chains are broken, fibrillar assembly occurs. Nearly all forms of light chain amyloidosis are composed of the N-terminus of an immunoglobulin light or heavy chain. Clinical differences have not been recognized on the basis of whether the amyloid is derived from the light or heavy chain. Single amino acid substitutions that predict amyloidogenicity with any accuracy have not been described, but the lambda VI subclass is always associated with amyloidosis, suggesting that this subclass of immunoglobulin light chain is uniquely predisposed to fibrillar confirmation.[11]

Other evidence of the intrinsic amyloidogenicity of certain light chains occurs when immunoglobulin light chains from humans are injected into mice. If the source of the light chain is a urinary Bence Jones protein from a patient with multiple myeloma, amyloid deposits do not develop. However, the light chains extracted from the urine of patients with amyloidosis will form amyloid deposits composed of those immunoglobulin light chains in mice.[12]

Other indirect evidence for a structural predisposition to amyloidogenesis is the fact that multiple myeloma and monoclonal gammopathy κ-immunoglobulin light chains account for two-thirds of the immunoglobulin proteins. In amyloidosis, λ immunoglobulin light chains represent three-fourths of the deposits, suggesting that λ light chains, as a whole, have a greater tendency to an amyloid confirmation.[13]

Patients with amyloidosis can also be subclassified into those with and without multiple myeloma. Typical criteria for multiple myeloma define its presence as the presence of lytic bone disease, multiple skeletal compression fractures, renal insufficiency due to myeloma cast nephropathy, not due to glomerular proteinuria, and significant plasmacytosis in the bone marrow. Overt symptomatic multiple myeloma is uncommon in AL and accounts for <10% of all patients. However, significant plasmacytosis of 20%-30% occurs in nearly 25% of patients. These patients generally do not share clinical features of patients with overt multiple myeloma. If a patient does not present with multiple myeloma when amyloidosis is diagnosed, the likelihood of subsequent myeloma is only 1 in 250.[14] The incidence of amyloidosis is eight per million per year, one-quarter of the incidence of multiple myeloma.[15] The median age of all amyloidosis patients seen in Olmsted County is 72 years. In summary, amyloidosis is a plasma cell dyscrasia with a small clonal number of plasma cells in the bone marrow, averaging 7%. Confusion with multiple myeloma is common, and proteinuria is seen in myeloma as well as amyloidosis. Primary therapy is directed against the plasma cell proliferative process.

DIAGNOSING AMYLOIDOSIS

The symptoms of amyloidosis are nonspecific and often result in multiple medical evaluations and consultations before an accurate diagnosis is established. The median age of AL is 72, but patients as young as 26 have been reported. One percent of patients are younger than age 40. Two-thirds of patients are men, suggesting a true male predisposition for this disorder for unknown reasons. This is in contrast to multiple myeloma where men account for 52% of patients. The most common symptoms seen in patients with AL are fatigue and weight loss. These are nonspecific complaints and are generally not helpful at arriving at an appropriate differential diagnosis that would include AL.[16] Many patients are investigated for occult malignancy and undergo extensive imaging, which is rarely helpful in this disorder unless significant hepatomegaly is present.[17] The most common cause of fatigue in amyloidosis has a cardiac basis, but the usual signs of heart disease (cardiomegaly on the chest radiograph, echocardiographic evidence of a reduced ejection fracture) are absent, so it is easy to incorrectly assume that there is no cardiac basis for the fatigue.[18] Patients frequently have lightheadedness. This is usually caused by orthostatic hypotension, a consequence of a reduced plasma volume in patients with nephrotic syndrome, or a reduced stroke volume in patients with restriction to diastolic blood flow into the myocardium. Syncope is often found in patients who have significant cardiac or renal amyloid and is also seen in those patients who have autonomic failure and defective regulatory contraction of the arterial wall upon standing.[19]

Just as the symptoms of amyloidosis are vague and nonspecific, the physical findings are insensitive. The most common are lower extremity edema, which hardly would call amyloidosis to mind. Periorbital purpura is diagnostic but is only seen in 15% of patients and often presents only as small petechial eruptions on the eyelids. We have seen patients misdiagnosed with "autoimmune

ophthalmopathy" or an indeterminate coagulation disorder when this represents vascular purpura, which in the old parlance was referred to as pinch purpura. The purpura is always above the nipple line involving eyelids, face, and webbing of the neck. We have seen dramatic purpura precipitated by endoscopic procedures, transesophageal echocardiography, and a simple spasm of coughing. Hepatomegaly is found in 15%-20% of patients, usually no greater than 5 cm below the right costal margin. This finding is usually taken as a sign of malignancy rather than a clue to amyloidosis.[20]

Enlargement of the tongue occurs and is diagnostic. Nonetheless, we have seen patients evaluated for acromegaly and carcinoma of the tongue. Biopsy of the tongue is exceedingly painful owing to the highly enriched sensory nerve plexus in the tongue. Macroglossia is often overlooked because the base of the tongue tends to enlarge before the anterior two-thirds, resulting in dental indentations on the underside of the tongue, which can be missed. The enlargement of the base of the tongue causes prominent submandibular salivary glands. These have been misdiagnosed as lymph nodes and biopsied, but without Congo red staining will be diagnosed as reactive. Occasional patients with amyloidosis present with symptoms of jaw claudication,[21] and temporal arteritis is diagnosed without a biopsy.[22] Empiric trials of corticosteroids result in no improvement. Vascular amyloid has been known to produce calf, shoulder, and buttock claudication. Very rarely, skeletal muscle pseudohypertrophy develops because of periarticular amyloid infiltration, the so-called shoulder-pad sign.[23] Dry mouth due to amyloid infiltration of the minor salivary glands is common. Sjögren's syndrome can be misdiagnosed.[24]

CLASSIFYING AMYLOIDOSIS

It is important that a patient seen with biopsy proof of amyloid deposits is not assumed to have systemic amyloidosis, and once systemic amyloidosis is confirmed, it should not be assumed that it is AL without specific confirmation. Ninety-nine percent of patients with AL will have a detectable monoclonal light chain in the serum or urine by immunofixation or an abnormal immunoglobulin free light chain ratio. Virtually all will have clonal populations of plasma cells in the bone marrow, by immunohistochemistry or immunofluorescence.[25] When immunohistochemistry is strongly positive, it confirms the light chain nature of amyloid, but a negative result does not exclude AL for two reasons.[26] The first is that commercially available antisera tend to recognize epitopes on the constant portion of the heavy and light chains. These epitopes frequently are not present in the amyloid subunit, which tends to represent the N-terminal fragment of the light chain. Therefore, commercially available antisera may not correctly identify deposits of AL. The second is that when an immunoglobulin light chain transforms from its native α-helical confirmation to the amyloid β-pleated sheet, previously exposed epitopes may no longer be available after the completion of the abnormal protein folding. A negative test does not exclude the diagnosis.

If a patient has no evidence of a plasma cell dyscrasia, they may have localized amyloidosis, or they may have systemic amyloidosis that is not AL in origin.[27] Localized amyloidosis is frequently recognized on the basis of the anatomic distribution of the amyloid deposits. When amyloid is recognized in the bladder, ureter, urethra, or renal pelvis, it is most likely to be localized genitourinary amyloid, and these patients are not candidates for systemic therapy. Other sites that are well recognized to be associated with localized disease include the larynx, vocal cords, and tracheobronchial tree. These patients do not benefit from systemic therapy, although reports of external beam radiation for localized tracheobronchial amyloid are in the literature.[28] Solitary pulmonary nodules that are usually resected to exclude malignancy can be pure amyloid[29] deposits and are not pulmonary plasmacytomas with exuberant amyloid production. These tend to be localized. Caution is required because diffuse interstitial pulmonary amyloid, which is a form of systemic AL, is well recognized. Many patients with cutaneous amyloid can have a localized form of amyloid, a consequence of the generation of keratin protein into β-pleated sheet conformation. It should be kept in mind that, in patients with AL proven to be systemic, skin biopsies will be positive in the majority of patients, so caution is required when making the distinction. Recently, localized amyloid deposits of the stomach and bowel have been reported.[30] It is known that rectal biopsies are positive in 80% of patients with systemic amyloid, and endoscopic gastric biopsies are positive in nearly 100%. As a consequence, the finding of a positive intestinal biopsy containing amyloid does not, in and of itself, clarify whether the amyloidosis is localized or systemic,

and further diagnostic investigation is required to make the distinction. Localized AL amyloid never becomes systemic.

One can be more certain when a patient presents with nephrotic syndrome, restrictive cardiomyopathy, and/or small fiber peripheral neuropathy that the amyloidosis is systemic in origin. A plasma cell dyscrasia must be recognized before confirming that the amyloid is AL in origin. If no monoclonal protein can be found in the serum or urine and no clonal population of plasma cells can be found in the bone marrow, the possibility of systemic AA or AF amyloidosis must be considered. AA is rare in the Western hemisphere with the widespread use of antibiotics but still can be seen in long-standing symmetric polyarthropathies, which include ankylosing spondylitis, psoriatic arthritis, and juvenile rheumatoid arthritis. These patients tend to have a long-standing history of an inflammatory arthropathy that can be present for 15 years before the development of renal amyloidosis.[31] The kidney is the target organ in the majority of patients with secondary amyloidosis. Secondary amyloidosis associated with tuberculosis, osteomyelitis, and inflammatory bowel disease is rare in the Western hemisphere. Patients with Castleman disease have been diagnosed with secondary amyloidosis, and this must be kept in mind when seeing a patient with nephrotic syndrome, amyloid in the kidney, and no plasma cell dyscrasia. In less well-developed countries, the presence of chronic infections including tuberculosis and leprosy makes AA an ongoing therapeutic challenge. Since there is only one amino acid sequence for AA, the commercially available antisera are quite good, and negative staining can usually exclude secondary amyloidosis from the differential diagnosis.

Familial amyloidosis is a greater diagnostic challenge. A family history is absent in over half of patients, and the absence of a family history cannot be used as an exclusion of the diagnosis and AF must be considered in those who do not have an obvious plasma cell dyscrasia. The clinical presentations of AF are quite similar to those of AL. Patients may present with progressive peripheral neuropathy.[32] These patients typically have a mutant transthyretin.[33] Amyloid nephrotic syndrome can be caused by mutations in the fibrinogen-A α chain. Hepatic amyloidosis due to lysozyme mutations[34] also exist, as do mutations of apolipoprotein A-I and A-II. The organ involvement and clinical phenotype are often indistinguishable from AL. Since monoclonal gammopathies in the serum are relatively common and are seen in 4% of patients 65 years and over, the question of familial amyloidosis with an incidental monoclonal gammopathy must be considered versus true AL.[35] We currently screen all new patients for mutations in exons 2-4 of the transthyretin gene.

An important form of amyloidosis is native transthyretin amyloidosis, formerly called senile systemic amyloidosis. This disorder manifests as cardiac amyloidosis in elderly patients. The echocardiographic criteria can be indistinguishable from AL.[36] These patients present with restrictive cardiomyopathy and mild to moderate congestive heart failure. Endomyocardial biopsy demonstrates typical amyloid deposits. The deposits tend to exhibit strong immunohistochemical staining with transthyretin, but no mutation is found with TTR gene sequencing.[37] A plasma cell dyscrasia does not exist. Patients with senile systemic amyloidosis have an inherently better prognosis, although no specific treatment is available. Remarkably, the extent of amyloid infiltration in the myocardium in TTR amyloidosis can produce septal thickness in excess of 20 mm. This finding is rare in cardiac AL since patients will usually succumb when the amyloid becomes that extensive. This suggests other mechanisms for the cardiac failure besides the amount of amyloid deposited in the myocardial wall.

AMYLOID SYNDROMES

There are dozens of possible clinical presentations for AL, but if a clinician is alert to the five most common, the majority of patients can be diagnosed with a simple algorithm.[38] The five most common presentations in decreasing order of frequency are as follows: nephrotic range proteinuria with or without renal insufficiency, restrictive cardiomyopathy with or without clinical congestive heart failure, unexplained hepatomegaly, progressive mixed axonal and demyelinating peripheral neuropathy, and atypical multiple myeloma (Table 10.2). When a patient is seen with a specific renal, cardiac, hepatic, or peripheral nerve presentation, the initial screening should include immunofixation of serum and urine and an immunoglobulin free light chain test.[39] By definition, all AL patients have a light chain producing clone of plasma cells; therefore, finding a monoclonal immunoglobulin protein is a powerful diagnostic clue. Since most patients with amyloidosis do not have an intact immunoglobulin in the serum, electrophoresis

TABLE 10.2 Syndromes in primary amyloidosis

Syndrome	Patients (%)
Nephrotic or nephrotic and renal failure	30
Hepatomegaly	24
Congestive heart failure	22
Carpal tunnel syndrome	21
Neuropathy	17
Orthostatic hypotension	12

alone is insufficient, and since the size of M-spikes are generally 0.5 g or less, the electrophoretic pattern will not be sufficiently sensitive to detect a peak. As a consequence, immunofixation of serum and urine and the more sensitive immunoglobulin free light chain assay is necessary for detection. Serum immunofixation is abnormal in 69% of amyloidosis patients. Urine immunofixation detects the light chain in 83% of patients. Combining serum and urine immunofixation will reveal an abnormal protein in 95%. The free light chain ratio will be abnormal in 91%, and when combining all three tests, 99% of patients will have a detectable immunoglobulin light chain abnormality.[40] The electrophoretic pattern of the urinary protein is helpful in distinguishing amyloidosis from multiple myeloma. Most myeloma patients have light chains detectable in the urine but actually have scant amounts of albumin. The electrophoretic pattern will show little or no albumin, with a discrete monoclonal peak in the β or γ region. On the contrary, amyloidosis has a very nonspecific urinary protein pattern. The electrophoresis looks similar to an ultrafiltration of the serum with a dominant albumin peak, and only occasionally will there be a discrete monoclonal peak seen in the urine. The excretion of large amounts of globulin in the urine often obscures the small amounts of free monoclonal light chain that may be present. The light chain can only be detected using immunofixation. The immunoglobulin free light chain assay has not been reliable for measurement of urinary light chain, and urinary light chain measurements should be considered to lack sensitivity. The introduction of the immunoglobulin free light chain has been important in amyloid diagnosis, prognosis, and assessment of therapy response.[41] Amyloidosis tends to be "nonsecretory" in a far greater proportion than patients with multiple myeloma. The immunoglobulin free light chain has reduced this to the 1% level,[42] and an abnormal free light chain ratio is not only consistent with AL amyloid but is also predictive of outcome[43] and is useful in assessing the impact of therapeutic interventions. The specificity of the free light chain test is high because most patients with AA and AF have normal free light chain ratios.[44]

DIAGNOSTIC CONFIRMATION OF AMYLOIDOSIS

The diagnosis of amyloidosis requires the demonstration of congophilic deposits in biopsy tissues. It is possible to confirm the diagnosis in renal, cardiac, hepatic, or peripheral nerve amyloid by performing direct biopsy of these organs. However, there is some risk associated with visceral biopsies in patients with amyloid as a consequence of impaired vascular integrity and acquired coagulopathy seen in these patients. So, if it is possible to perform a biopsy that is less invasive, it is preferable. Amyloid deposits can be demonstrated in vivo by scanning with radiolabeled amyloid-P component or aprotinin.[45] Amyloid deposits uniformly contain amyloid-P component, comprising 10% of the amyloid fibril by weight. The scans are highly specific for amyloid deposits, are incapable of recognizing trace deposits, and do poorly at visualizing cardiac amyloid deposits owing to the circulating blood pool. Although immensely helpful for monitoring the activity of the disease, the scan is not a substitute for histologic confirmation of the diagnosis.

Fortunately at diagnosis, amyloidosis is widespread through the vascular system. Any biopsy tissue that contains vascular structures will show endothelial amyloid deposits even when there is no clinical suspicion of amyloid at those sites. Common sources of amyloid in asymptomatic individuals include the minor salivary glands of the lip,[46] the skin, and the rectum. Salivary gland biopsies can show deposits in 85%. The rectal biopsy is positive in 80%. Upper endoscopic biopsies have been performed in patients with familial amyloidosis, with sensitivities approaching 100%.[47]

The practice at Mayo Clinic is to obtain simultaneous biopsies from the bone marrow and the subcutaneous fat.[48] Both will be positive in 55% of patients. The fat only will be positive in 22%, the marrow only in 10%, and both will be negative in 13%. Both of these procedures have the advantage that they carry minimal risk, bleeding is not an issue, and results are available in 24-48 h. Most patients require a bone marrow in any case to quantify the number of plasma cells and exclude multiple myeloma. In the remaining 13%

of patients, direct biopsy must be performed if the index of suspicion is high. Renal biopsies are particularly useful since electron microscopy can routinely be performed to determine whether fibrils are present, and immunoelectron microscopy has been used to permit accurate typing of the amyloid fibril. Equivocally, positive stains should be interpreted with caution because weak, nonspecific histologic staining may be seen. An enzyme-linked immunoabsorbent assay has been used to classify amyloidosis on fat biopsy specimens.[49] The type of amyloid was successfully characterized in 14 out of 15 positive fat biopsies. Difficulties in confirming amyloidosis by fat aspiration include interpretation of the Congo red stain due to pale staining of amyloid fibrils and collagen birefringence. In a large study, the fat aspirate was positive in 93% of patients, with a specificity of 100% in 45 controls. The additional value of a subsequent rectal biopsy in patients who had a negative fat aspirate was negligible.[47]

PROGNOSIS

When a patient presents with a syndrome compatible with amyloidosis, is found to have a monoclonal protein consistent with AL, and has histologic confirmation of the diagnosis, assessment of prognosis is the next step. Virtually all patients with amyloidosis succumb because of complications of cardiac involvement. This can be either progressive cardiomyopathy with intractable congestive heart failure or sudden death that can be mediated by ventricular fibrillation, ventricular systole, or unrecognized pulmonary emboli originating from thrombi in the left atrial appendage.[50]

The assessment of cardiac involvement in the 1960s and 1970s was primarily by clinical criteria—the presence of cardiomegaly on the chest radiograph; signs of impaired left ventricular filling; interstitial edema on the radiograph; and on the right side, elevated jugular venous pulse with typical clinical features of PND and orthopnea. This relatively crude method of assessing for cardiac involvement suggested that cardiac involvement was present in 20% of patients with a median survival of 3 to 6 months. In the 1980s and 1990s, clinical assessment was supplanted by two-dimensional echocardiography with Doppler.[51] This far more sensitive technique recognized cardiac involvement in nearly half of the patients by thickening of the interventricular septum and left ventricular free wall and Doppler studies that showed a reduced velocity of inflow during diastole. Most recently, strain echocardiography has enhanced the sensitivity of detection of impaired relaxation and contractility.[52] A deceleration time of 150 ms or less on Doppler echocardiography reflects restrictive physiology, and these patients have a 1-year survival probability of 49% versus 92% for those patients with a deceleration time >150 ms.

Echocardiography, however, may not be the most sensitive technique. In amyloidosis, the ejection fraction is preserved until late in the diagnosis. Most of the dysfunction is related to poor diastolic relaxation resulting in poor filling, low-end diastolic volumes, and low stroke volumes. The ejection fraction, however, is preserved. Significant dysfunction can be overlooked. In the past 5 years, the value of cardiac biomarkers in identifying patients with cardiac amyloidosis has come into routine use. The serum level of cardiac troponin has been shown to have a profound impact on survival, both in conventionally treated patients and in patients receiving high-dose therapy. It has been suggested that patients with troponin levels that are 0.06 ng/mL or greater are no longer suitable candidates for high-dose therapy owing to a high early mortality. Patients can be reliably separated into two prognostic groups by the level of serum troponin < 0.1 ng/mL and >0.1 ng/mL. The measurement of serum troponin has now become a routine evaluation for all newly diagnosed patients with amyloidosis.[53] The cardiac biomarker, brain natriuretic peptide (BNP), is a protein secreted into the serum when cardiac filling pressure increases, and it has also been shown to be an important prognostic variable for identifying cardiac amyloidosis. The BNP is so specific that normal levels generally indicate the absence of cardiac amyloidosis (Figure 10.1).

The troponin and the BNP can be combined into a staging system for amyloidosis with three stages where both are normal, both are abnormal, or only one of the two levels are abnormal. This results in groups of approximately equal size with vastly different prognosis: 26.4 months median for stage 1, 10.5 months for stage 2, and 3.5 months for stage 3.[54] In a multivariate analysis, the cardiac troponin T has a risk of death hazard ratio of 2.0 compared to the number of organ systems involved, which has a risk of 2.3. The cardiac troponin T, however, is more reproducible than the number of organ systems involved since it is oftentimes difficult to estimate whether an organ

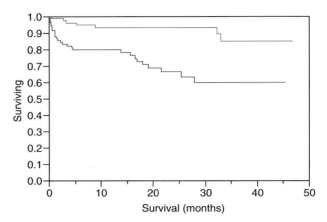

Figure 10.1. Survival of patients transplanted. The red line indicates patients with a BNP of <170 pg/mL. The blue line represents those with a BNP > 170 pg/mL. p = 0.001.

is involved. If the echocardiogram is equivocal or one cannot differentiate hepatic congestion due to high right-sided filling pressures from hepatic infiltration, organ involvement is uncertain. The serum β_2-microglobulin has a weak impact on survival with a hazard ratio of 1.2.[55]

When interpreting studies, there is always the risk of referral bias. Although the average of patients with amyloidosis in Olmsted County is 72 years, the median age of patients referred to the Mayo Clinic is 64, reflecting the increased willingness of younger patients to travel to a referral center. In addition, when patients are seen within 30 days of diagnosis, their median survival is 13 months compared to all patients seen where the median survival is 2 years, suggesting again a bias favoring patients physically able to travel to an amyloidosis treatment center.

Patients who present with isolated peripheral neuropathy appear to have a better prognosis than other patients. The median survival is 3 years. The level of the immunoglobulin free light chain is prognostic in patients having a stem cell transplantation. The higher the baseline free light chain level, the higher the risk of death. There is also a correlation between the free light chain level and the serum troponin T level. The suspicion is that high free light chain levels are associated with more advanced disease. Moreover, the absolute level of the free light chain achieved after high-dose therapy is predictive of survival. A hematologic complete response is predictive of an organ response. Normalization of the free light chain level is predictive of an organ response, and survival is better than

TABLE 10.3. Criteria for amyloid-related organ responses to treatment*

Response	Progression
Heart	
Decrease of ≥2 mm in mean left ventricular wall thickness from baseline thickness > 11 mm	Increase ≥ 2 mm in wall thickness
Two class improvement in NYHA class	Two class worsening in NYHA class
Kidneys	
Decrease of >50% in daily proteinuria without progressive renal insufficiency	Increase of >50% in daily proteinuria
	Progressive renal insufficiency
Liver	
A decrease in liver span of >50%	An increase in liver span of >25%
A concomitant decrease of alkaline phosphatase by 50%	An increase of alkaline phosphatase by 50%
Nervous system	
Autonomic: normalization of orthostatic vital signs and symptoms, resolution of gastric atony	Autonomic: progression of orthostatic vital signs and symptoms, increasing gastric atony
Peripheral neuropathy: resolution of symptoms	Peripheral neuropathy: progression of symptoms

*If organ function neither improves nor worsens, it is graded as stable.
Source: NYHA, New York Heart Association.

those patients who have a 50% reduction and substantially better than those who fail to show evidence of a light chain response.[56] The free light chain level should be measured serially in patients undergoing therapy for amyloidosis.

Unintentional weight loss occurs in over half the patients with amyloidosis. The percentage of weight loss is significantly greater in patients with cardiac involvement. The serum albumin has also been demonstrated to be a measure of survival, presumably reflecting the patients' nutritional status. Malnutrition is known to be prominent in AL patients, and nutritional variables associated with survival should be part of the clinical assessment.[57]

ASSESSING RESPONSE IN AMYLOIDOSIS

Familiarity with the response criteria in amyloidosis patients is helpful in interpreting the data on therapy. Responses in amyloidosis can be organ based or hematologic. Consensus criteria exist for response in amyloidosis, including response criteria for each specific visceral organ (Table 10.3). These response criteria are time dependent, often taking more than a year to be achieved, so specific time end points are, by their nature, inaccurate. Assessment of amyloid peripheral neuropathy, soft tissue

amyloid, and pulmonary amyloid are exceedingly difficult and notoriously unreliable.[58]

Hematologic responses are very similar to those reported for multiple myeloma patients, and hematologic response requires a 50% reduction in the size of the M protein when measurable or in the amount of involved immunoglobulin light chain. Bone marrow assessment is not required to assess outcome since the number of plasma cells are small to begin with, and visual estimates of a 50% reduction would be inherently unreliable. It has been demonstrated that patients who fulfill these response criteria have a longer survival than nonresponders, and this is true even when corrected for early treatment-related mortality by a landmark analysis.[56] Patients who have a free light chain level > 10 mcg/mL can be serially monitored for hematologic response. For those patients who are <10 mcg/mL, it is a bit more difficult to be certain that a 50% reduction is a true reduction in tumor mass rather than variability of the test itself. A complete response requires immunofixation negativity of the serum and urine, and a normalization of the free light chain level and its ratio. From a clinical standpoint, patients have the greatest benefit when their response is organ based. Our experience suggested that those patients who have an organ-defined response almost invariably had a hematologic response, although it does not necessarily have to be a complete response. For patients who have light chains that are not highly amyloidogenic, it is conceivable that moderate reductions in precursor protein level (the light chain) can shift the equilibrium from fibril deposition to resolubilization of the light chain, which ultimately can lead to improvement in organ function.

TREATMENT OF AMYLOIDOSIS

Supportive care

Because mortality in amyloidosis is so heavily dependent on the degree of cardiac involvement, managing cardiac symptomatology and physiology is an important part of supportive care. The cornerstone of supportive management of cardiac amyloidosis is diuretic therapy.[59] Orthostatic hypotension with intravascular volume contraction from nephrotic syndrome can limit the ability to administer adequate doses of diuretics.[60] Recurrent syncope can benefit from the implantation of a pacemaker. The role of an implantable cardiac defibrillator in amyloidosis has not been thoroughly investigated. Afterload reduction with angiotensin converting enzyme inhibitors is a standard in the management of heart failure, but the high frequency of hypotension makes administration of therapeutic doses challenging. Calcium channel blockers have been reported to aggravate the heart failure associated with amyloidosis. β-Blockers are used to reduce the heart rate and, therefore, improve diastolic filling time, but the impact on contractility can exacerbate symptoms in patients with AL. Cardiac transplantation has been used to manage AL. Long-term survivors have been reported. A select group of patients underwent cardiac transplantation followed by high-dose chemotherapy with stem cell reconstitution in an effort to prevent recurrent amyloid deposits. This was performed in five patients, and after a median follow-up of 95 months, three patients were well without evidence of recurrent cardiac amyloid, and two died of progressive amyloidosis 33 and 90 months after heart transplantation with hematologic relapse of their plasma cell dyscrasia.[61]

Supportive care for renal amyloid includes the use of diuretics. The continuous urinary protein loss related to the glomerular amyloid deposits will result in end-stage renal failure if not impacted by therapeutic intervention. The median time from the diagnosis of renal amyloidosis to dialysis is 14 months.[62] Median survival from the start of dialysis is 8 months, with cardiac failure being the most common cause of death. Dialyzing patients with end-stage renal disease in AL can be difficult since the concomitant cardiac amyloid leads to dialysis-induced hypotension. The survival of patients with AL end-stage renal disease is shorter compared to patients who dialyzed because of a primary renal disorder. In 61 patients with amyloidosis, 18 died within a month after starting dialysis and 15 out of 43 were alive at a median of 61 months. Patients with renal AL have been transplanted.[63] It is unclear whether it is better to administer high-dose chemotherapy with stem cell transplantation before a renal transplant or to perform it after a renal transplant. Patients who receive a kidney before receiving high-dose chemotherapy tolerate the transplant better, but because of concomitant antirejection therapy are at higher risk of peritransplant infections. In patients who have received a kidney and do not achieve a complete response after transplant, there is a significant risk of recurrent amyloid in the allograft. In one group of 15 patients who had renal transplantation from 42 to 216 months after diagnosis, there were 10 in whom the underlying amyloid had been treated first and they remain stable. Amyloid in the graft was identified in 4 out of 10; and in all four, the precursor protein had not been diminished. Where chemotherapy resulted in eradication of the free light chain in two, both have normal renal function after more than 4 years of follow-up.[64] Sequential heart and stem cell transplantation has also been applied to patients with amyloidosis.[65]

CHEMOTHERAPY FOR AMYLOIDOSIS

Alkylating agents

Since most patients are not candidates for high-dose therapy followed by stem cell transplantation, lower intensity chemotherapy is necessary. Melphalan-based therapy combined with prednisone has been used for amyloidosis for more than 30 years. It provides a survival advantage with very low toxicity. The median survival for patients receiving melphalan-containing regimens is 17 months compared to 8.5 months for colchicine alone.[66] Virtually any patient with amyloidosis would tolerate appropriate dosing of melphalan and prednisone. Therefore, virtually all patients are candidates for a therapeutic trial, and although the response rates are low, approximately 20%, it would be inappropriate to deny a therapeutic trial for most patients.

Dexamethasone

Nine patients with biopsy-proven AL were treated with dexamethasone followed by maintenance interferon.[67] Improvement in at least one organ was seen in eight of nine, and in the seven with nephrotic range proteinuria, the proteinuria decreased in six. Time to response was rapid at a median of 4 months, and the responses were durable. In follow-up of two cohorts of patients from Mayo Clinic, dexamethasone as a single agent produced a 10% 10-year survival rate.[68,69] A lower dose and frequency of dexamethasone administration that is better tolerated produces responses in 35% of patients, again with a median time of 4 months.[70] A Southwest Oncology Group Cooperative Trial enrolled 93 patients with AL receiving induction with dexamethasone followed by maintenance interferon.[71] Complete hematologic responses were seen in 24%. Improved organ function was seen in 45%. The median survival was 31%, with a 2-year overall survival of 60%. Predictors of adverse outcomes were heart failure and serum β_2-microglobulin levels. Dexamethasone as a single agent can produce reversal of amyloid-related organ dysfunction.

Melphalan and dexamethasone

The group from Pavia, Italy, has reported on the use of melphalan plus high-dose dexamethasone in the management of amyloidosis. All patients were selected on the basis of ineligibility for high-dose melphalan and stem cell transplantation. Of 46 patients, a hematologic response was seen in 31, and a hematologic complete response was seen in 15 (33%). Improvement in organ function was seen in 22 patients (48%). The 100-day mortality was only 4%, and cardiac failure resolved in 6 of 32 patients.[72] The median time to response was 4.5 months, and only 11% showed adverse effects. A 5-year update of these results was recently published, and the outcomes were maintained.[73] Projected survival with follow-ups in excess of four years gave a median overall survival of nearly 6 years, and a progression-free survival median of almost 4 years. Median survival for the 30 responders has not been reached and was just over 2 years in the 11 nonresponding patients.

IMIDS

After it was demonstrated to have high activity in the treatment of multiple myeloma, thalidomide was used in the management of amyloidosis as a single agent and in combination with dexamethasone. In a protocol of 12 patients who received thalidomide, 8 had renal and 4 had cardiac involvement.[74] Ten patients had previous stem cell transplantation. The median maximal tolerated dose of thalidomide was 500 mg. This dose appears to be excessively high in amyloid patients. No patient had more than a 50% reduction in M component value. Three had disease progression. In a study from Mayo Clinic, significant toxicity was seen.[75] The median time on thalidomide was only 72 days with a median dose of 50 mg. When combined with dexamethasone as second-line treatment for AL, thalidomide produced a hematologic response in 48%, complete responses in 19%, a median time to response of 3.6 months, but severe adverse effects were seen in 65% and symptomatic bradycardia in 26%.[76] Thalidomide is not as well tolerated as it is in patients with myeloma, has serious adverse effects, and the median tolerated dose is between 50 and 100 mg.

Lenalidomide, a thalidomide analog with greater antiangiogenic potency, has been reported from two groups. In one, 8 out of 13 had a measurable response, 4 to lenalidomide alone.[77] Nine additional patients responded when dexamethasone was added. In a Mayo Clinic study, 22 patients were treated. However, only 12 were evaluable for response.[78] Only one patient had a response to lenalidomide alone. The remainder required the addition of dexamethasone, but in this cohort, the overall response rate was 83%. Of interest, the cardiac troponin T was predictive of which patients would succumb to their disease before becoming evaluable for a response and also predicted those that would be able to tolerate 4 months of induction therapy. Cardiac troponin T may be an important criteria for protocol eligibility in future studies.

Bortezomib

The proteasome inhibitor bortezomib has been reported by two groups for activity in AL amyloidosis. The National Amyloidosis Research Center in Great Britain reported on 18 patients with relapsed amyloidosis.[79] Hematologic responses were seen in 14 for an overall response rate of 77%. There were three complete responses (16%), 11 partial responses (61%), and five organ responses (27%). An abstract from the Princess Margaret Hospital also reported on bortezomib therapy for patients in a phase I-II design.[80] The ultimate dose was 1.6 mg/m^2 on days 1, 4, 8, and 11. The Greek Myeloma Study Group reported 18 patients who were treated with bortezomib and dexamethasone. Ninety-four percent had a hematologic response, and 44% had a complete hematologic response, including five patients who had not responded to prior high-dose dexamethasone alone. Five patients (28%) had a response in at least one affected organ, with a median time to hematologic response of 0.9 months. The schedule of bortezomib was typical: 1.3 mg/m^2 on days 1, 4, 8, 11 and dexamethasone 40 mg for 4 days every 21 days with a maximum of six cycles.[81]

ORGAN TRANSPLANTATION

Cardiac transplantation followed by stem cell transplantation to suppress the light chain production and delay recurrence of disease was reported in five patients with AL and dominant cardiomyopathy. The patients were followed for a median of 95 months after diagnosis, and three of the five were well without evidence of cardiac amyloid.[61] Two patients died of progressive amyloidosis at 33 and 90 months, respectively, after heart transplantation. At Mayo Clinic, 11 patients had stem cell transplant following a heart transplant for amyloid cardiomyopathy. Median survival for the entire group is 76 months.[65] Five of the eleven patients remain alive. Five-year survival is 80%.

STEM CELL TRANSPLANTATION

Indications for stem cell transplantation

Given the results obtained with stem cell transplantation in multiple myeloma with improved complete response rates and improved median survival in randomized studies, it was inevitable that the technique would be applied to patients with amyloidosis. Patients who have a hematologic malignancy and who receive a transplant have significant bone marrow dysfunction usually manifest by cytopenias. These patients generally have adequate visceral function with normal renal, hepatic, cardiac, and pulmonary functions, and most transplant protocols require that these organs have adequate reserve before considering myeloablative chemotherapy. Patients with amyloidosis present with the opposite findings. These patients are generally normal hematologically. Anemia is uncommon in the absence of active bleeding or renal insufficiency, but amyloidosis patients regularly have cardiac, hepatic, renal, and neuropathic problems that uniquely distinguish them from other groups of patients receiving high-dose chemotherapy.[82]

The current therapeutic approach to treatment at Mayo Clinic is to stratify patients on the basis of their eligibility for stem cell transplantation. Patients with an adequate performance status (Eastern Cooperative Oncology Group 0-2), no major comorbidities, less than three organs significantly involved, and no greater than moderate cardiac amyloidosis are offered participation in a phase 3 clinical trial of melphalan/dexamethasone compared with stem cell transplant. Patients who decline randomization but are otherwise eligible are offered high-dose therapy with stem cell transplantation. Amyloidosis appears to be an ideal model for stem cell transplantation because the patients with multiple myeloma who have the best outcomes appear to have the lowest tumor burden[83] pretransplant and have indolent plasma cell kinetics (low percentage of cells in S phase), features that are typical of patients with AL. In multiple myeloma, however, treatment-related mortality rates should not exceed 1%-2%. Because of amyloidosis-related widespread organ dysfunction, reported mortalities can range from 6% to 27% related to a wide range of complications including renal, cardiac, and hepatic failure.

Of the first 270 AL patients treated at Mayo Clinic, 59% were men with a median age of 57. Ten percent of patients had a serum creatinine > 1.8 mg/dL, and 75% had a creatinine that was 1.3 mg/dL or less. The serum albumin level median was 2.8 and represents the high proportion of patients who have nephrotic range proteinuria. Urine protein excretion was in the nephrotic range (>3 g) in 54% of patients. The percentage of patients with one-, two-, and three-organ involvement was 48%, 38%, and 14%, respectively. Alkaline phosphatase, a surrogate marker for liver involvement, was twice the normal level in 19% of patients.[82]

There is no evidence that induction therapy after diagnosis improves outcomes after high-dose therapy, and one study of pretransplant melphalan and prednisone did not result in improved outcomes.[84] Therefore, patients are regularly collected and transplanted immediately after diagnosis. At Mayo Clinic, the median time from diagnosis to day 0 of the transplant is 4.2 months; 25% are transplanted within 3 months, and 75% within 7 months of diagnosis. All patients who are transplanted have biopsy-verified amyloidosis, with liver, endoscopic, cardiac, and renal biopsies positive in over 95% of patients, bone marrow amyloid deposits demonstrable in 75%, and subcutaneous fat in 71%. Cardiac amyloid was seen in 51% of patients defined by echocardiography. The median septal thickness was 12 mm but was <14 mm in 75%, suggesting that this cohort has milder cardiac involvement than groups of patients with amyloidosis at large. The median ejection fraction was 65% but was <60% in 25% of the entire patient group.

Transplantation requires the mobilization of peripheral blood progenitor cells, and this is done using growth factor alone.[85] The median number of aphereses is three. The median number of collected CD34 cells was 6.5 × 10^6. It is practice at Mayo Clinic not to administer growth factor after stem cell infusion on day 0 because it causes significant morbidity in terms of fluid retention. Median time to 500 neutrophils was 14 days, with a range of 7-116 days. Twenty-five percent of patients engraft before day 13, 75% by day 16, and 90% by day 22. A platelet count of 20 000 is achieved at a median of 14 days; 25%, however, achieve 20 000 by day 12, 75% by day 19, and 90% by day 28. A platelet count of 50 000 is achieved at a median of 18 days, 25% by day 14, and 75% by day 28; 90% of patients achieve 50 000 platelets by day 52. The number of CD34 cells infused is critical to safe, prompt engraftment.[86] A minimum of 3 × 10^6 CD34 cells/kg is required. If between two and three million cells are infused, the time to engraftment is significantly longer.

The standard conditioning chemotherapy for transplant is melphalan as a single agent. In the Mayo cohort, 62% received melphalan 200 mg/m², 26% melphalan at 140 mg/m², and the remainder lower doses due to advanced cardiac amyloid, advanced age, or elevated creatinine.

The intensity of chemotherapy administered is critical to outcome. Patients receiving full-dose melphalan have better outcomes than patients who are transplanted at a lower dose.[87] The day-100 mortality at Mayo Clinic is 11%. Achieving a low day-100 mortality is important since it would be impossible to demonstrate any benefit of the technique if up-front treatment-related deaths are high. In the Mayo group, the median actuarial survival is 75 months. Mortality rates are declining with time. Before 2004, 12% of stem cell recipients at Mayo died by day 100, but it has now fallen to 9.3%. The cause of death in patients transplanted before day 100 include ventricular tachycardia, refractory cardiac failure, multiorgan failure following oliguric renal failure, and exsanguinating hemorrhage associated with factor X deficiency. The median duration of hospitalization for patients is 9 days, but 18% of patients are never hospitalized, and 75% are hospitalized for durations of 17 days or less. Patients who received an infusion of less than three million CD34 cells per/kg did not achieve a platelet count of 20 000 until a median of 25 days; 75% reached 20 000 platelets by 33 days; 75% achieved a platelet count of 50 000 by 70 days. This is significantly longer compared to patients who received an infusion of more than 3 × 10^6 CD34 cells that achieved 50 000 platelets at a median of 18 days and 75% by 27 days.[87] The number of stem cells infused, however, had no impact on the median hospital duration (11.5 versus 8 days, p = NS). Bacteremia was documented in 45% of all patients, although 28% of these patients, or 80, had a coagulase-negative staphylococcal bacteremia. All other bacteremias occurred in 16%. In total, 27 patients, or 10% of our entire cohort, died before day 100. However, the serum troponin level appears to predict treatment-related mortality, with 28% of 40 patients with a troponin level of 0.06 mcg/L or higher succumbing before day 100 compared to only 16 of 231 patients (7%) with a troponin level < 0.06 mcg/L. Most deaths were attributable to cardiac complications, and the pretransplant troponin may be a useful exclusionary criterion for patients that should not be considered for high-dose therapy. A risk-adapted approach where patients at higher risk are given lower doses of chemotherapy did not reduce the mortality risk in patients with elevated troponin level. Patients with high troponin levels had a reduced dose of melphalan in 78%, yet still had the unacceptably high mortality rate of 28%. Troponin T can be used in studies comparing stem cell transplant to conventional therapy by stratifying randomized arms and should be measured in all patients in the pretransplantation evaluation.

Response assessment indicates that hematologic response does translate into improved survival. Among our first 282 patients, 201 achieved a hematologic response, and 93 of these were complete.[56] Eighty-one patients were considered nonresponders. Median survival in nonresponders was only 10.3 months and has not been reached in the CR and PR group but will be >70 months. A landmark analysis performed excluding those patients who were early deaths and that could not be considered evaluable for hematologic response showed significant survival differences between hematologic complete responders and partial responders. Achievement of a hematologic response is a predictor of improved survival following stem cell transplant and should be the initial goal of therapy. These results also apply to patients with echocardiographic evidence of cardiac amyloidosis. It does not answer, however, whether patients who achieve a partial response should receive post-transplant maintenance therapy in order to attempt to achieve a complete response.[88]

The American Bone Marrow Transplant Registry reported 107 patients from 48 transplant centers with a 30-day treatment-related mortality of 18% (7.4% at day 30 at Mayo Clinic).[89] However, high response rates were reported with only 11% of patients progressing after stem cell transplantation. The median survival in this study was 47 months, with a response rate of 34% and 33% stable. The most important predictor of survival was the level of experience at the center with those having been transplanted within the past 5 years faring significantly better. This does raise a question as to whether this form of transplantation should only be performed in specialized centers with extensive experience.[90]

One may not conclude that stem cell transplantation is a superior therapy. A French Multi-Center Randomized Trial did not demonstrate a survival benefit for patients receiving high-dose therapy compared to melphalan/dexamethasone. This was a trial that randomly assigned 100 patients to either melphalan/dexamethasone or stem cell transplant. The median actuarial survivals were 56.9 and 22.2 months for melphalan/dexamethasone versus transplantation, respectively.[91] Hematologic response rates for the two groups were 65% and 64%. Median follow-up was 24 months, and the treatment-related mortality for the transplanted group was 24%. Only 26 of the 100 patients received

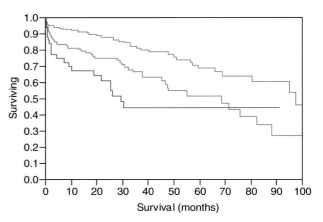

Figure 10.2. Amyloid transplant $n = 270$ survival by organ number. The red line indicates one-organ involvement; the green line, two-organ involvement; and the blue line, three-organ involvement.

the stem cell transplant and were evaluable at day 100 for response. This makes it difficult to draw firm conclusions.

Patients who are transplanted are selected since their candidacy inherently makes them better patients to begin with. At Mayo Clinic, approximately 25% of patients evaluated actually receive high-dose therapy. Patients selected for stem cell transplant but who are treated conventionally have a median survival of 45 months, reflecting their inherently better prognosis. In a case-matched control study of stem cell transplant and conventionally treated patients, stem cell transplant patients had an overall survival advantage.[92]

Factors that affect survival post-transplant include the absolute lymphocyte count at day 15 after stem cell transplant[93] and the number of organs involved in amyloidosis. Patients with two-organ involvement have a median survival of 55 months compared to 25.5 months for those patients with three-organ involvement (Figure 10.2).

The counting of organs, however, is more of an art than a science since it is often difficult to interpret the echocardiographic findings in patients with borderline wall thickening or the interpretation of an elevated alkaline phosphatase in a patient with right-sided cardiac failure. Multivariate analyses have shown that serum creatinine levels, serum troponin T, BNP, and septal thickness have all been predictive of survival following high-dose therapy.[53] Excessive fluid accumulation during mobilization and a weight gain in excess of 2% also predicts a higher mortality rate.[Leung94] BNP presumably impacts survival because of its ability to reflect the severity of cardiac failure in AL. Using a breakpoint of BNP of 170 pg/mL, a benefit was recognized for those with lower BNP levels.

Overall survival is also linked to the pretransplant free light chain level and number of organs involved.[43] As noted, treatment-related mortality ranges from 6% to 40%, hematologic responses from 15% to 60%, and organ responses from 30% to 65%. Organ responses are time dependent and can be delayed up to 36 months after transplantation.[95]

A quality-of-life questionnaire administered to patients over an 8-year period demonstrated that transplant recipients who achieved a hematologic complete response had normalization of their quality-of-life index. The treatment of AL patients with high-dose therapy produces measurable sustained improvement in quality of life, particularly for those who achieve a hematologic complete response.[96] A reduction of more than 90% in the free light chain level was associated with a similarly high likelihood of clinical improvement and prolonged survival whether or not patients achieved a complete response. Organ responses including complete resolution of nephrotic syndrome, improvement in echocardiographic evidence of amyloid, resolution of pseudo-obstruction, and regression of symptomatic peripheral neuropathy have been reported.

In one study, six patients under the age of 60 with renal amyloidosis were transplanted. One died of septicemia and five experienced severe toxicity, including a gastrointestinal perforation, and a splenic rupture. Acute renal failure developed in four, and this reflects the reality of the toxicity that can be associated with stem cell transplantation.[97]

A second autologous stem cell transplant in tandem has been shown to be feasible. Patients who have a relapse after an initial response can be remobilized, but the ultimate benefits of a second cycle of high-dose therapy have not been determined.[98]

CONCLUSION

The diagnosis of amyloidosis should be considered in nondiabetic patients with nephrotic range proteinuria, infiltrative cardiomyopathy in the absence of coronary artery disease or hypertension, patients with unexplained hepatomegaly, peripheral neuropathy in nondiabetics, and "atypical" myeloma. When a patient is seen with a compatible clinical syndrome, immunofixation of the serum and urine and an immunoglobulin free light chain assay should be performed. Histologic confirmation of the diagnosis is required in all patients. Any site may be appropriate in a given situation, but the simplest would be biopsy of the subcutaneous fat and the bone marrow. For assessment of prognosis, echocardiography combined with the troponin and BNP level is essential. The available treatment and the most appropriate first-line therapy remains controversial but includes melphalan/prednisone, dexamethasone, melphalan/dexamethasone, cyclophosphamide/thalidomide/dexamethasone, bortezomib, stem cell transplantation, and organ transplantation followed by stem cell transplantation. Prioritization of the first appropriate therapy remains to be defined.

REFERENCES

1. Bely M, Makovitzky J. Sensitivity and specificity of Congo red staining according to Romhanyi. Comparison with Puchtler's or Bennhold's methods. *Acta Histochem* 2006;108:175-80.
2. Puchtler H, Sweat F. Congo red as a stain for fluorescence microscopy of amyloid. *J Histochem Cytochem* 1965;13:693-4.
3. Ishii W, Matsuda M, Nakamura N, et al. Phenol Congo red staining enhances the diagnostic value of abdominal fat aspiration biopsy in reactive AA amyloidosis secondary to rheumatoid arthritis. *Intern Med* 2003;42:400-5.
4. Pras M, Schubert M, Zucker-Franklin D, Rimon A, Franklin EC. The characterization of soluble amyloid prepared in water. *J Clin Invest* 1968;47:924-33.
5. Benson MD. Ostertag revisited: the inherited systemic amyloidoses without neuropathy. *Amyloid* 2005;12:75-87.
6. Sipe JD, Cohen AS. Review: history of the amyloid fibril. *J Struct Biol* 2000;130:88-98.
7. Peng S, Glennert J, Westermark P. Medin-amyloid: a recently characterized age-associated arterial amyloid form affects mainly arteries in the upper part of the body. *Amyloid* 2005;12:96-102.
8. Rocken C, Shakespeare A. Pathology, diagnosis and pathogenesis of AA amyloidosis. *Virchows Arch* 2002;440:111-22.
9. van der Hilst JC, Simon A, Drenth JP. Hereditary periodic fever and reactive amyloidosis. *Clin Exp Med* 2005;5:87-98.
10. Pepys MB. Pathogenesis, diagnosis and treatment of systemic amyloidosis. *Philos Trans R Soc Lond B Biol Sci* 2001;356:203-10; discussion 210-11.
11. Pokkuluri PR, Solomon A, Weiss DT, Stevens FJ, Schiffer M. Tertiary structure of human lambda 6 light chains. *Amyloid* 1999;6:165-71.
12. Solomon A, Weiss DT, Pepys MB. Induction in mice of human light-chain-associated amyloidosis. *Am J Pathol* 1992;140:629-37.
13. Rajkumar SV, Dispenzieri A, Kyle RA. Monoclonal gammopathy of undetermined significance, Waldenstrom macroglobulinemia,

AL amyloidosis, and related plasma cell disorders: diagnosis and treatment. *Mayo Clin Proc* 2006;81:693-703.

14. Rajkumar SV, Gertz MA, Kyle RA. Primary systemic amyloidosis with delayed progression to multiple myeloma. *Cancer* 1998;82:1501-5.

15. Kyle RA, Linos A, Beard CM, et al. Incidence and natural history of primary systemic amyloidosis in Olmsted County, Minnesota, 1950 through 1989. *Blood* 1992;79:1817-22.

16. Palladini G, Perfetti V, Merlini G. Therapy and management of systemic AL (primary) amyloidosis. *Swiss Med Wkly* 2006;136:715-20.

17. Park MA, Mueller PS, Kyle RA, Larson DR, Plevak MF, Gertz MA. Primary (AL) hepatic amyloidosis: clinical features and natural history in 98 patients. *Medicine (Baltimore)* 2003; 82:291-8.

18. Shah KB, Inoue Y, Mehra MR. Amyloidosis and the heart: a comprehensive review. *Arch Intern Med* 2006;166:1805-13.

19. Rodriguez RJ, Iglesias CG, Rubin J. Primary amyloidosis and syncope. *Int J Cardiol* 1997;58:185-7.

20. Pan WH, Li NP. Clinical pathological feature of early tongue amyloidosis. *Chin Med Sci J* 2006;21:104-6.

21. Gertz MA, Kyle RA, Griffing WL, Hunder GG. Jaw claudication in primary systemic amyloidosis. *Medicine (Baltimore)* 1986;65:173-9.

22. Ing EB, Woolf IZ, Younge BR, Bjornsson J, Leavitt JA. Systemic amyloidosis with temporal artery involvement mimicking temporal arteritis. *Ophthalmic Surg Lasers* 1997;28:328-31.

23. Guerreiro de Moura CG, Pinto de Souza S. Images in clinical medicine. "Shoulder pad" sign. *N Engl J Med* 2004;351:e23.

24. Jardinet D, Westhovens R, Peeters J. Sicca syndrome as an initial symptom of amyloidosis. *Clin Rheumatol* 1998;17:546-8.

25. Hasserjian RP, Goodman HJ, Lachmann HJ, Muzikansky A, Hawkins PN. Bone marrow findings correlate with clinical outcome in systemic AL amyloidosis patients. *Histopathology* 2007;50:567-73.

26. Picken MM, Herrera GA. The burden of "sticky" amyloid: typing challenges. *Arch Pathol Lab Med* 2007;131:850-1.

27. Comenzo RL, Zhou P, Fleisher M, Clark B, Teruya-Feldstein J. Seeking confidence in the diagnosis of systemic AL (Ig light-chain) amyloidosis: patients can have both monoclonal gammopathies and hereditary amyloid proteins. *Blood* 2006;107:3489-91.

28. Neben-Wittich MA, Foote RL, Kalra S. External beam radiation therapy for tracheobronchial amyloidosis. *Chest* 2007;132:262-7.

29. Gaurav K, Panda M. An uncommon cause of bilateral pulmonary nodules in a long-term smoker. *J Gen Intern Med* 2007;22:1617-20.

30. Lesslauer W. On the structure of agglutinated sheep red blood cell membranes. *Biochim Biophys Acta* 1976;436:25-37.

31. Lachmann HJ, Goodman HJ, Gilbertson JA, et al. Natural history and outcome in systemic AA amyloidosis. *N Engl J Med* 2007;356:2361-71.

32. Moon WK, Kim SH, Im JG, Yeon KM, Han MC. Castleman disease with renal amyloidosis: imaging findings and clinical significance. *Abdom Imaging* 1995;20:376-8.

33. Hou X, Aguilar MI, Small DH. Transthyretin and familial amyloidotic polyneuropathy. Recent progress in understanding the molecular mechanism of neurodegeneration. *FEBS J* 2007;274:1637-50.

34. Granel B, Valleix S, Serratrice J, et al. Lysozyme amyloidosis: report of 4 cases and a review of the literature. *Medicine (Baltimore)* 2006;85:66-73.

35. Lachmann HJ, Booth DR, Booth SE, et al. Misdiagnosis of hereditary amyloidosis as AL (primary) amyloidosis. *N Engl J Med* 2002;346:1786-91.

36. Ng B, Connors LH, Davidoff R, Skinner M, Falk RH. Senile systemic amyloidosis presenting with heart failure: a comparison with light chain-associated amyloidosis. *Arch Intern Med* 2005;165:1425-29.

37. Kyle RA, Spittell PC, Gertz MA, et al. The premortem recognition of systemic senile amyloidosis with cardiac involvement. *Am J Med* 1996;101:395-400.

38. Kyle RA, Gertz MA. Primary systemic amyloidosis: clinical and laboratory features in 474 cases. *Semin Hematol* 1995;32:45-59.

39. Morris KL, Tate JR, Gill D, et al. Diagnostic and prognostic utility of the serum free light chain assay in patients with AL amyloidosis. *Intern Med J* 2007;37:456-63.

40. Abraham RS, Katzmann JA, Clark RJ, Bradwell AR, Kyle RA, Gertz MA. Quantitative analysis of serum free light chains. A new marker for the diagnostic evaluation of primary systemic amyloidosis. *Am J Clin Pathol* 2003;119:274-8.

41. Leung N, Dispenzieri A, Lacy MQ, et al. Severity of baseline proteinuria predicts renal response in immunoglobulin light chain-associated amyloidosis after autologous stem cell transplantation. *Clin J Am Soc Nephrol* 2007;2:440-4.

42. Mayo MM, Johns GS. Serum free light chains in the diagnosis and monitoring of patients with plasma cell dyscrasias. *Contrib Nephrol* 2007;153:44-65.

43. Dispenzieri A, Lacy MQ, Katzmann JA, et al. Absolute values of immunoglobulin free light chains are prognostic in patients with primary systemic amyloidosis undergoing peripheral blood stem cell transplantation. *Blood* 2006;107:3378-83.

44. Akar H, Seldin DC, Magnani B, et al. Quantitative serum free light chain assay in the diagnostic evaluation of AL amyloidosis. *Amyloid* 2005;12:210-15.

45. Hazenberg BP, van Rijswijk MH, Lub-de Hooge MN, et al. Diagnostic performance and prognostic value of extravascular retention of ^{123}I-labeled serum amyloid P component in systemic amyloidosis. *J Nucl Med* 2007;48:865-72.

46. Lechapt-Zalcman E, Authier FJ, Creange A, Voisin MC, Gherardi RK. Labial salivary gland biopsy for diagnosis of amyloid polyneuropathy. *Muscle Nerve* 1999;22:105-7.

47. Yoshimatsu S, Ando Y, Terazaki H, et al. Endoscopic and pathological manifestations of the gastrointestinal tract in familial amyloidotic polyneuropathy type I (Met30). *J Intern Med* 1998;243:65-72.

48. Guy CD, Jones CK. Abdominal fat pad aspiration biopsy for tissue confirmation of systemic amyloidosis: specificity, positive predictive value, and diagnostic pitfalls. *Diagn Cytopathol* 2001;24:181-5.

49. Olsen KE, Sletten K, Westermark P. The use of subcutaneous fat tissue for amyloid typing by enzyme-linked immunosorbent assay. *Am J Clin Pathol* 1999;111:355-62.

50. Palladini G, Malamani G, Co F, et al. Holter monitoring in AL amyloidosis: prognostic implications. *Pacing Clin Electrophysiol* 2001;24:1228-33.

51. Lindqvist P, Olofsson BO, Backman C, Suhr O, Waldenstrom A. Pulsed tissue Doppler and strain imaging discloses early signs of infiltrative cardiac disease: a study on patients with familial amyloidotic polyneuropathy. *Eur J Echocardiogr* 2006;7:22-30.

52. Bellavia D, Abraham TP, Pellikka PA, et al. Detection of left ventricular systolic dysfunction in cardiac amyloidosis with strain rate echocardiography. *J Am Soc Echocardiogr* 2007;20:1194-202.

53. Dispenzieri A, Gertz MA, Kyle RA, et al. Serum cardiac troponins and N-terminal pro-brain natriuretic peptide: a staging system for primary systemic amyloidosis. *J Clin Oncol* 2004;22:3751-7.

54. Dispenzieri A, Gertz MA, Kyle RA, et al. Prognostication of survival using cardiac troponins and N-terminal pro-brain natriuretic peptide in patients with primary systemic amyloidosis undergoing peripheral blood stem cell transplantation. *Blood* 2004;104:1881-7.

55. Zerbini CA, Anderson JJ, Kane KA, et al. Beta 2 microglobulin serum levels and prediction of survival in AL amyloidosis. *Amyloid* 2002;9:242-6.

56. Gertz MA, Lacy MQ, Dispenzieri A, et al. Effect of hematologic response on outcome of patients undergoing transplantation for primary amyloidosis: importance of achieving a complete response. *Haematologica* 2007;92:1415-18.b.

57. Caccialanza R, Palladini G, Klersy C, et al. Nutritional status of outpatients with systemic immunoglobulin light-chain amyloidosis 1. *Am J Clin Nutr* 2006;83:350-4.

58. Gertz MA, Comenzo R, Falk RH, et al. Definition of organ involvement and treatment response in immunoglobulin light chain amyloidosis (AL): a consensus opinion from the 10th International Symposium on Amyloid and Amyloidosis, Tours, France, 18-22 April 2004. *Am J Hematol* 2005;79:319-28.

59. Sanchorawala V. Light-chain (AL) amyloidosis: diagnosis and treatment. *Clin J Am Soc Nephrol* 2006;1:1331-41.

60. Mukai S, Lipsitz LA. Orthostatic hypotension. *Clin Geriatr Med* 2002;18:253-68.

61. Gillmore JD, Goodman HJ, Lachmann HJ, et al. Sequential heart and autologous stem cell transplantation for systemic AL amyloidosis. *Blood* 2006;107:1227-9.

62. Gertz MA, Kyle RA, O'Fallon WM. Dialysis support of patients with primary systemic amyloidosis. A study of 211 patients. *Arch Intern Med* 1992;152:2245-50.

63. Leung N, Griffin MD, Dispenzieri A, et al. Living donor kidney and autologous stem cell transplantation for primary systemic amyloidosis (AL) with predominant renal involvement. *Am J Transplant* 2005;5:1660-70.

64. Gillmore JD, Madhoo S, Pepys MB, Hawkins PN. Renal transplantation for amyloid end-stage renal failure—insights from serial serum amyloid P component scintigraphy. *Nucl Med Commun* 2000;21:735-40.

65. Lacy MQ, Dispenzieri A, Hayman SR, et al. Sequential heart and autologous stem cell transplantation for AL amyloidosis (Abstract 3092). *Blood* (*ASH Annual Meeting Abstracts*) 2006;108:3092.

66. Kyle RA, Gertz MA, Greipp PR, et al. A trial of three regimens for primary amyloidosis: colchicine alone, melphalan and prednisone, and melphalan, prednisone, and colchicine. *N Engl J Med* 1997;336:1202-7.

67. Dhodapkar MV, Jagannath S, Vesole D, et al. Treatment of AL-amyloidosis with dexamethasone plus alpha interferon. *Leuk Lymphoma* 1997;27:351-6.

68. Gertz MA, Lacy MQ, Lust JA, Greipp PR, Witzig TE, Kyle RA. Phase II trial of high-dose dexamethasone for previously treated immunoglobulin light-chain amyloidosis. *Am J Hematol* 1999;61:115-19.

69. Gertz MA, Lacy MQ, Lust JA, Greipp PR, Witzig TE, Kyle RA. Phase II trial of high-dose dexamethasone for untreated patients with primary systemic amyloidosis. *Med Oncol* 1999;16:104-9.

70. Palladini G, Anesi E, Perfetti V, et al. A modified high-dose dexamethasone regimen for primary systemic (AL) amyloidosis. *Br J Haematol* 2001;113:1044-6.

71. Dhodapkar MV, Hussein MA, Rasmussen E, et al. Clinical efficacy of high-dose dexamethasone with maintenance dexamethasone/alpha interferon in patients with primary systemic amyloidosis: results of United States Intergroup Trial Southwest Oncology Group (SWOG) S9628. *Blood* 2004;104:3520-6.

72. Palladini G, Perfetti V, Obici L, et al. Association of melphalan and high-dose dexamethasone is effective and well tolerated in patients with AL (primary) amyloidosis who are ineligible for stem cell transplantation. *Blood* 2004;103:2936-8.

73. Palladini G, Russo P, Nuvolone M, et al. Treatment with oral melphalan plus dexamethasone produces long-term remissions in AL amyloidosis. *Blood* 2007;110:787-8.

74. Seldin DC, Choufani EB, Dember LM, et al. Tolerability and efficacy of thalidomide for the treatment of patients with light chain-associated (AL) amyloidosis. *Clin Lymphoma* 2003;3:241-6.

75. Dispenzieri A, Lacy MQ, Rajkumar SV, et al. Poor tolerance to high doses of thalidomide in patients with primary systemic amyloidosis. *Amyloid* 2003;10:257-61.

76. Palladini G, Perfetti V, Perlini S, et al. The combination of thalidomide and intermediate-dose dexamethasone is an effective but toxic treatment for patients with primary amyloidosis (AL). *Blood* 2005;105:2949-51.

77. Sanchorawala V, Wright DG, Rosenzweig M, et al. Lenalidomide and dexamethasone in the treatment of AL amyloidosis: results of a phase 2 trial. *Blood* 2007;109:492-6.

78. Dispenzieri A, Lacy MQ, Zeldenrust SR, et al. The activity of lenalidomide with or without dexamethasone in patients with primary systemic amyloidosis. *Blood* 2007;109:465-70.

79. Wechalekar AD, Gillmore JD, Lachmann HJ, Offer M, Hawkins PN. Efficacy and safety of bortezomib in systemic AL amyloidosis—a preliminary report (Abstract). *Blood* (*ASH Annual Meeting Abstracts*) 2006;108:29.

80. Reece DE, Sanchorawala V, Hegenbart U, et al. Phase I/II study of bortezomib (B) in patients with systemic AL-amyloidosis (AL) (Abstract 8050). *J Clin Oncol* (*Meeting Abstracts*) 2006;25:8050.

81. Kastritis E, Anagnostopoulos A, Roussou M, et al. Treatment of light chain (AL) amyloidosis with the combination of bortezomib and dexamethasone. *Haematologica* 2007;92:1351-8.

82. Gertz MA, Lacy MQ, Dispenzieri A, Hayman SR, Kumar S. Transplantation for amyloidosis. *Curr Opin Oncol* 2007;19: 136-41.

83. Gertz MA, Lacy MQ, Dispenzieri A, Hayman SR. Amyloidosis. *Best Pract Res Clin Haematol* 2005;18:709-27.

84. Sanchorawala V, Wright DG, Seldin DC, et al. High-dose intravenous melphalan and autologous stem cell transplantation as initial therapy or following two cycles of oral chemotherapy for the treatment of AL amyloidosis: results of a prospective randomized trial. *Bone Marrow Transplant* 2004;33:381-8.

85. Comenzo RL, Sanchorawala V, Fisher C, et al. Intermediate-dose intravenous melphalan and blood stem cells mobilized with sequential GM+G-CSF or G-CSF alone to treat AL (amyloid light chain) amyloidosis. *Br J Haematol* 1999;104:553-9.

86. Gertz MA, Lacy MQ, Dispenzieri A, et al. Transplantation without growth factor: engraftment kinetics after stem cell transplantation for primary systemic amyloidosis (AL). *Bone Marrow Transplant* 2007;40:989-3.

87. Gertz MA, Lacy MQ, Dispenzieri A, et al. Risk-adjusted manipulation of melphalan dose before stem cell transplantation in patients with amyloidosis is associated with a lower response rate. *Bone Marrow Transplant* 2004;34:1025-31.

88. Cohen AD, Zhou P, Chou J, et al. Risk-adapted autologous stem cell transplantation with adjuvant dexamethasone ± thalidomide for systemic light-chain amyloidosis: results of a phase II trial. *Br J Haematol* 2007;139:224-33.

89. Vesole DH, Perez WS, Akasheh M, Boudreau C, Reece DE, Bredeson CN. High-dose therapy and autologous hematopoietic stem cell transplantation for patients with primary systemic amyloidosis: a Center for International Blood and Marrow Transplant Research Study. *Mayo Clin Proc* 2006;81:880-8.

90. Gertz MA, Blood E, Vesole DH, Abonour R, Lazarus HM, Greipp PR. A multicenter phase 2 trial of stem cell transplantation for immunoglobulin light-chain amyloidosis (E4A97): an Eastern Cooperative Oncology Group Study. *Bone Marrow Transplant* 2004;34:149-54.

91. Jaccard A, Moreau P, Leblond V, et al. High-dose melphalan versus melphalan plus dexamethasone for AL amyloidosis. *N Engl J Med* 2007;357:1083-93.

92. Dispenzieri A, Kyle RA, Lacy MQ, et al. Superior survival in primary systemic amyloidosis patients undergoing peripheral blood stem cell transplantation: a case-control study. *Blood* 2004;103:3960-3.

93. Porrata LF, Gertz MA, Litzow MR, et al. Early lymphocyte recovery predicts superior survival after autologous hematopoietic stem cell transplantation for patients with primary systemic amyloidosis. *Clin Cancer Res* 2005;11:1210-18.

94. Leung N, Leung TR, Cha SS, Dispenzieri A, Lacy MQ, Gertz MA. Excessive fluid accumulation during stem cell mobilization: a novel prognostic factor of first-year survival after stem cell transplantation in AL amyloidosis patients. *Blood* 2005;106:3353-7.

95. Leung N, Dispenzieri A, Fervenza FC, et al. Renal response after high-dose melphalan and stem cell transplantation is a favorable marker in patients with primary systemic amyloidosis. *Am J Kidney Dis* 2005;46:270-7.

96. Seldin DC, Anderson JJ, Sanchorawala V, et al. Improvement in quality of life of patients with AL amyloidosis treated with high-dose melphalan and autologous stem cell transplantation. *Blood* 2004;104:1888-93.

97. Schonland SO, Perz JB, Hundemer M, et al. Indications for high-dose chemotherapy with autologous stem cell support in patients with systemic amyloid light chain amyloidosis. *Transplantation* 2005;80:S160-3.

98. Sanchorawala V, Wright DG, Quillen K, et al. Tandem cycles of high-dose melphalan and autologous stem cell transplantation increases the response rate in AL amyloidosis. *Bone Marrow Transplant* 2007;40:607.

11 Waldenström Macroglobulinemia/Lymphoplasmacytic Lymphoma

Steven P. Treon and Giampaolo Merlini

INTRODUCTION

Waldenström macroglobulinemia (WM) is a distinct clinicopathological entity resulting from the accumulation, predominantly in the bone marrow, of clonally related lymphocytes, lymphoplasmacytic cells, and plasma cells that secrete a monoclonal immunoglobulin M (IgM) protein (Figure 11.1).[1] This condition is considered to correspond to the lymphoplasmacytic lymphoma (LPL) as defined by the Revised European American Lymphoma (REAL) and World Health Organization classification systems.[2,3] Most cases of LPL are WM, with less than 5% of cases made up of IgA, IgG, and nonsecreting LPL.

EPIDEMIOLOGY AND ETIOLOGY

WM is an uncommon disease, with a reported age-adjusted incidence rate of 3.4 per million among males and 1.7 per million among females in the United States, and a geometrical increase with age.[4,5] The incidence rate for WM is higher among Caucasians, with African descendants representing only 5% of all patients. Genetic factors appear to be an important factor to the pathogenesis of WM. Approximately 20% of WM patients have an Ashkenazi (Eastern European) Jewish ethnic background, and there have been numerous reports of familiar disease, including multigenerational clustering of WM and other B-cell lymphoproliferative diseases.[6-10] In a recent study, approximately 20% of 257 serial WM patients presenting to a tertiary referral had a first degree relative with either WM or another B-cell disorder.[7] Frequent familiar association with other immunological disorders in healthy relatives, including hypogammaglobulinemia and hypergammaglobulinemia (particularly polyclonal IgM), autoantibody (particularly to thyroid) production, and manifestation of hyperactive B cells have also been reported.[9,10] Increased expression of the *bcl-2* gene with enhanced B-cell survival may underlie the increased immunoglobulin synthesis in familial WM.[9] The role of environmental factors in WM remains to be clarified, but chronic antigenic stimulation from infections, certain drug and agent orange exposures remain suspect. An etiological role for hepatitis C virus (HCV) infection has been suggested, though in a recent study examining 100 consecutive WM patients, no association could be established using both serological and molecular diagnostic studies for HCV infection.[11-13]

BIOLOGY

Cytogenetic findings

Several studies, usually performed on limited series of patients, have been published on cytogenetic findings in WM demonstrating a great variety of numerical and structural chromosome abnormalities. Numerical losses involving chromosomes 17, 18, 19, 20, 21, 22, X, and Y have been commonly observed, though gains in chromosomes 3, 4, and 12 have also been reported.[7,14-19] Chromosome 6q deletions encompassing 6q21-22 have been observed in up to half of WM patients, and at a comparable frequency among patients with and without a familial history.[7,19] Several candidate tumor suppressor genes in this region including *BLIMP-1*, a master regulatory gene implicated in lymphoplasmacytic differentiation, are under study. Notable, however, is the absence of IgH switch region rearrangements in WM, a finding that may be used to discern cases of IgM myeloma where IgH switch region rearrangements are a predominant feature.[20]

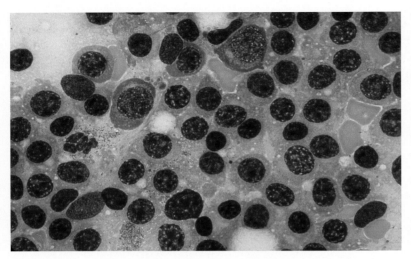

Figure 11.1. Aspirate from a patient with Waldenström macroglobulinemia demonstrating excess mature lymphocytes, lymphoplasmacytic cells, and plasma cells. *Source*: Courtesy of Marvin Stone, MD.

indication is further strengthened by the results of the analysis of the nature (silent or amino acid replacing) and distribution (in framework or CDR regions) of somatic mutations in Ig heavy- and light-chain variable regions performed in patients with WM.[28,29] This analysis showed a high rate of replacement mutations, compared with the closest germline genes, clustering in the CDR regions and without intraclonal variation. Subsequent studies showed a strong preferential usage of *VH3/JH4* gene families, no intraclonal variation, and no evidence for any isotype-switched transcripts.[30,31] These data indicate that WM may originate from a IgM⁺ and/or IgM⁺ IgD⁺ memory B cell. Normal IgM⁺ memory B cells localize in bone marrow, where they mature to IgM-secreting cells.[32]

Nature of the clonal cell

The WM bone marrow B-cell clone shows intraclonal differentiation from small lymphocytes with large focal deposits of surface immunoglobulins, to lymphoplasmacytic cells, to mature plasma cells that contain intracytoplasmic immunoglobulins.[21] Clonal B cells are detectable among blood B lymphocytes, and their number increases in patients who fail to respond to therapy or who progress.[22] These clonal blood cells present the peculiar capacity to differentiate spontaneously, in in vitro culture, to plasma cells. This is through an interleukin-6 (IL-6)-dependent process in IgM monoclonal gammopathy of undetermined significance (MGUS) and mostly an IL-6-independent process in WM patients.[23] All these cells express the monoclonal IgM present in the blood, and a variable percentage of them also express surface IgD. The characteristic immunophenotypic profile of the lymphoplasmacytic cells in WM includes the expression of the pan B-cell markers CD19, CD20, CD22, CD79, and FMC7.2.[24-26] The expression of CD5, CD10, and CD23 may be found in 10%-20% of cases, and does not exclude the diagnosis of WM.[27]

The phenotype of lymphoplasmacytic cells in WM cell suggests that the clone is a postgerminal center B cell. This

Bone marrow microenvironment

Increased numbers of mast cells are found in the bone marrow of WM patients, wherein they are usually admixed with tumor aggregates.[26,33] Recent studies have helped clarify the role of mast cells in WM. Co-culture of primary autologous or mast cell lines with WM LPC resulted in dose-dependent WM cell proliferation and/or tumor colony, primarily through CD40 ligand (CD40L) signaling. Furthermore, WM cells through elaboration of soluble CD27 (sCD27) induced the upregulation of CD40L on mast cells derived from WM patients and mast cell lines.[34]

CLINICAL FEATURES

The clinical and laboratory findings at the time of diagnosis of WM in one large institutional study[7] are presented in Table 11.1. Unlike most indolent lymphomas, splenomegaly and lymphadenopathy are prominent in only a minority of patients (<15%). Purpura is frequently associated with cryoglobulinemia and more rarely with AL amyloidosis, while hemorrhagic manifestations and neuropathies are multifactorial (see later). The morbidity associated with WM is caused by the concurrence of two

TABLE 11.1. Clinical and laboratory findings for 149 consecutive newly diagnosed patients with the consensus panel diagnosis of WM presenting to the Dana Farber Cancer Institute

	Median	Range	Institutional normal reference range
Age (years)	59	34-84	NA
Gender (male/female)	85/64		NA
Bone marrow involvement	30%	5%-95%	NA
Adenopathy	16%		NA
Splenomegaly	10%		NA
IgM (mg/dL)	2 870	267-12 400	40-230
IgG (mg/dL)	587	47-2 770	700-1 600
IgA (mg/dL)	47	8-509	70-400
Serum viscosity (cp)	2.0	1.4-6.6	1.4-1.9
Hct (%)	35.0%	17.2%-45.4%	34.8-43.6
Plt (×10^9/L)	253	24-649	155-410
WBC (×10^9/L)	6.0	0.3-13	3.8-9.2
B$_2$M (mg/dL)	3.0	1.3-13.7	0-2.7
LDH	395	122-1 131	313-618

B2M, β$_2$-microglobulin; Hct, hematocrit; LDH, lactate dehydrogenase; NA, not applicable; Plt, platelet count; WBC, white blood cell.

TABLE 11.2. Physicochemical and immunological properties of the monoclonal IgM protein in Waldenström macroglobulinemia

Properties of IgM monoclonal protein	Diagnostic condition	Clinical manifestations
Pentameric structure	Hyperviscosity	Headaches, blurred vision, epistaxis, retinal hemorrhages, leg cramps, impaired mentation, intracranial hemorrhage
Precipitation on cooling	Cryoglobulinemia (type 1)	Raynaud's phenomenon, acrocyanosis, ulcers, purpura, cold urticaria
Auto-antibody activity to myelin-associated glycoprotein (MAG), ganglioside M1 (GM1), sulfatide moieties on peripheral nerve sheaths	Peripheral neuropathies	Sensorimotor neuropathies, painful neuropathies, ataxic gait, bilateral foot drop
Auto-antibody activity to IgG	Cryoglobulinemia (type 2)	Purpura, arthralgias, renal failure, sensorimotor neuropathies
Auto-antibody activity to red blood cell antigens	Cold agglutinins	Hemolytic anemia, Raynaud phenomenon, acrocyanosis, livedo reticularis
Tissue deposition as amorphous aggregates	Organ dysfunction	Skin: bullous skin disease, papules, Schnitzler syndrome; GI: diarrhea, malabsorption, bleeding; Kidney: proteinuria, renal failure (light chain component)
Tissue deposition as amyloid fibrils (light chain component most commonly)	Organ dysfunction	Fatigue, weight loss, edema, hepatomegaly, macroglossia, organ dysfunction of involved organs: heart, kidney, liver, peripheral sensory and autonomic nerves

main components: tissue infiltration by neoplastic cells and, more importantly, the physicochemical and immunological properties of the monoclonal IgM. As shown in Table 11.2, the monoclonal IgM can produce clinical manifestations through several different mechanisms related to its physicochemical properties, nonspecific interactions with other proteins, antibody activity, and tendency to deposit in tissues.[35-37]

MORBIDITY MEDIATED BY THE EFFECTS OF IGM

Hyperviscosity syndrome

Blood hyperviscosity is effected by increased serum IgM levels leading to hyperviscosity-related complications.[38] The mechanisms behind the marked increase in the resistance to blood flow and the resulting impaired transit through the microcirculatory system are rather complex.[38-40] The main determinants are (1) a high concentration of monoclonal IgMs, which may form aggregates and may bind water through their carbohydrate component; and (2) their interaction with blood cells. Monoclonal IgMs increase red cell aggregation (rouleaux formation) and red cell internal viscosity while also reducing deformability. The possible presence of cryoglobulins can contribute to increasing blood viscosity as well as to the tendency to induce erythrocyte aggregation. Serum viscosity is proportional to IgM concentration up to 30 g/L; it then increases sharply at higher levels. Plasma viscosity and hematocrit are directly regulated by the body. Increased plasma viscosity may also contribute to inappropriately low erythropoietin production, which is the major reason for anemia in these patients.[41] Clinical manifestations are related to circulatory disturbances that can be best appreciated by ophthalmoscopy, which shows distended and tortuous retinal veins, hemorrhages, and papilledema[42] (Figure 11.2). Symptoms usually occur when the monoclonal IgM concentration exceeds 50 g/L or when serum viscosity is >4.0 centipoises (cp), but there is a great individual variability, with some patients showing no evidence of hyperviscosity even at 10 cp.[38] The most common symptoms are oronasal bleeding, visual disturbances due to retinal bleeding, and dizziness that may rarely lead to coma. Heart failure can be aggravated, particularly in the elderly, owing to increased blood viscosity, expanded plasma volume, and anemia. Inappropriate transfusion can exacerbate hyperviscosity and may precipitate cardiac failure.

Cryoglobulinemia

In up to 20% of WM patients, the monoclonal IgM can behave as a cryoglobulin (type 1), but it is symptomatic in 5% or less of the cases.[43] Cryoprecipitation is mainly dependent on the concentration of monoclonal IgM; for this reason, plasmapheresis or plasma exchange are commonly

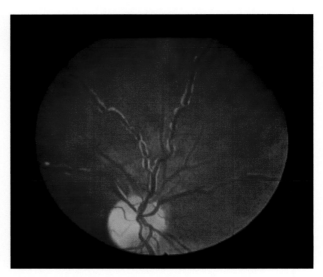

Figure 11.2. Funduscopic examination of a patient with Waldenström macroglobulinemia demonstrating hyperviscosity-related changes including dilated retinal vessels, peripheral hemorrhages, and "venous sausaging." *Source*: Courtesy of Marvin Stone, MD.

effective in this condition. Symptoms result from impaired blood flow in small vessels and include Raynaud phenomenon, acrocyanosis, and necrosis of the regions most exposed to cold (tip of the nose, ears, fingers, and toes), malleolar ulcers, purpura, and cold urticaria. Renal manifestations may occur but are infrequent.

Autoantibody activity

Monoclonal IgM may exert its pathogenic effects through specific recognition of autologous antigens, the most notable being nerve constituents, immunoglobulin determinants, and red blood cell (RBC) antigens.

IgM-related neuropathy

In a series of 215 patients with WM, Merlini et al.[43] reported the clinical presence of peripheral neuropathy in 24% of WM patients, although prevalence rates ranging from 5% to 38% have been reported in other series.[44,45] An estimated 6.5%-10% of idiopathic neuropathies are associated with a monoclonal gammopathy, with a preponderance of IgM (60%) followed by IgG (30%) and IgA (10%) (reviewed in Nemni et al.[46] and Ropper and Gorson[47]). In WM patients, the nerve damage is mediated by diverse pathogenetic mechanisms: IgM antibody activity toward nerve constituents causing demyelinating polyneuropathies; endoneurial granulofibrillar deposits of IgM without antibody activity, associated with axonal polyneuropathy; occasionally, by tubular deposits in the endoneurium associated with IgM cryoglobulin and, rarely, by amyloid deposits or by neoplastic cell infiltration of nerve structures.[48] Half of the patients with IgM neuropathy have a distinctive clinical syndrome that is associated with antibodies against a minor 100-kDa glycoprotein component of nerve, myelin-associated glycoprotein (MAG). Anti-MAG antibodies are generally monoclonal IgMκ, and usually also exhibit reactivity with other glycoproteins or glycolipids that share antigenic determinants with MAG.[49-51] The anti-MAG-related neuropathy is typically distal and symmetrical, affecting both motor and sensory functions; it is slowly progressive with a long period of stability.[45,52] Most patients present with sensory complaints (paresthesias, aching discomfort, dysesthesias, or lancinating pains), imbalance and gait ataxia, owing to lack of proprioception, and leg muscles atrophy in advanced stage. Patients with predominantly demyelinating sensory neuropathy in association with monoclonal IgM to gangliosides with disialosyl moieties, such as GD1b, GD3, GD2, GT1b, and GQ1b, have also been reported.[53,54] Anti-GD1b and anti-GQ1b antibodies were significantly associated with predominantly sensory ataxic neuropathy. These antiganglioside monoclonal IgMs present core clinical features of chronic ataxic neuropathy with variably present ophthalmoplegia and/or RBC cold agglutinating activity. The disialosyl epitope is also present on RBC glycophorins, thereby accounting for the red cell cold agglutinin activity of anti-Pr2 specificity.[55,56] Monoclonal IgM proteins that bind to gangliosides with a terminal trisaccharide moiety, including GM2 and GalNac-GD1A, are associated with chronic demyelinating neuropathy and severe sensory ataxia, unresponsive to corticosteroids.[57] Antiganglioside IgM proteins may also cross-react with lipopolysaccharides of *Campylobacter jejuni*, whose infection is known to precipitate the Miller Fisher syndrome, a variant of the Guillain–Barré syndrome.[58] This finding indicates that molecular mimicry may play a role in this condition. Antisulfatide monoclonal IgM proteins, associated with sensory/sensorimotor neuropathy, have been detected in 5% of patients with IgM monoclonal gammopathy and neuropathy.[59]

Motor neuron disease has been reported in patients with WM, and monoclonal IgM in patients with anti-GM1 and sulfoglucuronyl paragloboside activity.[60] POEMS (polyneuropathy, organomegaly, endocrinopathy, M-protein, and skin changes) syndrome is rarely associated with WM.[61]

Cold agglutinin hemolytic anemia

Monoclonal IgM may present with cold agglutinin activity, that is, it can recognize specific red cell antigens at temperatures below physiological, and produce hemolytic anemia. This disorder occurs in <10% of WM patients[62] and is associated with cold agglutinin titers >1:1000 in most cases. The monoclonal component is usually an IgMκ and reacts most commonly with I/i antigens, with complement fixation and activation.[63,64] Mild chronic hemolytic anemia can be exacerbated after cold exposure but rarely does hemoglobin drop below 70 g/L. The hemolysis is usually extravascular (removal of C3b opsonized cells by the reticuloendothelial system, primarily in the liver) and rarely intravascular from complement destruction of RBC membrane. The agglutination of RBCs in the cooler peripheral circulation also causes Raynaud syndrome, acrocyanosis, and livedo reticularis. Macroglobulins with the properties of both cryoglobulins and cold agglutinins with anti-Pr specificity have been reported. These properties may have as a common basis the immune binding of the sialic acid–containing carbohydrate present on RBC glycophorins and on Ig molecules. Several other macroglobulins with various antibody activities toward autologous antigens (i.e. phospholipids, tissue and plasma proteins, etc.) and foreign ligands have also been reported.

Tissue deposition

The monoclonal protein can deposit in several tissues as amorphous aggregates. Linear deposition of monoclonal IgM along the skin basement membrane is associated with bullous skin disease.[65] Amorphous IgM deposits in the dermis determine the so-called IgM storage papules on the extensor surface of the extremities–macroglobulinemia cutis.[66] Deposition of monoclonal IgM in the lamina propria and/or submucosa of the intestine may be associated with diarrhea, malabsorption, and gastrointestinal bleeding.[67,68] It is well known that kidney involvement is less common and less severe in WM than in multiple myeloma, probably because the amount of light chain excreted in the urine is generally lower in WM than in myeloma and because of the absence of contributing factors, such as hypercalcemia, although cast nephropathy has also been described in WM.[69] On the other hand, the IgM macromolecule is more susceptible to being trapped in the glomerular loops where ultrafiltration presumably contributes to its precipitation, forming subendothelial deposits of aggregated IgM proteins that occlude the glomerular capillaries.[70] Mild and reversible proteinuria may result and most patients are asymptomatic. The deposition of monoclonal light chain as fibrillar amyloid deposits (AL amyloidosis) is uncommon in patients with WM.[71] Clinical expression and prognosis are similar to those of other AL patients with involvement of heart (44%), kidneys (32%), liver (14%), lungs (10%), peripheral/autonomic nerves (38%), and soft tissues (18%). However, the incidence of cardiac and pulmonary involvement is higher in patients with monoclonal IgM than with other immunoglobulin isotypes. The association of WM with reactive amyloidosis (AA) has been documented rarely.[72,73] Simultaneous occurrence of fibrillary glomerulopathy, characterized by glomerular deposits of wide noncongophilic fibrils and amyloid deposits, has been reported in WM.[74]

Manifestations related to tissue infiltration by neoplastic cells

Tissue infiltration by neoplastic cells is rare and can involve various organs and tissues, from the bone marrow (described later) to the liver, spleen, lymph nodes, and possibly the lungs, gastrointestinal tract, kidneys, skin, eyes, and central nervous system. Pulmonary involvement in the form of masses, nodules, diffuse infiltrate, or pleural effusions is relatively rare, since the overall incidence of pulmonary and pleural findings reported for WM is only 3%-5%.[75-77] Cough is the most common presenting symptom, followed by dyspnea and chest pain. Chest radiographic findings include parenchymal infiltrates, confluent masses, and effusions. Malabsorption, diarrhea, bleeding, or obstruction may indicate involvement of the gastrointestinal tract at the level of the stomach, duodenum, or small intestine.[78-81] In contrast to multiple myeloma, infiltration of the kidney interstitium with lymphoplasmacytoid cell has been reported in WM,[82] while renal or perirenal masses are not uncommon.[83] The skin can be the site of dense lymphoplasmacytic infiltrates, similar to that seen in the liver, spleen, and lymph nodes, forming cutaneous plaques and, rarely, nodules.[84] Chronic urticaria and IgM gammopathy are the two cardinal features of the Schnitzler syndrome, which is not usually associated initially with clinical features of WM,[85] although evolution to WM is not uncommon. Thus, close follow-up of these patients is warranted. Invasion of articular and periarticular structures by WM malignant cells is rarely reported.[86] The neoplastic cells can infiltrate the periorbital structures, lacrimal gland, and retro-orbital lymphoid tissues, resulting in ocular nerve palsies.[87,88] Direct infiltration of the central nervous system by monoclonal lymphoplasmacytic cells as infiltrates or as tumors constitutes the rarely observed Bing–Neel syndrome, characterized clinically by confusion, memory loss, disorientation, and motor dysfunction (reviewed in Ref. 89).

LABORATORY INVESTIGATIONS AND FINDINGS

Hematological abnormalities

Anemia is the most common finding in patients with symptomatic WM and is caused by a combination of factors: mild decrease in red cell survival, impaired erythropoiesis, hemolysis, moderate plasma volume expansion, and blood loss from the gastrointestinal tract. Blood smears are usually normocytic and normochromic, and rouleaux formation is often pronounced. Electronically measured mean corpuscular volume may be elevated spuriously owing to erythrocyte aggregation. In addition, the hemoglobin estimate can be inaccurate, that is, falsely high, because of interaction between the monoclonal protein and the diluent used in some automated analyzers.[90] Leukocyte and platelet counts are usually within the reference range at presentation, although patients may occasionally present with severe thrombocytopenia. As reported above, monoclonal B lymphocytes expressing surface IgM and late-differentiation B-cell markers are uncommonly detected in blood by using flow cytometry. A raised erythrocyte sedimentation rate is almost constantly observed in WM and may be the first clue to the presence of the macroglobulin. The clotting abnormality detected most frequently is the prolongation of thrombin time. AL amyloidosis should be suspected in all patients with nephrotic syndrome, cardiomyopathy, hepatomegaly, or peripheral neuropathy. Diagnosis requires the demonstration of green birefringence under polarized light of amyloid deposits stained with Congo red.

Biochemical investigations

High-resolution electrophoresis combined with immunofixation of serum and urine are recommended for the identification and characterization of the IgM monoclonal protein. The light chain of the monoclonal IgM is κ in 75%-80% of patients. A few WM patients have more than one M-component. The concentration of the serum monoclonal protein is very variable but in most cases lies within the range of 15-45 g/L. Densitometry should be adopted to determine IgM levels for serial evaluations because nephelometry is unreliable and shows large intralaboratory as well as interlaboratory variation. The presence of cold agglutinins or cryoglobulins may affect the determination of IgM levels and, therefore, testing for cold agglutinins and cryoglobulins should be performed at diagnosis. If present, subsequent serum samples should be analyzed under warm conditions for the determination of serum monoclonal IgM level. Although Bence Jones proteinuria is frequently present, it exceeds 1 g/24 hours in only 3% of cases. While IgM levels are elevated in WM patients, IgA and IgG levels are most often depressed and do not demonstrate recovery even after successful treatment.[91] In recent studies by Hunter et al.,[92] mutations in the receptor TACI were demonstrated in WM patients similar to those demonstrated in patients with common variable deficiency disorder (CVID), suggesting a possible CVID background for WM patients.

Serum viscosity

Because of its large size (almost 1 000 000 Daltons), most IgM molecules are retained within the intravascular compartment and can exert an undue effect on serum viscosity. Therefore, serum viscosity should be measured if the patient has signs or symptoms of hyperviscosity syndrome. Fundoscopy remains an excellent indicator of clinically relevant hyperviscosity. Among the first clinical signs of hyperviscosity are the appearance of peripheral and mid-peripheral dot and blotlike hemorrhages in the retina, which are best appreciated with indirect ophthalmoscopy and scleral depression.[42] In more severe cases of hyperviscosity, dot-, blot-, and flame-shaped hemorrhages can appear in the macular area along with markedly dilated and tortuous veins with focal constrictions resulting in "venous sausaging," as well as papilledema.

Bone marrow findings

The bone marrow is always involved in WM. Central to the diagnosis of WM is the demonstration, by trephine biopsy, of bone marrow infiltration by a lymphoplasmacytic cell population constituted by small lymphocytes with evidence of plasmacytoid/plasma cell differentiation (Figure 11.1). The pattern of bone marrow infiltration may be diffuse, interstitial, or nodular, showing usually an intertrabecular pattern of infiltration. A solely paratrabecular pattern of infiltration is unusual and should raise the possibility of follicular lymphoma.[1] The bone marrow infiltration should routinely be confirmed by immunophenotypic studies (flow cytometry and/or immunohistochemistry) showing the following profile: sIgM+CD19+CD20+CD22+CD79+.[24-26] Up to 20% of cases may express either CD5, CD10, or CD23.[27] In these cases, care should be taken to satisfactorily exclude chronic lymphocytic leukemia and mantle cell lymphoma.[1] "Intranuclear" periodic acid-Schiff (PAS)-positive inclusions (Dutcher-Fahey bodies; see Fig. 10)[93] consisting of IgM deposits in the perinuclear space, and sometimes in intranuclear vacuoles, may be seen occasionally in lymphoid cells in WM. An increase in the number of mast cells, usually in association with the lymphoid aggregates is commonly found in WM, and their presence may help in differentiating WM from other B-cell lymphomas.[2,3]

Other investigations

Magnetic resonance imaging (MRI) of the spine in conjunction with computed tomography (CT) of the abdomen and pelvis are useful in evaluating the disease status in WM.[94] Bone marrow involvement can be documented by MRI studies of the spine in over 90% of patients, while CT of the abdomen and pelvis demonstrated enlarged nodes in 43% of WM patients.[94] Lymph node biopsy may show preserved architecture or replacement by infiltration of neoplastic cells with lymphoplasmacytoid, lymphoplasmacytic, or polymorphous cytological patterns. The residual disease after high-dose chemotherapy with allogeneic or autologous stem cell rescue can be monitored by polymerase chain reaction (PCR)-based methods using primers specific for the monoclonal Ig variable regions.

PROGNOSIS

WM typically presents as an indolent disease, although considerable variability in prognosis can be seen. The median survival reported in several large series has ranged from 5 to 10 years.[95-101] Age is consistently an important prognostic factor (>60-70 years),[95,96,98,101] but this factor is often impacted by unrelated morbidities. Anemia, which reflects both marrow involvement and the serum level of the IgM monoclonal protein (due to the impact of IgM on intravascular fluid retention), has emerged as a strong adverse prognostic factor, with hemoglobin levels of <9-12 g/dL associated with decreased survival in several series.[95-98,101] Cytopenias have also been regularly identified as a significant predictor of survival.[96] However, the precise level of cytopenias with prognostic significance remains to be determined.[98] Some series have identified a platelet count

of <100-150 $\times$ 10^9/L and a granulocyte count of <1.5 $\times$ 10^9/L as independent prognostic factors.[95,96,98,101] The number of cytopenias in a given patient has been proposed as a strong prognostic factor.[96] Serum albumin levels have also correlated with survival in WM patients in certain but not all studies using multivariate analyses.[96,98,99] High β_2-microglobulin levels (>3-3.5 g/dL),[97-101] as well as both high (>7 g/dL) and low (<4 g/dL) serum IgM M-protein,[99,101] and the presence of cryoglobulins[95] have been reported as adverse factors in WM patients. A few scoring systems have been proposed on the basis of these analyses (Table 11.3).

TREATMENT OF WALDENSTRÖM MACROGLOBULINEMIA

As part of the 2nd International Workshop on Waldenström macroglobulinemia, a consensus panel was organized to recommend criteria for the initiation of therapy in patients

TABLE 11.3. Prognostic scoring systems in Waldenström macroglobulinemia

Study	Adverse prognostic factors	Number of groups	Survival
Gobbi et al.[95]	Hb < 9 g/dL Age >70 years Weight loss Cryoglobulinemia	Prognostic factors 2-4 Prognostic factors	Median: 48 months Median: 80 months
Morel et al.[96]	Age ≥ 65 years Albumin <4 g/dL Number of cytopenias: Hb <12 g/dL Platelets < 150 $\times$ 10^9/L WBC < 4 $\times$ 10^9/L	Prognostic factors 2 Prognostic factors 3-4 Prognostic factors	5 years: 87% 5 years: 62% 5 years: 25%
Dhodapkar et al.[97]	β_2M ≥ 3 g/dL Hb < 12 g/dL IgM < 4 g/dL	β_2M < 3 mg/dL + Hb ≥ 12 g/dL β_2M < 3 mg/dL + Hb < 12 g/dL β_2M≥ 3 mg/dL + IgM ≥ 4 g/dL β_2M ≥ 3 mg/dL + IgM < 4 g/dL	5 years: 87% 5 years: 63% 5 years: 53% 5 years: 21%
Application of International Staging System criteria for myeloma to WM Dimopoulos et al.[99]	Albumin ≤ 3.5 g/dL β_2M ≥ 3.5 mg/L	Albumin ≥ 3.5 g/dL + β_2M < 3.5 mg/dL Albumin ≤ 3.5 g/dL + β_2M < 3.5 or β_2M 3.5-5.5 mg/dL β_2M > 5.5 mg/dL	Median: NR Median: 116 months Median: 54 months
International Prognostic Scoring System for WM Morel et al.[101]	Age > 65 years Hb < 11.5 g/dL Platelets < 100 $\times$ 10^9/L β_2M > 3 mg/L IgM > 7 g/dL	Prognostic factors* 2 Prognostic factors† 3-5 Prognostic factors	5 years: 87% 5 years: 68% 5 years: 36%

*Excluding age or †age >65.

with WM.[98] The panel recommended that initiation of therapy should not be based on the IgM level per se, since this may not correlate with the clinical manifestations of WM. The consensus panel, however, agreed that the initiation of therapy was appropriate for patients with constitutional symptoms, such as recurrent fever, night sweats, fatigue due to anemia, or weight loss. The presence of progressive symptomatic lymphadenopathy or splenomegaly provides additional reasons to begin therapy. The presence of anemia with a hemoglobin value of <10 g/dL or a platelet count $<100 \times 10^9$/L owing to marrow infiltration also justifies treatment. Certain complications, such as hyperviscosity syndrome, symptomatic sensorimotor peripheral neuropathy, systemic amyloidosis, renal insufficiency, or symptomatic cryoglobulinemia, may also be indications for therapy.[98]

Frontline therapy

While a precise therapeutic algorithm for the therapy of WM remains to be defined, given the paucity of randomized clinical trials, consensus panels composed of experts who treat WM were organized as part of the 2nd and 3rd International Workshop on Waldenström macroglobulinemia and have formulated recommendations for both frontline and salvage therapy of WM based on the best available clinical trials' evidence. Among frontline options, the panels considered alkylator agents (e.g. chlorambucil), nucleoside analogues (cladribine or fludarabine), the monoclonal antibody rituximab as well as combinations thereof as reasonable choices for the upfront therapy of WM.[102,103] Of importance, the panel felt that individual patient considerations, including the presence of cytopenias, need for more rapid disease control, age, and candidacy for autologous transplant therapy should be taken into account in making the choice of a first-line agent. For patients who are candidates for autologous transplant therapy, and in whom such therapy is seriously considered, the panel recommended that exposure to alkylator or nucleoside analogue therapy should be limited.

Alkylator-based therapy
Oral alkylating drugs, alone and in combination therapy with steroids, have been extensively evaluated in

the upfront treatment of WM. The greatest experience with oral alkylator therapy has been with chlorambucil, which has been administered on both a continuous (i.e. daily dose schedule) and an intermittent schedule. Patients receiving chlorambucil on a continuous schedule typically receive 0.1 mg/kg for 1 day, whilst on the intermittent schedule patients will typically receive 0.3 mg/kg for 7 days, every 6 weeks. In a prospective randomized study, Kyle et al.[104] reported no significant difference in the overall response rate between these schedules, although interestingly the median response duration was greater for patients receiving intermittent versus continuously dosed chlorambucil (46 vs. 26 months). Despite the favorable median response duration in this study for use of the intermittent schedule, no difference in the median overall survival was observed. Moreover, an increased incidence for the development of myelodysplasia and acute myelogenous leukemia with the intermittent (3 of 22 patients) versus the continuous (0 of 24 patients) chlorambucil schedule prompted the authors of this study to express preference for the use of continuous chlorambucil dosing. The use of steroids in combination with alkylator therapy has also been explored. Dimopoulos and Alexanian[105] evaluated chlorambucil (8 mg/m²) along with prednisone (40 mg/m²) given orally for 10 days, every 6 weeks, and reported a major response (i.e. reduction of IgM by greater than 50%) in 72% of patients. Nonchlorambucil-based alkylator regimens employing melphalan and cyclophosphamide in combination with steroids have also been examined by Petrucci et al.[106] and Case et al.,[107] producing slightly higher overall response rates and response durations, although the benefit of these more complex regimens over chlorambucil remains to be demonstrated. Facon et al.[108] have evaluated parameters predicting for response to alkylator therapy. Their studies in patients receiving single-agent chlorambucil demonstrated that age 60, male sex, symptomatic status, and cytopenias (but, interestingly, not high tumor burden and serum IgM levels) were associated with poor response to alkylator therapy. Additional factors to be taken into account in considering alkylator therapy for patients with WM include necessity for more rapid disease control given the slow nature of response to alkylator therapy, as well as consideration for preserving stem cells in patients who are candidates for autologous transplant therapy.

Nucleoside analogue therapy

Both cladribine and fludarabine have been extensively evaluated in untreated as well as previously treated WM patients. Cladribine administered as a single agent by continuous intravenous infusion, by 2-hour daily infusion, or by subcutaneous bolus injections for 5-7 days has resulted in major responses in 40%-90% of patients who received primary therapy, whilst in the salvage setting responses have ranged from 38% to 54%.[108-115] Median time to achievement of response in responding patients following cladribine ranged from 1.2 to 5 months. The overall response rate with daily infusional fludarabine therapy administered mainly on 5-day schedules in previously untreated and treated WM patients has ranged from 38% to 100% and 30%-40%, respectively,[116-121] which are on par with the response data for cladribine. Median time to achievement of response for fludarabine was also on par with cladribine at 3-6 months. In general, response rates and durations of responses have been greater for patients receiving nucleoside analogues as first-line agents, although in several of the above studies wherein both untreated and previously treated patients were enrolled, no substantial difference in the overall response rate was reported. Myelosuppression commonly occurred following prolonged exposure to either of the nucleoside analogues, as did lymphopenia with sustained depletion of both $CD4^+$ and $CD8^+$ T lymphocytes observed in WM patients 1 year following initiation of therapy.[108,110] Treatment-related mortality due to myelosuppression and/or opportunistic infections attributable to immunosuppression occurred in up to 5% of all treated patients in some series with either nucleoside analogue. Factors predicting for response to nucleoside analogues in WM included age at start of treatment (<70 years), pretreatment hemoglobin > 95 g/L, platelets >75 000/mm³, disease relapsing off therapy, patients with resistant disease within the first year of diagnosis, and a long interval between first-line therapy and initiation of a nucleoside analogue in relapsing patients.[108,114,120] There are limited data on the use of an alternate nucleoside analogue to salvage patients whose disease relapsed or demonstrated resistance off cladribine or fludarabine therapy.[122,123] Three of four (75%) patients responded to cladribine to salvage patients who progressed following an unmaintained remission to fludarabine, whereas only 1 out of 10 (10%) with disease resistant to fludarabine responded to cladribine.[122] However, Lewandowski et al.[123]

reported a response in two of six patients (33%) and disease stabilization in the remaining patients to fludarabine, in spite of an inadequate response or progressive disease following cladribine therapy. The long-term safety of nucleoside analogues in WM was recently examined by Leleu et al.[124] in a large series of WM patients. A 7-fold increase in transformation to an aggressive lymphoma, and a 3-fold increase in the development of acute myelogenous leukemia/myelodysplasia was observed among patients who received a nucleoside analogue versus other therapies for their WM.

CD20-directed antibody therapy

Rituximab is a chimeric monoclonal antibody that targets CD20, a widely expressed antigen on lymphoplasmacytic cells in WM.[125] Several retrospective and prospective studies have indicated that rituximab, when used at standard dosimetry (i.e. 4 weekly infusions at 375 mg/m²), induced major responses in approximately 27-35% of previously treated and untreated patients.[126-132] Furthermore, it was shown in some of these studies that patients who achieved minor responses or even stable disease benefited from rituximab, as evidenced by improved hemoglobin and platelet counts, and reduction of lymphadenopathy and/or splenomegaly. The median time to treatment failure in these studies was found to range from 8 to 27+ months. Studies evaluating an extended rituximab schedule consisting of 4 weekly courses at 375 mg/m²/week, repeated 3 months later by another 4-week course have demonstrated major response rates of 44%-48%, with time to progression estimates of 16+ to 29+ months.[132,133]

In many WM patients, a transient increase of serum IgM may be noted immediately following initiation of treatment. Such an increase does not herald treatment failure, and while most patients will return to their baseline serum IgM level by 12 weeks, some continue to show prolonged spiking despite demonstrating a reduction in their bone marrow tumor load.[134-136] However, patients with baseline serum IgM levels of >50 g/dL or serum viscosity of >3.5 cp may be particularly at risk for a hyperviscosity-related event, and in such patients plasmapheresis should be considered in advance of rituximab therapy.[135] Because of the decreased likelihood of response in patients with higher IgM levels, as well as the possibility that serum IgM and viscosity levels may abruptly rise, rituximab monotherapy should not be used as sole therapy for the treatment of patients at risk for hyperviscosity symptoms.

Time to response after rituximab is slow and exceeds 3 months on the average. The time to best response in one study was 18 months.[133] Patients with baseline serum IgM levels of <60 g/dL are more likely to respond, irrespective of the underlying bone marrow involvement by tumor cells.[132,133] A recent analysis of 52 patients who were treated with single-agent rituximab has indicated that the objective response rate was significantly lower in patients who had either low serum albumin (<35 g/L) or elevated serum monoclonal protein (>40 g/L M-spike). Furthermore, the presence of both adverse prognostic factors was related with a short time to progression (3.6 months). Moreover, patients who had normal serum albumin and relatively low serum monoclonal protein levels derived a substantial benefit from rituximab, with a time to progression exceeding 40 months.[137]

The genetic background of patients may also be important for determining response to rituximab. In particular, a correlation between polymorphisms at position 158 in the Fc gamma RIIIa receptor (CD16), an activating Fc receptor on important effector cells that mediate antibody-dependent cell-mediated cytotoxicity (ADCC), and rituximab response was observed in WM patients. Individuals may encode either the amino acid valine or phenylalanine at position 158 in the FcγRIIIa receptor. WM patients who carried the valine amino acid (either in a homozygous or in a heterozygous pattern) had a fourfold higher major response rate (i.e. 50% decline in serum IgM levels) to rituximab versus those patients who expressed phenylalanine in a homozygous pattern.[138]

Combination therapies

Because rituximab is an active and a nonmyelosuppressive agent, its combination with chemotherapy has been explored in WM patients. Weber et al.[139] administered rituximab along with cladribine and cyclophosphamide to 17 previously untreated patients with WM. At least a partial response was documented in 94% of WM patients including a complete response in 18%. With a median follow-up of 21 months no patient has relapsed. In a study by the Waldenström Macroglobulinemia Clinical Trials Group (WMCTG), the combination of rituximab and fludarabine was evaluated in 43 WM patients, 32 (75%) of whom were previously untreated.[140] Ninety-one percent of patients

demonstrated at least a 25% decrease in serum IgM levels, and response rates were as follows: CR: 7%; PR: 74.4%, and MR: 9.3%. Hematological toxicity was common with grade III, IV neutropenia observed in 58% of patients. Two deaths occurred in this study, which may have been related to therapy-induced immunosuppression. With a median follow-up of 17 months, 34/39 (87%) remain in remission. The addition of rituximab to fludarabine and cyclophosphamide has also been explored in the salvage setting by Tam et al., wherein 4 of 5 patients demonstrated a response.[141] In another combination study with rituximab, Hensel et al.[142] administered rituximab along with pentostatin and cyclophosphamide to 13 patients with untreated and previously treated WM or LPL. A major response was observed in 77% of patients. In a study by Dimopoulos et al., the combination of rituximab, dexamethasone, and cyclophosphamide was used as primary therapy to treat 72 patients with WM.[143] On an intent to treat basis, at least a major response was observed in 74% of patients. With a median follow-up of 24 months, 67% of patients are progression free. Therapy was well tolerated, although one patient died of interstitial pneumonia.

In addition to nucleoside analogue–based trials with rituximab, two studies have examined CHOP (cyclophosphamide, doxorubicin, vincristine, prednisone) in combination with rituximab (CHOP-R). In a randomized frontline study by the German Low Grade Lymphoma Study Group (GLSG) involving 72 patients (71% of whom had LPL), a significantly higher response rate (94% vs. 69%) was observed among patients receiving CHOP-R versus CHOP, respectively.[144] Treon et al.[145] have also evaluated CHOP-R in 13 WM patients, 8 and 5 of whom were relapsed or refractory to nucleoside analogues and single-agent rituximab, respectively. Among 13 evaluable patients, 10 patients achieved a major response (77%) including 3 CR and 7 PR, and 2 patients achieved a minor response.

The addition of alkylating agents to nucleoside analogues has also been explored in WM. Weber et al.[139] administered two cycles of oral cyclophosphamide along with subcutaneous cladribine to 37 patients with previously untreated WM. At least a partial response was observed in 84% of patients, and the median duration of response was 36 months. Dimopoulos et al.[146] examined fludarabine in combination with intravenous cyclophosphamide and observed partial responses in 6 of 11 (55%) WM patients with primary refractory disease or who had relapsed on treatment. The combination of fludarabine plus cyclos-phosphamide was also evaluated in a recent study by Tamburini et al.[147] involving 49 patients, 35 of whom were previously treated. Seventy-eight percent of the patients in this study achieved a response, and median time to treatment failure was 27 months. Hematological toxicity was commonly observed, and three patients died of treatment-related toxicities. Two interesting findings in this study was the development of acute leukemia in two patients, histologic transformation to diffuse large cell lymphoma in one patient, and two cases of solid malignancies (prostate and melanoma), as well as failure to mobilize stem cells in four of six patients.

In view of the above data, the consensus panel on therapeutics amended its original recommendations for the therapy of WM to include the use of combination therapy with either nucleoside analogues and alkylator agents or rituximab in combination with nucleoside analogues, nucleoside analogues plus alkylator agents, or combination chemotherapy such as CHOP as reasonable therapeutics options for the treatment of WM.[103]

Salvage therapy including novel agents

For patients in relapse or who have refractory disease, the consensus panels recommended the use of an alternative first-line agent as defined above, with the caveat that for those patients for whom autologous transplantation was being seriously considered, further exposure to stem cell damaging agents (i.e. many alkylator agents and nucleoside analogue drugs) should be avoided, and a non–stem cell toxic agent should be considered if stem cells had not previously been harvested.[102,103] Recent studies have also demonstrated activity for several novel agents including bortezomib, thalidomide alone or in combination, and alemtuzumab and can be considered in the treatment of relapsed/refractory WM. Finally, autologous stem cell transplant remains an option for the salvage therapy of WM, particularly among younger patients who have had multiple relapses, or have primary refractory disease.

Proteasome inhibitor

Bortezomib, a stem cell sparing agent,[148,149] is a proteasome inhibitor that induces apoptosis of primary WM lymphoplasmacytic cells, as well as the WM-WSU WM cell line at pharmacologically achievable levels.[150] Moreover,

bortezomib may also impact on bone marrow microenvironmental support for lymphoplasmacytic cells.[151] In a multicenter study of the Waldenström Macroglobulinemia Clinical Trials Group (WMCTG),[152] 27 patients received up to 8 cycles of bortezomib at 1.3 mg/m^2 on days 1, 4, 8, and 11. All but one patient had relapsed/or refractory disease. Following therapy, median serum IgM levels declined from 4660 mg/dL to 2092 mg/dL (p < 0.0001). The overall response rate was 85%, with 10 and 13 patients achieving a minor (<25% decrease in IgM) and major (<50% decrease in IgM) response. Responses were prompt, and occurred at median of 1.4 months. The median time to progression for all responding patients in this study was 7.9 (range 3-21.4+) months, and the most common grade III/IV toxicities occurring in >5% of patients were sensory neuropathies (22.2%); leukopenia (18.5%); neutropenia (14.8%); dizziness (11.1%); and thrombocytopenia (7.4%). Of importance, sensory neuropathies resolved or improved in nearly all patients following cessation of therapy. As part of an NCI-Canada study, Chen et al.[153] treated 27 patients with both untreated (44%) and previously treated (56%) disease. Patients in this study received bortezomib utilizing the standard schedule until they demonstrated either progressive disease or two cycles beyond a complete response or stable disease. The overall response rate in this study was 78%, with major responses observed in 44% of patients. Sensory neuropathy occurred in 20 patients, 5 with grade > 3, and it occurred following 2-4 cycles of therapy. Among the 20 patients developing a neuropathy, 14 patients resolved and one patient demonstrated a one-grade improvement at 2-13 months. In addition to the above experiences with bortezomib monotherapy in WM, Dimopoulos et al.[154] observed major responses in 6 of 10 (60%) previously treated WM patients, whereas Goy et al.[155] observed a major response in one of two WM patients included in a series of relapsed or refractory patients with non-Hodgkin's lymphoma (NHL). In view of the single-agent activity of bortezomib in WM, Treon et al.[156] have examined the combination of bortezomib, dexamethasone, and rituximab (BDR) as primary therapy in patients with WM. An overall response rate of 95% and a major response rate of 70% were observed with the BDR combination. The incidence of grade 3 neuropathy was about 30% in this study, but was reversible in most patients following discontinuation of therapy. An increased incidence of herpes zoster was also observed, prompting the prophylactic use of antiviral therapy with BDR. Alternative schedules for the administration of bortezomib (i.e. once weekly at higher doses) in combination with rituximab are also being examined by Ghobrial et al.[157] and Agathocleous et al.[158] in patients with WM with overall response rates of 80%-90%. The impact of these schedules on the development of bortezomib-related peripheral neuropathy remains to be clarified, although in one study appeared diminished.[157]

CD52-directed antibody therapy

Alemtuzumab is a humanized monoclonal antibody that targets CD52, an antigen widely expressed on bone marrow LPC in WM patients, as well as on mast cells that are increased in the BM of patients with WM and provide growth and survival signals to WM LPC through several TNF family ligands (CD40L, APRIL, BLYS). As part of a WMCTG effort,[159] 28 subjects with the REAL/WHO clinico-pathological diagnosis of LPL, including 27 patients with IgM (WM) and one with IgA monoclonal gammopathy, were enrolled in this prospective, multicenter study. Five patients were untreated and 23 were previously treated, all of whom had previously received rituximab. Patients received three daily test doses of alemtuzumab (3, 10, and 30 mg IV) followed by 30 mg alemtuzumab IV three times a week for up to 12 weeks. All patients received acyclovir and bactrim or equivalent prophylaxis for the duration of therapy plus 8 weeks following the last infusion of alemtuzumab. Among 25 patients evaluable for response, the overall response rate was 76%, which included 8 (32%) major responders and 11 (44%) minor responders. Hematological toxicities were common among previously treated (but not untreated) patients and included grade 3/4 neutropenia 39%; thrombocytopenia 18%; anemia 7%. Grade 3/4 non-hematological toxicity for all patients included dermatitis 11%; fatigue 7%; and infection 7%. CMV reactivation and infection was commonly seen among previously treated patients and may have been etiological for one death on study. With a median follow-up of 8.5+ months, 11/19 responding patients remain free of progression. High rates of response with the use of alemtuzumab as salvage therapy have also been reported by Owen et al.[160] in a small series of heavily pretreated WM patients (with a median prior therapies of 4) who received up to 12 weeks of therapy (at 30 mg IV TIW) following initial dose escalation. Among the seven patients receiving alemtuzumab, five patients achieved a partial response, and one patient a complete response. Infectious complications were common, with CMV reactivation occurring in three patients requiring ganciclovir therapy and hospitalization for three patients for bacterial infections. Opportunistic infections occurred in two patients and was responsible for their deaths. An upfront study by the WMCTG examining the role of alemtuzumab in combination with rituximab is anticipated given the efficacy results of the above studies.

Thalidomide and lenalidomide

Thalidomide as a single agent, and in combination with dexamethasone and clarithromycin, has also been examined in patients with WM, in view of the success of these regimens in patients with advanced multiple myeloma. Dimopoulos et al.[161] demonstrated a major response in 5 out of 20 (25%) previously untreated and treated patients who received single-agent thalidomide. Dose escalation from the thalidomide start dose of 200 mg daily was hindered by the development of side effects, including the development of peripheral neuropathy in five patients obligating discontinuation or dose reduction. Low doses of thalidomide (50 mg orally daily) in combination with dexamethasone (40 mg orally once a week) and clarithromycin (250 mg orally twice a day) have also been examined, with 10 out of 12 (83%) previously treated patients demonstrating at least a major response.[162] However, in a follow-up study by Dimopoulos et al.[163] using a higher thalidomide dose (200 mg orally daily) along with dexamethasone (40 g orally once a week) and clarithromycin (500 mg orally twice a day), only 2 out of 10 (20%) previously treated patients responded. In a previous study, the immunomodulators thalidomide and its analogue lenalidomide significantly augmented rituximab-mediated antibody-dependent cell-mediated cytotoxicity (ADCC) against lymphoplasmacytic cells.[164] Moreover, an expansion of natural killer cells has been observed with thalidomide, which in previous studies have been shown to be associated with rituximab response.[165,166] In view of these data, the WMCTG conducted two phase 2 clinical trials in symptomatic patients with WM combining thalidomide or lenalidomide with rituximab.[167] Intended therapy for patients on the phase 2 study of thalidomide plus rituximab consisted of thalidomide administered at 200 mg daily for 2 weeks, followed by 400 mg daily thereafter for 1 year. Patients received four weekly infusions of rituximab at 375 mg/m² beginning 1 week after the initiation of thalidomide, followed by four additional weekly infusions of rituximab at 375 mg/m^2 beginning at week 13. Twenty-three of twenty-five patients were evaluable in this study, and responses included CR ($n = 1$); PR ($n = 15$); MR ($n = 2$); SD ($n = 1$) for an overall (ORR) and a major response rate of 78% and 70%, respectively. Median serum IgM levels decreased from 3670 (924-8610 mg/dL) to 1590 (36-5230 mg/dL) (p < 0.001), while the median hematocrit rose from 33.0 (23.6%-42.6%) to 37.6 (29.3%-44.3%) (p = 0.004) at best response. With a median follow-up of 42+ months, the median TTP for evaluable patients on this study was 35 months, and 38+ months for responders. Responses were associated with a median cumulative thalidomide dose: CR/PR/MR (29 275 mg) versus SD/NR (7400 mg); p = 0.004. Responses were unaffected by FcγRIIIA-158 polymorphism status (81% vs. 71% for VV/FV vs. FF); IgM (78% vs. 80% for <6000 vs. >6000 mg/dL); and B$_2$M (71% vs. 89% for <3 vs. >3 g/dL). Dose reduction of thalidomide occurred in all patients and led to discontinuation in 11 patients. Among 11 patients experiencing grade > 2 neuroparesthesias, 10 demonstrated resolution to grade 1 ($n = 3$) or complete resolution ($n = 7$) at a median of 6.7 (range 0.4-22.5 months).

In a phase 2 study of lenalidomide and rituximab in WM,[168] patients were initiated on lenalidomide at 25 mg daily on a syncopated schedule wherein therapy was administered for 3 weeks, followed by a 1 week pause for an intended duration of 48 weeks. Patients received 1 week of therapy with lenalidomide, after which rituximab (375 mg/m^2) was administered weekly on weeks 2-5, and then 13-16. Twelve of sixteen patients were evaluable and responses included PR ($n = 4$); MR ($n = 4$); SD ($n = 3$); NR ($n = 1$) for an overall and a major response rate of 67% and 33%, respectively, and a median TTP of 15.6 months. In two patients with bulky disease, significant reduction in node/spleen size was observed. Acute decreases in hematocrit were observed during first 2 weeks of lenalidomide therapy in 13/16 (81%) patients, with a median hematocrit decrease of 4.4% (1.7%-7.2%), resulting in hospitalization in four patients. Despite reduction of initiation doses to 5 mg daily, anemia continued to be problematic without evidence of hemolysis or more general myelosuppression. Therefore, the mechanism for pronounced anemia in WM patients receiving lenalidomide remains to be determined and the use of this agent among WM patients remains investigational.

High-dose therapy and stem cell transplantation

The use of transplant therapy has also been explored in WM patients. Desikan et al.[169] reported their initial experience of high-dose chemotherapy and autologous stem cell transplant, which has more recently been updated by Munshi et al.[170] Their studies involved eight previously treated WM patients between the ages of 45 and 69 years, who received either melphalan at 200 mg/m^2 ($n = 7$) or melphalan at 140 mg/m^2 along with total body irradiation. Stem cells were successfully collected in all eight patients, although a second collection procedure was required for two patients who had extensive previous nucleoside analogue exposure. There were no transplant-related mortalities and toxicities were manageable. All eight patients responded, with seven out of eight patients achieving a major response, and one patient achieving a complete response with durations of response ranging from 5+ to 77+ months. Dreger et al.[171] investigated the use of the DEXA-BEAM (dexamethasone, BCNU, etoposide, cytarabine, melphalan) regimen followed by myeloablative therapy with cyclophosphamide, and total body irradiation and autologous stem cell transplantation in seven WM patients, which included four untreated patients. Serum IgM levels declined by >50% following DEXA-BEAM and myeloablative therapy for six out of seven patients, with progression-free survival ranging from 4+ to 30+ months. All three evaluable patients, who were previously treated, also attained a major response in a study by Anagnostopoulos et al.[172] in which WM patients received various preparative regimens and showed event-free survivals of 26+, 31, and 108+ months. Tournilhac et al.[173] recently reported the outcome of 18 WM patients in France who received high-dose chemotherapy followed by autologous stem cell transplantation. All patients were previously treated with a median of three (range 1-5) prior regimens. Therapy was well tolerated, with an improvement in response status observed for seven patients (six PR to CR; one SD to PR), while only one patient demonstrated progressive disease. The median event-free survival for all nonprogressing patients was 12 months. Tournilhac et al.[173] have also reported the outcome of allogeneic transplantation in 10 previously treated WM patients (ages 35-46), who received a median of three prior therapies, including three patients with progressive disease despite therapy. Two out of three patients with progressive disease responded, and an improvement in response status was observed in five patients. The median event-free survival for nonprogressing, evaluable patients was 31 months. Of concern in this series was the death of three patients owing to transplantation-related toxicity. Anagnostopoulos et al.[174] have also reported on a retrospective review of WM patients who underwent either autologous or allogeneic transplantation, and whose outcomes were reported to the Center for International Blood and Marrow Transplant Research. Seventy-eight percent of patients in this cohort had two or more previous therapies, and 58% of them were resistant to their previous therapy. The relapse rate at 3 years was 29% in the allogeneic group and 24% in the autologous group. Nonrelapse mortality, however, was 40% in the allogeneic group and 11% in the autologous group in this series. In view of the high rate of nonrelapse mortality associated with high-dose chemotherapy and allogeneic transplantation, Maloney et al.[175] have evaluated the use of nonmyeloablative allogeneic transplantation in five patients with refractory WM. In this series, three of three evaluable patients (all of whom had matched sibling donors) responded with two CR and one in PR at 1-3 years post-transplant. In view of the above data, the consensus panel on therapeutics for WM has recommended that autologous transplantation in WM be considered in the relapsed setting, particularly among younger patients who have had multiple relapses or primary refractory disease, whereas allogeneic and mini-allogeneic transplantation should be undertaken ideally in the context of a clinical trial.[102,103]

RESPONSE CRITERIA IN WALDENSTRÖM MACROGLOBULINEMIA

Assessment of response to treatment of WM has been widely heterogeneous. As a consequence, studies using the same regimen have reported significantly different response rates. As part of the second and third International Workshops on WM, consensus panels developed guidelines for uniform response criteria in WM.[176,177] The category of minor response was adopted at the Third International Workshop of WM, given that clinically meaningful responses were observed with newer biological agents and is based on >25% to <50% decrease in serum IgM level, which is used as a surrogate marker of disease in WM. In distinction, the term major response is used to denote a response of >50% in serum IgM levels, and includes partial and complete responses.[174] Response categories and criteria for progressive disease in WM based on consensus recommendations are summarized in Table 11.4. An important concern with the use of IgM as a surrogate marker of disease is that it can fluctuate, independent of tumor cell killing, particularly with newer biologically targeted agents such as rituximab and bortezomib.[134-136,152,178] Rituximab induces a spike or flare in serum IgM levels that can last for months, whereas bortezomib can suppress IgM levels independent of tumor cell killing in certain patients. In circumstances where the serum IgM levels appear out of context with the clinical progress of the patient, a bone marrow biopsy

TABLE 11.4. Summary of updated response criteria from the 3rd International Workshop on Waldenström macroglobulinemia[173]		
Complete response	CR	Disappearance of monoclonal protein by immunofixation; no histological evidence of bone marrow involvement, and resolution of any adenopathy/organomegaly (confirmed by CT scan), along with no signs or symptoms attributable to WM. Reconfirmation of the CR status is required at least 6 weeks apart with a second immunofixation
Partial response	PR	A ≥50% reduction of serum monoclonal IgM concentration on protein electrophoresis and ≥50% decrease in adenopathy/organomegaly on physical examination or on CT scan. No new symptoms or signs of active disease
Minor response	MR	A ≥25% but <50% reduction of serum monoclonal IgM by protein electrophoresis. No new symptoms or signs of active disease
Stable disease	SD	A <25% reduction and <25% increase of serum monoclonal IgM by electrophoresis without progression of adenopathy/organomegaly, cytopenias, or clinically significant symptoms due to disease and/or signs of WM
Progressive disease	PD	A ≥25% increase in serum monoclonal IgM by protein electrophoresis confirmed by a second measurement or progression of clinically significant findings due to disease (i.e. anemia, thrombocytopenia, leukopenia, bulky adenopathy/organomegaly) or symptoms (unexplained recurrent fever ≥ 38.4°C, drenching night sweats, ≥10% body weight loss, or hyperviscosity, neuropathy, symptomatic cryoglobulinemia, or amyloidosis) attributable to WM

should be considered in order to clarify the patient's underlying disease burden. Soluble CD27 is currently being investigated by Ho et al.[34] as an alternative surrogate marker in WM.

REFERENCES

1. Owen RG, Treon SP, Al-Katib A, et al. Clinicopathological definition of Waldenström's macroglobulinemia: Consensus Panel Recommendations from the Second International Workshop on Waldenström's macroglobulinemia. *Semin Oncol* 2003;30:110-15.

2. Harris NL, Jaffe ES, Stein H, et al. A revised European-American classification of lymphoid neoplasms: a proposal from the International Lymphoma Study Group. *Blood* 1994; 84:1361-92.

3. Harris NL, Jaffe ES, Diebold J, et al. The World Health Organization classification of neoplastic diseases of the hematopoietic and lymphoid tissues. Report of the Clinical Advisory Committee meeting, Airlie House, Virginia, November, 1997. *Ann Oncol* 1999;10:1419-32.

4. Groves FD, Travis LB, Devesa SS, Ries LA, Fraumeni JF Jr. Waldenström's macroglobulinemia: incidence patterns in the United States, 1988-1994. *Cancer* 1998;82:1078-81.

5. Herrinton LJ, Weiss NS. Incidence of Waldenström's macroglobulinemia. *Blood* 1993;82:3148-50.

6. Bjornsson OG, Arnason A, Gudmunosson S, Jensson O, Olafsson S, Valimarsson H. Macroglobulinaemia in an Icelandic family. *Acta Med Scand* 1978;203:283-8.

7. Treon SP, Hunter ZR, Aggarwal A, et al. Characterization of familial Waldenstrom's Macroglobulinemia. *Ann Oncol* 2006;17:488-94.

8. Renier G, Ifrah N, Chevailler A, Saint-Andre JP, Boasson M, Hurez D. Four brothers with Waldenström's macroglobulinemia. *Cancer* 1989;64:1554-9.

9. Ogmundsdottir HM, Sveinsdottir S, Sigfusson A, Skaftadottir I, Jonasson JG, Agnarsson BA. Enhanced B cell survival in familial macroglobulinaemia is associated with increased expression of Bcl-2. *Clin Exp Immunol* 1999;117:252-60.

10. Linet MS, Humphrey RL, Mehl ES, Brown LM, Pottern LM, Bias WB, et al. A case-control and family study of Waldenström's macroglobulinemia. *Leukemia* 1993;7:1363-9.

11. Santini GF, Crovatto M, Modolo ML, et al. Waldenström macroglobulinemia: a role of HCV infection? *Blood* 1993;82:2932.

12. Silvestri F, Barillari G, Fanin R, et al. Risk of hepatitis C virus infection, Waldenström's macroglobulinemia, and monoclonal gammopathies. *Blood* 1996;88:1125-6.

13. Leleu X, O'Connor K, Ho A, et al. Hepatitis C viral infection is not associated with Waldenstrom's macroglobulinemia. *Am J Hematol* 2007;82: 83-4.

14. Carbone P, Caradonna F, Granata G, Marceno R, Cavallaro AM, Barbata G. Chromosomal abnormalities in Waldenstrom's macroglobulinemia. *Cancer Genet Cytogenet* 1992;61:147-51.

15. Mansoor A, Medeiros LJ, Weber DM, et al. Cytogenetic findings in lymphoplasmacytic lymphoma/Waldenström macroglobulinemia. Chromosomal abnormalities are associated with the polymorphous subtype and an aggressive clinical course. *Am J Clin Pathol* 2001;116:543-9.

16. Han T, Sadamori N, Takeuchi J, et al. Clonal chromosome abnormalities in patients with Waldenstrom's and CLL-associated macroglobulinemia: significance of trisomy 12. *Blood* 1983;62:525-31.

17. Rivera AI, Li MM, Beltran G, Krause JR. Trisomy 4 as the sole cytogenetic abnormality in a Waldenstrom macroglobulinemia. *Cancer Genet Cytogenet* 2002;133:172-3.

18. Wong KF, So CC, Chan JC, Kho BC, Chan JK. Gain of chromosome 3/3q in B-cell chronic lymphoproliferative disorder is associated with plasmacytoid differentiation with or without IgM overproduction. *Cancer Genet Cytogenet* 2002;136:82-5.

19. Schop RF, Kuehl WM, Van Wier SA, et al. Waldenström macroglobulinemia neoplastic cells lack immunoglobulin heavy chain locus translocations but have frequent 6q deletions. *Blood* 2002;100:2996-3001.

20. Avet-Loiseau H, Garand R, Lode L, Robillard N, Bataille R. 14q32 translocations discriminate IgM multiple myeloma from Waldenstrom's macroglobulinemia. *Semin Oncol* 2003;30:153-5.

21. Preud'homme JL, Seligmann M. Immunoglobulins on the surface of lymphoid cells in Waldenström's macroglobulinemia. *J Clin Invest* 1972;51:701-5.

22. Smith BR, Robert NJ, Ault KA. In Waldenstrom's macroglobulinemia the quantity of detectable circulating monoclonal B lymphocytes correlates with clinical course. *Blood* 1983; 61:911-14.

23. Levy Y, Fermand JP, Navarro S, et al. Interleukin 6 dependence of spontaneous in vitro differentiation of B cells from patients with IgM gammopathy. *Proc Natl Acad Sci USA* 1990;87:3309-13.

24. Owen RG, Barrans SL, Richards SJ, et al. Waldenström macroglobulinemia. Development of diagnostic criteria and identification of prognostic factors. *Am J Clin Pathol* 2001;116:420-8.

25. Feiner HD, Rizk CC, Finfer MD, et al. IgM monoclonal gammopathy/Waldenström's macroglobulinemia: a morphological and immunophenotypic study of the bone marrow. *Mod Pathol* 1990;3:348-56.

26. San Miguel JF, Vidriales MB, Ocio E, et al. Immunophenotypic analysis of Waldenstrom's macroglobulinemia. *Semin Oncol* 2003;30:187-95.

27. Hunter ZR, Branagan AR, Manning R, et al. CD5, CD10, CD23 expression in Waldenstrom's Macroglobulinemia. *Clin Lymph* 2005;5:246-9.

28. Wagner SD, Martinelli V, Luzzatto L. Similar patterns of V kappa gene usage but different degrees of somatic mutation in hairy cell leukemia, prolymphocytic leukemia, Waldenström's macroglobulinemia, and myeloma. *Blood* 1994;83:3647-53.

29. Aoki H, Takishita M, Kosaka M, Saito S. Frequent somatic mutations in D and/or JH segments of Ig gene in Waldenström's macroglobulinemia and chronic lymphocytic leukemia

(CLL) with Richter's syndrome but not in common CLL. *Blood* 1995;85:1913-19.

30. Shiokawa S, Suehiro Y, Uike N, Muta K, Nishimura J. Sequence and expression analyses of mu and delta transcripts in patients with Waldenström's macroglobulinemia. *Am J Hematol* 2001;68:139-43.

31. Sahota SS, Forconi F, Ottensmeier CH, et al. Typical Waldenström macroglobulinemia is derived from a B-cell arrested after cessation of somatic mutation but prior to isotype switch events. *Blood* 2002;100:1505-7.

32. Paramithiotis E, Cooper MD. Memory B lymphocytes migrate to bone marrow in humans. *Proc Natl Acad Sci USA* 1997;94:208-12.

33. Tournilhac O, Santos DD, Xu L, et al. Mast cells in Waldenstrom's Macroglobulinemia support lymphoplasmacytic cell growth through CD154/CD40 signaling. *Ann Oncol* 2006;17:1275-82.

34. Ho A, Leleu X, Hatjiharissi E, et al. CD27-CD70 interactions in the pathogenesis of Waldenstrom's Macroglobulinemia. *Blood* 2008; Epub ahead of print.

35. Merlini G, Farhangi M, Osserman EF. Monoclonal immunoglobulins with antibody activity in myeloma, macroglobulinemia and related plasma cell dyscrasias. *Semin Oncol* 1986;13:350-65.

36. Farhangi M, Merlini G. The clinical implications of monoclonal immunoglobulins. *Semin Oncol* 1986;13:366-79.

37. Marmont AM, Merlini G. Monoclonal autoimmunity in hematology. *Haematologica* 1991;76:449-59.

38. Mackenzie MR, Babcock J. Studies of the hyperviscosity syndrome. II. Macroglobulinemia. *J Lab Clin Med* 1975;85:227-34.

39. Gertz MA, Kyle RA. Hyperviscosity syndrome. *J Intens Care Med* 1995;10:128-41.

40. Kwaan HC, Bongu A. The hyperviscosity syndromes. *Semin Thromb Hemost* 1999;25:199-208.

41. Singh A, Eckardt KU, Zimmermann A, et al. Increased plasma viscosity as a reason for inappropriate erythropoietin formation. *J Clin Invest* 1993;91:251-6.

42. Menke MN, Feke GT, McMeel JW, Branagan A, Hunter Z, Treon SP. Hyperviscosity-related retinopathy in Waldenstrom's Macroglobulinemia. *Arch Opthalmol* 2006;124:1601-6.

43. Merlini G, Baldini L, Broglia C, et al. Prognostic factors in symptomatic Waldenström's macroglobulinemia. *Semin Oncol* 2003;30:211-15.

44. Dellagi K, Dupouey P, Brouet JC, et al. Waldenström's macroglobulinemia and peripheral neuropathy: a clinical and immunologic study of 25 patients. *Blood* 1983;62:280-5.

45. Nobile-Orazio E, Marmiroli P, Baldini L, et al. Peripheral neuropathy in macroglobulinemia: incidence and antigen-specificity of M proteins. *Neurology* 1987;37:1506-14.

46. Nemni R, Gerosa E, Piccolo G, Merlini G. Neuropathies associated with monoclonal gammopathies. *Haematologica* 1994;79:557-66.

47. Ropper AH, Gorson KC. Neuropathies associated with paraproteinemia. *N Engl J Med* 1998;338:1601-7.

48. Vital A. Paraproteinemic neuropathies. *Brain Pathol* 2001;11:399-407.

49. Latov N, Braun PE, Gross RB, Sherman WH, Penn AS, Chess L. Plasma cell dyscrasia and peripheral neuropathy: identification of the myelin antigens that react with human paraproteins. *Proc Natl Acad Sci USA* 1981;78:7139-42.

50. Chassande B, Leger JM, Younes-Chennoufi AB, et al. Peripheral neuropathy associated with IgM monoclonal gammopathy: correlations between M-protein antibody activity and clinical/electrophysiological features in 40 cases. *Muscle Nerve* 1998;21:55-62.

51. Weiss MD, Dalakas MC, Lauter CJ, Willison HJ, Quarles RH. Variability in the binding of anti-MAG and anti-SGPG antibodies to target antigens in demyelinating neuropathy and IgM paraproteinemia. *J Neuroimmunol* 1999;95:174-84.

52. Latov N, Hays AP, Sherman WH. Peripheral neuropathy and anti-MAG antibodies. *Crit Rev Neurobiol* 1988;3:301-32.

53. Dalakas MC, Quarles RH. Autoimmune ataxic neuropathies (sensory ganglionopathies): are glycolipids the responsible autoantigens? *Ann Neurol* 1996;39:419-22.

54. Eurelings M, Ang CW, Notermans NC, Van Doorn PA, Jacobs BC, Van den Berg LH. Antiganglioside antibodies in polyneuropathy associated with monoclonal gammopathy. *Neurology* 2001;57:1909-12.

55. Ilyas AA, Quarles RH, Dalakas MC, Fishman PH, Brady RO. Monoclonal IgM in a patient with paraproteinemic polyneuropathy binds to gangliosides containing disialosyl groups. *Ann Neurol* 1985;18:655-9.

56. Willison HJ, O'Leary CP, Veitch J, et al. The clinical and laboratory features of chronic sensory ataxic neuropathy with anti-disialosyl IgM antibodies. *Brain* 2001;124:1968-77.

57. Lopate G, Choksi R, Pestronk A. Severe sensory ataxia and demyelinating polyneuropathy with IgM anti-GM2 and GalNAc-GD1A antibodies. *Muscle Nerve* 2002;25:828-36.

58. Jacobs BC, O'Hanlon GM, Breedland EG, Veitch J, Van Doorn PA, Willison HJ. Human IgM paraproteins demonstrate shared reactivity between *Campylobacter jejuni* lipopolysaccharides and human peripheral nerve disialylated gangliosides. *J Neuroimmunol* 1997;80:23-30.

59. Nobile-Orazio E, Manfredini E, Carpo M, et al. Frequency and clinical correlates of antineural IgM antibodies in neuropathy associated with IgM monoclonal gammopathy. *Ann Neurol* 1994;36:416-24.

60. Gordon PH, Rowland LP, Younger DS, et al. Lymphoproliferative disorders and motor neuron disease: an update. *Neurology* 1997;48:1671-8.

61. Pavord SR, Murphy PT, Mitchell VE. POEMS syndrome and Waldenström's macroglobulinaemia. *J Clin Pathol* 1996;49:181-2.

62. Crisp D, Pruzanski W. B-cell neoplasms with homogeneous cold-reacting antibodies (cold agglutinins). *Am J Med* 1982;72:915-22.

63. Pruzanski W, Shumak KH. Biologic activity of cold-reacting autoantibodies (first of two parts). *N Engl J Med* 1977;297:538-42.

64. Pruzanski W, Shumak KH. Biologic activity of cold-reacting autoantibodies (second of two parts). *N Engl J Med* 1977;297:583-9.

65. Whittaker SJ, Bhogal BS, Black MM. Acquired immunobullous disease: a cutaneous manifestation of IgM macroglobulinaemia. *Br J Dermatol* 1996;135:283-6.

66. Daoud MS, Lust JA, Kyle RA, Pittelkow MR. Monoclonal gammopathies and associated skin disorders. *J Am Acad Dermatol* 1999;40:507-35.

67. Gad A, Willen R, Carlen B, Gyland F, Wickander M. Duodenal involvement in Waldenström's macroglobulinemia. *J Clin Gastroenterol* 1995;20:174-6.

68. Case records of the Massachusetts General Hospital. Weekly clinicopathological exercises. Case 3-1990. A 66-year-old woman with Waldenström's macroglobulinemia, diarrhea, anemia, and persistent gastrointestinal bleeding. *N Engl J Med* 1990;322:183-92.

69. Isaac J, Herrera GA. Cast nephropathy in a case of Waldenström's macroglobulinemia. *Nephron* 2002;91:512-15.

70. Morel-Maroger L, Basch A, Danon F, Verroust P, Richet G. Pathology of the kidney in Waldenström's macroglobulinemia. Study of sixteen cases. *N Engl J Med* 1970;283:123-9.

71. Gertz MA, Kyle RA, Noel P. Primary systemic amyloidosis: a rare complication of immunoglobulin M monoclonal gammopathies and Waldenström's macroglobulinemia. *J Clin Oncol* 1993;11:914-20.

72. Moyner K, Sletten K, Husby G, Natvig JB. An unusually large (83 amino acid residues) amyloid fibril protein AA from a patient with Waldenström's macroglobulinaemia and amyloidosis. *Scand J Immunol* 1980;11:549-54.

73. Gardyn J, Schwartz A, Gal R, Lewinski U, Kristt D, Cohen AM. Waldenström's macroglobulinemia associated with AA amyloidosis. *Int J Hematol* 2001;74:76-8.

74. Dussol B, Kaplanski G, Daniel L, Brunet P, Pellissier JF, Berland Y. Simultaneous occurrence of fibrillary glomerulopathy and AL amyloid. *Nephrol Dial Transplant* 1998;13:2630-2.

75. Rausch PG, Herion JC. Pulmonary manifestations of Waldenström macroglobulinemia. *Am J Hematol* 1980;9:201-9.

76. Fadil A, Taylor DE. The lung and Waldenström's macroglobulinemia. *South Med J* 1998;91:681-5.

77. Kyrtsonis MC, Angelopoulou MK, Kontopidou FN, et al. Primary lung involvement in Waldenström's macroglobulinaemia: report of two cases and review of the literature. *Acta Haematol* 2001;105:92-6.

78. Kaila VL, El-Newihi HM, Dreiling BJ, Lynch CA, Mihas AA. Waldenström's macroglobulinemia of the stomach presenting with upper gastrointestinal hemorrhage. *Gastrointest Endosc* 1996;44:73-5.

79. Yasui O, Tukamoto F, Sasaki N, et al. Malignant lymphoma of the transverse colon associated with macroglobulinemia. *Am J Gastroenterol* 1997;92:2299-301.

80. Rosenthal JA, Curran WJ Jr, Schuster SJ. Waldenström's macroglobulinemia resulting from localized gastric lymphoplasmacytoid lymphoma. *Am J Hematol* 1998;58:244-5.

81. Recine MA, Perez MT, Cabello-Inchausti B, Lilenbaum RC, Robinson MJ. Extranodal lymphoplasmacytoid lymphoma (immunocytoma) presenting as small intestinal obstruction. *Arch Pathol Lab Med* 2001;125:677-9.

82. Veltman GA, van Veen S, Kluin-Nelemans JC, Bruijn JA, van Es LA. Renal disease in Waldenström's macroglobulinaemia. *Nephrol Dial Transplant* 1997;12:1256-9.

83. Moore DF Jr, Moulopoulos LA, Dimopoulos MA. Waldenström macroglobulinemia presenting as a renal or perirenal mass: clinical and radiographic features. *Leuk Lymphoma* 1995;17:331-4.

84. Mascaro JM, Montserrat E, Estrach T, et al. Specific cutaneous manifestations of Waldenström's macroglobulinaemia. A report of two cases. *Br J Dermatol* 1982;106:17-22.

85. Schnitzler L, Schubert B, Boasson M, Gardais J, Tourmen A. Urticaire chronique, lésions osseuses, macroglobulinémie IgM: Maladie de Waldenström? *Bull Soc Fr Dermatol Syphiligr* 1974;81:363-8.

86. Roux S, Fermand JP, Brechignac S, Mariette X, Kahn MF, Brouet JC. Tumoral joint involvement in multiple myeloma and Waldenström's macroglobulinemia – report of 4 cases. *J Rheumatol* 1996;23:2175-8.

87. Orellana J, Friedman AH. Ocular manifestations of multiple myeloma, Waldenström's macroglobulinemia and benign monoclonal gammopathy. *Surv Ophthalmol* 1981;26:157-69.

88. Ettl AR, Birbamer GG, Philipp W. Orbital involvement in Waldenström's macroglobulinemia: ultrasound, computed tomography and magnetic resonance findings. *Ophthalmologica* 1992;205:40-5.

89. Civit T, Coulbois S, Baylac F, Taillandier L, Auque J. [Waldenström's macroglobulinemia and cerebral lymphoplasmocytic proliferation: Bing and Neel syndrome. Apropos of a new case.] *Neurochirurgie* 1997;43:245-9.

90. McMullin MF, Wilkin HJ, Elder E. Inaccurate haemoglobin estimation in Waldenström's macroglobulinaemia. *J Clin Pathol* 1995;48:787.

91. Treon SP, Branagan AR, Hunter Z, et al. IgA and IgG hypogammaglobulinemia persists in most patients with Waldenstrom's macroglobulinemia despite therapeutic responses, including complete remissions. *Blood* 2004;104:306b.

92. Hunter Z, Leleu X, Hatjiharissi E, et al. IgA and IgG hypogammaglobulinemia are associated with mutations in the APRIL/BLYS receptor TACI in Waldenstrom's macroglobulinemia (WM). *Blood* 2006;108:228.

93. Dutcher TF, Fahey JL. The histopathology of macroglobulinemia of Waldenström. *J Natl Cancer Inst* 1959;22:887-917.

94. Moulopoulos LA, Dimopoulos MA, Varma DG, et al. Waldenström macroglobulinemia: MR imaging of the spine and CT of the abdomen and pelvis. *Radiology* 1993;188:669-73.

95. Gobbi PG, Bettini R, Montecucco C, et al. Study of prognosis in Waldenström's macroglobulinemia: a proposal for a simple binary classification with clinical and investigational utility. *Blood* 1994;83:2939-45.

96. Morel P, Monconduit M, Jacomy D, et al. Prognostic factors in Waldenström macroglobulinemia: a report on 232 patients with

the description of a new scoring system and its validation on 253 other patients. *Blood* 2000;96:852-8.

97. Dhodapkar MV, Jacobson JL, Gertz MA, et al. Prognostic factors and response to fludarabine therapy in patients with Waldenström macroglobulinemia: results of United States intergroup trial (Southwest Oncology Group S9003). *Blood* 2001;98:41-8.

98. Kyle RA, Treon SP, Alexanian R, et al. Prognostic markers and criteria to initiate therapy in Waldenström's macroglobulinemia: Consensus Panel Recommendations from the Second International Workshop on Waldenström's macroglobulinemia. *Semin Oncol* 2003;30:116-20.

99. Dimopoulos M, Gika D, Zervas K, et al. The international staging system for multiple myeloma is applicable in symptomatic Waldenstrom's macroglobulinemia. *Leuk Lymph* 2004;45:1809-13.

100. Anagnostopoulos A, Zervas K, Kyrtsonis M, et al. Prognostic value of serum beta2-microglobulin in patients with Waldenstrom's macroglobulinemia requiring therapy. *Clin Lymph Myeloma* 2006;7:205-9.

101. Morel P, Duhamel A, Gobbi P, et al. International prognostic scoring system (IPSS) for Waldenstrom's macroglobulinemia. *Blood* 2006;108:42a.

102. Gertz M, Anagnostopoulos A, Anderson KC, et al. Treatment recommendations in Waldenström's macroglobulinemia: Consensus Panel Recommendations from the Second International Workshop on Waldenström's macroglobulinemia. *Semin Oncol* 2003;30:121-6.

103. Treon SP, Gertz MA, Dimopoulos M, et al. Update on treatment recommendations from the Third International Workshop on Waldenstrom's Macroglobulinemia. *Blood* 2006;107:3442-6.

104. Kyle RA, Greipp PR, Gertz MA, et al. Waldenström's macroglobulinaemia: a prospective study comparing daily with intermittent oral chlorambucil. *Br J Haematol* 2000;108:737-42.

105. Dimopoulos MA, Alexanian R. Waldenström's macroglobulinemia. *Blood* 1994;83:1452-9.

106. Petrucci MT, Avvisati G, Tribalto M, Giovangrossi P, Mandelli F. Waldenström's macroglobulinaemia: results of a combined oral treatment in 34 newly diagnosed patients. *J Intern Med* 1989;226:443-7.

107. Case DC Jr, Ervin TJ, Boyd MA, Redfield DL. Waldenström's macroglobulinemia: long-term results with the M-2 protocol. *Cancer Invest* 1991;9:1-7.

108. Facon T, Brouillard M, Duhamel A, et al. Prognostic factors in Waldenström's macroglobulinemia: a report of 167 cases. *J Clin Oncol* 1993;11:1553-8.

109. Dimopoulos MA, Kantarjian H, Weber D, et al. Primary therapy of Waldenström's macroglobulinemia with 2-chlorodeoxyadenosine. *J Clin Oncol* 1994;12:2694-8.

110. Delannoy A, Ferrant A, Martiat P, Bosly A, Zenebergh A, Michaux JL. 2-Chlorodeoxyadenosine therapy in Waldenström's macroglobulinaemia. *Nouv Rev Fr Hematol* 1994;36:317-20.

111. Fridrik MA, Jager G, Baldinger C, Krieger O, Chott A, Bettelheim P. First-line treatment of Waldenström's disease with cladribine.

Arbeitsgemeinschaft Medikamentose Tumortherapie. *Ann Hematol* 1997;74:7-10.

112. Liu ES, Burian C, Miller WE, Saven A. Bolus administration of cladribine in the treatment of Waldenström macroglobulinaemia. *Br J Haematol* 1998;103:690-5.

113. Hellmann A, Lewandowski K, Zaucha JM, Bieniaszewska M, Halaburda K, Robak T. Effect of a 2-hour infusion of 2-chlorodeoxyadenosine in the treatment of refractory or previously untreated Waldenström's macroglobulinemia. *Eur J Haematol* 1999;63:35-41.

114. Betticher DC, Hsu Schmitz SF, Ratschiller D, et al. Cladribine (2-CDA) given as subcutaneous bolus injections is active in pretreated Waldenström's macroglobulinaemia. Swiss Group for Clinical Cancer Research (SAKK). *Br J Haematol* 1997;99:358-63.

115. Dimopoulos MA, Weber D, Delasalle KB, Keating M, Alexanian R. Treatment of Waldenström's macroglobulinemia resistant to standard therapy with 2-chlorodeoxyadenosine: identification of prognostic factors. *Ann Oncol* 1995;6:49-52.

116. Dimopoulos MA, O'Brien S, Kantarjian H, et al. Fludarabine therapy in Waldenström's macroglobulinemia. *Am J Med* 1993;95:49-52.

117. Foran JM, Rohatiner AZ, Coiffier B, et al. Multicenter phase II study of fludarabine phosphate for patients with newly diagnosed lymphoplasmacytoid lymphoma, Waldenström's macroglobulinemia, and mantle-cell lymphoma. *J Clin Oncol* 1999;17:546-53.

118. Thalhammer-Scherrer R, Geissler K, Schwarzinger I, et al. Fludarabine therapy in Waldenström's macroglobulinemia. *Ann Hematol* 2000;79:556-9.

119. Dhodapkar MV, Jacobson JL, Gertz MA, et al. Prognostic factors and response to fludarabine therapy in patients with Waldenström macroglobulinemia: results of United States intergroup trial (Southwest Oncology Group S9003). *Blood* 2001;98:41-8.

120. Zinzani PL, Gherlinzoni F, Bendandi M, et al. Fludarabine treatment in resistant Waldenström's macroglobulinemia. *Eur J Haematol* 1995;54:120-3.

121. Leblond V, Ben Othman T, Deconinck E, et al. Activity of fludarabine in previously treated Waldenström's macroglobulinemia: a report of 71 cases. Groupe Cooperatif Macroglobulinemie. *J Clin Oncol* 1998;16:2060-4.

122. Dimopoulos MA, Weber DM, Kantarjian H, Keating M, Alexanian R. 2Chlorodeoxyadenosine therapy of patients with Waldenström macroglobulinemia previously treated with fludarabine. *Ann Oncol* 1994;5:288-9.

123. Lewandowski K, Halaburda K, Hellmann A. Fludarabine therapy in Waldenström's macroglobulinemia patients treated previously with 2-chlorodeoxyadenosine. *Leuk Lymphoma* 2002;43:361-3.

124. Leleu XP, Manning R, Soumerai JD, et al. Increased incidence of disease transformation and development of MDS/AML in Waldenstrom's Macroglobulinemia patients treated with nucleoside analogues. *Proc Am Soc Clin Oncol* 2007;25:445s.

125. Treon SP, Kelliher A, Keele B, et al. Expression of serotherapy target antigens in Waldenstrom's macroglobulinemia: Therapeutic applications and considerations. *Semin Oncol* 2003;30:248-52.

126. Treon SP, Shima Y, Preffer FI, et al. Treatment of plasma cell dyscrasias with antibody-mediated immunotherapy. *Semin Oncol* 1999;26(Suppl 14):97-106.

127. Byrd JC, White CA, Link B, et al. Rituximab therapy in Waldenstrom's macroglobulinemia: preliminary evidence of clinical activity. *Ann Oncol* 1999;10:1525-7.

128. Weber DM, Gavino M, Huh Y, et al. Phenotypic and clinical evidence supports rituximab for Waldenstrom's macroglobulinemia. *Blood* 1999;94:125a.

129. Foran JM, Rohatiner AZ, Cunningham D, et al. European phase II study of rituximab (chimeric anti-CD20 monoclonal antibody) for patients with newly diagnosed mantle-cell lymphoma and previously treated mantle-cell lymphoma, immunocytoma, and small B-cell lymphocytic lymphoma. *J Clin Oncol* 2000;18:317-24.

130. Treon SP, Agus DB, Link B, et al. CD20-directed antibody-mediated immunotherapy induces responses and facilitates hematologic recovery in patients with Waldenstrom's macroglobulinemia. *J Immunother* 2001;24:272-9.

131. Gertz MA, Rue M, Blood E, et al. Multicenter phase 2 trial of rituximab for Waldenstrom macroglobulinemia (WM): An Eastern Cooperative Oncology Group Study (E3A98). *Leuk Lymphoma* 2004;45:2047-55.

132. Dimopoulos MA, Zervas C, Zomas A, et al. Treatment of Waldenstrom's macroglobulinemia with rituximab. *J Clin Oncol* 2002;20:2327-33.

133. Treon SP, Emmanouilides C, Kimby E, et al. Extended rituximab therapy in Waldenström's Macroglobulinemia. *Ann Oncol* 2005;16:132-8.

134. Donnelly GB, Bober-Sorcinelli K, Jacobson R, Portlock CS. Abrupt IgM rise following treatment with rituximab in patients with Waldenstrom's macroglobulinemia. *Blood* 2001;98:240b.

135. Treon SP, Branagan AR, Anderson KC. Paradoxical increases in serum IgM levels and serum viscosity following rituximab therapy in patients with Waldenstrom's macroglobulinemia. *Blood* 2003;102:690a.

136. Ghobrial IM, Fonseca R, Greipp PR, et al. The initial "flare" of IgM level after rituximab therapy in patients diagnosed with Waldenstrom Macroglobulinemia: An Eastern Cooperative Oncology Group Study. *Blood* 2003;102:448a.

137. Dimopoulos MA, Anagnostopoulos A, Zervas C, et al. Predictive factors for response to rituximab in Waldenstrom's macroglobulinemia. *Clin Lymphoma* 2005;5:270-2.

138. Treon SP, Hansen M, Branagan AR, et al. Polymorphisms in FcγRIIIA (CD16) receptor expression are associated with clinical responses to Rituximab in Waldenstrom's Macroglobulinemia. *J Clin Oncol* 2005;23:474-81.

139. Weber DM, Dimopoulos MA, Delasalle K, et al. 2-Chlorodeoxyadenosine alone and in combination for previously untreated Waldenstrom's macroglobulinemia. *Semin Oncol* 2003;30:243-7.

140. Treon SP, Branagan A, Wasi P, et al. Combination therapy with Rituximab and Fludarabine in Waldenstrom's macroglobulinemia. *Blood* 2004;104:215a.

141. Tam CS, Wolf MM, Westerman D, et al. Fludarabine combination therapy is highly effective in first-line and salvage treatment of patients with Waldenstrom's macroglobulinemia. *Clin Lymphoma Myeloma* 2005;6:136-9.

142. Hensel M, Villalobos M, Kornacker M, et al. Pentostatin/cyclophosphamide with or without rituximab: an effective regimen for patients with Waldenstrom's macroglobulinemia/lymphoplasmacytic lymphoma. *Clin Lymphoma Myeloma* 2005;6:131-5.

143. Dimopoulos MA, Anagnostopoulos A, Kyrtsonis MC, et al. Primary treatment of Waldenstrom's macroglobulinemia with Dexamethasone, Rituximab and Cyclophosphamide. *J Clin Oncol* 2007;25:3344-9.

144. Buske C, Dreyling MH, Eimermacher H, et al. Combined immuno-chemotherapy (R-CHOP) results in significantly superior response rates and time to treatment failure in first line treatment of patients with lymphoplasmacytoid/ic immunocytoma. Results of a prospective randomized trial of the German Low Grade Lymphoma Study Group. *Blood* 2004;104:162a.

145. Treon SP, Hunter Z, Branagan A. CHOP plus rituximab therapy in Waldenström's Macroglobulinemia. *Clin Lymphoma Myeloma* 2005;5:273-7.

146. Dimopoulos MA, Hamilos G, Efstathiou E, et al. Treatment of Waldenstrom's macroglobulinemia with the combination of fludarabine and cyclophosphamide. *Leuk Lymphoma* 2003;44:993-6.

147. Tamburini J, Levy V, Chateilex C, et al. Fludarabine plus cyclophosphamide in Waldenstrom's macroglobulinemia: results in 49 patients. *Leukemia* 2005;19:1831-4.

148. Jagannath S, Durie BG, Wolf J, et al. Bortezomib therapy alone and in combination with dexamethasone for previously untreated symptomatic multiple myeloma. *Br J Haematol* 2005;129:776-83.

149. Oakervee HE, Popat R, Curry N, et al. PAD combination therapy (PS-341/bortezomib, doxorubicin and dexamethasone) for previously untreated patients with multiple myeloma. *Br J Haematol* 2005;129:755-62.

150. Harousseau JL, Attal M, Leleu X, et al. Bortezomib plus dexamethasone as induction treatment prior to autologous stem cell transplantation in patients with newly diagnosed multiple myeloma. Preliminary results of an IFM Phase II Study. *Blood* 2004;104:416a.

151. Mitsiades CS, Mitsiades N, McMullan CJ, et al. The proteasome inhibitor bortezomib (PS-341) is active against Waldenstrom's macroglobulinemia. *Blood* 2003;102:181a.

152. *Treon SP, Hunter ZR, Matous J, et al.* Multicenter clinical trial of bortezomib in relapsed/refractory Waldenstrom's macroglobulinemia: results of WMCTG Trial 03-248. *Clin Cancer Res* 2007;13:3320-5.

153. Chen CI, Kouroukis CT, White D, et al. Bortezomib is active in patients with untreated or relapsed Waldenstrom's

macroglobulinemia: a phase II study of the National Cancer Institute of Canada Clinical Trials Group. *J Clin Oncol* 2007;25:1570-5.

154. Dimopoulos MA, Anagnostopoulos A, Kyrtsonis MC, et al. Treatment of relapsed or refractory Waldenstrom's macroglobulinemia with bortezomib. *Haematologica* 2005;90:1655-7.

155. Goy A, Younes A, McLaughlin P, et al. Phase II study of proteasome inhibitor bortezomib in relapsed or refractory B-cell non-Hodgkin's lymphoma. *J Clin Oncol* 2005;23:667-75.

156. Treon SP, Ioakimidis L, Soumerai JD, et al. Primary Therapy of Waldenstrom's Macroglobulinemia with Bortezomib, Dexamethasone and Rituximab: Results of WMCTG Clinical Trial 05-180. *J Clin Oncol* 2008;26(suppl):abstr 8519.

157. Ghobrial IM, Padmanabhan S, Badros A, et al. Phase II trial of combination of bortezomib and rituximab in relapsed and/or refractory Waldenstrom's Macroglobulinemia: preliminary results. *Blood* 2007; 110;195b.

158. Agathocleous A, Rule S, Johson P. Preliminary results of a phase I/LL study of weekly or twice weekly bortezomib in combination with rituximab in patients with follicular lymphoma, mantle cell lymphoma, and Waldenstrom's macroglobulinemia. *Blood* 2007;110:754a.

159. Hunter ZR, Boxer M, Kahl B, et al. Phase II study of alemtuzumab in lymphoplasmacytic lymphoma: results of WMCTG trial 02-079. *Proc Am Soc Clin Oncol* 2006;24:427s.

160. Owen RG, Rawstron AC, Osterborg A, Lundin J, Svensson G, Hillmen P. Activity of alemtuzumab in relapsed/refractory Waldenstrom's macroglobulinemia. *Blood* 2003;102:644a.

161. Dimopoulos MA, Zomas A, Viniou NA, et al. Treatment of Waldenström's macroglobulinemia with thalidomide. *J Clin Oncol* 2001;19:3596-601.

162. Coleman C, Leonard J, Lyons L, Szelenyi H, Niesvizky R. Treatment of Waldenström's macroglobulinemia with clarithromycin, low-dose thalidomide and dexamethasone. *Semin Oncol* 30:270-4.

163. Dimopoulos MA, Zomas K, Tsatalas K, et al. Treatment of Waldenström's macroglobulinemia with single agent thalidomide or with combination of clarithromycin, thalidomide and dexamethasone. *Semin Oncol* 2003;30:265-9.

164. Hayashi T, Hideshima T, Akiyama M, et al. Molecular mechanisms whereby immunomodulatory drugs activate natural killer cells: clinical application. *Br J Haematol* 2005;128:192-203.

165. Davies FE, Raje N, Hideshima T, et al. Thalidomide and immunomodulatory derivatives augment natural killer cell cytotoxicity in multiple myeloma. *Blood* 2001;98:210-16.

166. Janakiraman N, McLaughlin P, White CA, et al. Rituximab: correlation between effector cells and clinical activity in NHL. *Blood* 1998;92:337a.

167. Soumerai JD, Branagan AR, Patterson CJ, et al. Long term responses to thalidomide and rituximab in Waldenstrom's Macroglobulinemia. *Proc Am Soc Clin Oncol* 2007;25:445s.

168. **Treon S**, Patterson C, Hunter Z, Branagan A. Phase II study of CC-5013 (revlimid) and rituximab in Waldenström's macroglobulinemia: preliminary safety and efficacy results. *Blood* 2005;106:2443.

169. Desikan R, Dhodapkar M, Siegel D, et al. High-dose therapy with autologous haemopoietic stem cell support for Waldenström's macroglobulinaemia. *Br J Haematol* 1999;105:993-6.

170. Munshi NC, Barlogie B. Role for high dose therapy with autologous hematopoietic stem cell support in Waldenström's macroglobulinemia. *Semin Oncol* 2003;30:282-5.

171. Dreger P, Glass B, Kuse R, et al. Myeloablative radiochemotherapy followed by reinfusion of purged autologous stem cells for Waldenström's macroglobulinaemia. *Br J Haematol* 1999;106:115-18.

172. Anagnostopoulos A, Dimopoulos MA, Aleman A, et al. High-dose chemotherapy followed by stem cell transplantation in patients with resistant Waldenström's macroglobulinemia. *Bone Marrow Transplant* 2001;27:1027-9.

173. Tournilhac O, Leblond V, Tabrizi R, et al. Transplantation in Waldenström's macroglobulinemia – the French Experience. *Semin Oncol* 2003;30:291-6.

174. Anagnostopoulos A, Hari PN, Perez WS, et al. Autologous or allogeneic stem cell transplantation in patients with Waldenström's macroglobulinemia. *Biol Blood Marrow Transplant* 2006;12:845-54.

175. Maloney DG, Sandmaier B, Maris M, Storb R. The use of nonmyeloablative allogeneic hematopoietic cell transplantation for patients with refractory Waldenström's macroglobulinemia: replacing high-dose cytotoxic therapy with graft versus tumor effects. *Proceedings of the Second International Workshop on Waldenström's Macroglobulinemia*, 2002, Athens, Greece.

176. Weber D, Treon SP, Emmanouilides C, et al. Uniform response criteria in Waldenstrom's macroglobulinemia: consensus panel recommendations from the Second International Workshop on Waldenstrom's Macroglobulinemia. *Semin Oncol* 2003;30:127-31.

177. Kimby E, Treon SP, Anagnostopoulos A, et al. Update on recommendations for assessing response from the Third International Workshop on Waldenstrom's Macroglobulinemia. *Clin Lymphoma Myeloma* 2006;6:380-3.

178. Strauss SJ, Maharaj L, Hoare S, et al. Bortezomib therapy in patients with relapsed or refractory lymphoma: potential correlation of in vitro sensitivity and tumor necrosis factor alpha response with clinical activity. *J Clin Oncol* 2006;24:2105-12.

12 Diagnosis, Risk-stratification, and Management of Solitary Plasmacytoma

Meletios A. Dimopoulos and Efstathios Kastritis

INTRODUCTION

Plasma cell dyscrasias include a wide variety of diseases characterized by the abnormal accumulation of plasma cells resulting in various systemic symptoms and signs. Plasma cells are usually widespread throughout the bone marrow; however, in a minority of patients malignant plasma cells may form a single lesion. These lesions are usually confined to the bone and, less frequently, in extramedullary sites. They are composed of monoclonal plasma cells that are otherwise identical to plasma cells found in myeloma. However, these patients do not have evidence of systemic multiple myeloma (MM), and an extensive work up shows no other foci of disease. When this solitary lesion is confined to bone it is characterized as a solitary bone plasmacytoma (SBP) while when this lesion is confined to extraosseous sites it is characterized as a solitary extramedullary plasmacytoma (SEP).

DEFINITIONS

According to criteria reported by the International Myeloma Working Group,[1] diagnosis of **solitary plasmacytoma of bone** is based on histological evidence of a tumor consisting of monoclonal plasma cells identical to those seen in MM (Table 12.1). In addition, complete skeletal radiographs must show no other lesions of MM. Magnetic resonance imaging (MRI) has significantly increased sensitivity over conventional radiographs, especially in the imaging of the axial skeleton, and an MRI of the spine and pelvis may show unsuspected and asymptomatic skeletal lesions. Patients with multiple lesions in MRI should be considered as having myeloma and not SBP even if conventional radiographs show no other evidence of skeletal involvement.[2] Thus a normal MRI of spine and

pelvis is also included in the diagnostic criteria of SBP. Over the past years positron emission tomography (PET) scanning has emerged as a sensitive and reliable imaging technique; however, it has not been prospectively evaluated in SBP patients. It probably has increased sensitivity over MRI owing to wider field of view, and patients showing positive findings in more than one site in a PET scan should be diagnosed as having myeloma and not SBP.[3,4] However, it should be noted that this technique has false positive results.

Bone marrow should not have evidence of typical myeloma involvement, although in some older series patients with up to 10% bone marrow plasma cells were included.[2] According to the latest criteria the bone marrow

---

TABLE 12.1. Diagnostic criteria for SBP and SEP

Solitary bone plasmacytoma (all required)
- Single area of bone destruction due to monoclonal plasma cells
- Histologically normal bone marrow aspirate and trephine biopsy
- Normal skeletal survey
- No additional lesion on MRI scan of the spine and pelvis
- No related tissue impairment or organ damage other than solitary bone lesion, absent or low levels of serum or urinary monoclonal immunoglobulin and preserved levels of uninvolved immunoglobulins

Solitary extramedullary plasmacytoma
- Single extramedullary mass due to monoclonal plasma cells
- Histologically normal bone marrow aspirate and trephine biopsy
- Normal results on skeletal survey, including radiology of long bones
- No anemia, hypercalcemia, or renal impairment due to plasma cell dyscrasias
- Absent or low levels of serum($<$3 g/dL) or urinary monoclonal immunoglobulin ($<$0.7 g/dL) and preserved levels of uninvolved immunoglobulins

aspirate and biopsy may contain only a few plasma cells but not consistent with MM. More sensitive techniques such as flow cytometry studies and molecular detection of heavy- and light-chain gene rearrangements may reveal clonal plasma cells in the bone marrow of some patients who have no evidence of infiltration on light microscopy;[5] however, these have not been adequately studied.

Immunofixation of the serum and concentrated urine may show no M-protein, but approximately 50% or more of patients do have a small M-protein in the serum or urine. Usually patients with a M-protein > 3 g/dL are not included in SBP series and are considered as patients with myeloma. Recently, the introduction of free light chain assay has increased the sensitivity of detection of monoclonal proteins. In a recent series 40% of patients with negative serum or urine immunofixation had an abnormal FLC ratio. Levels of uninvolved immunoglobulins are almost always normal. According to the aforementioned criteria there should be no evidence of end-organ damage such as anemia, hypercalcemia, or renal insufficiency related to the plasmacytoma.[21]

CLINICAL PRESENTATION, LABORATORY, AND IMAGING

SBP accounts for less than 5% of plasma cell dyscrasias, and the introduction of new, more sensitive, imaging techniques is expected to further reduce its incidence. Males are affected more commonly than females (65% vs 35%) and the age of onset is about one decade earlier than in patients with MM.[2]

Axial skeleton is most commonly affected; other common sites include pelvis, ribs, sternum, skull, humerus, femur, tibia, and jaw; however, any bone can be involved (Table 12.2). Primary malignant tumors of the spine are rare and SBP is the commonest among these neoplasms accounting for about one-third of them.[6] The most common presenting symptom in SBP patients is pain at the site of the lesion. When vertebrae are involved, symptoms due to spinal cord or nerve root compression may be the first manifestation, while in the case of long bone involvement a fracture may be the initial presentation. Involvement of the base of the skull may present with cranian nerve palsies.[7-9] Localized light chain amyloidosis has been detected within the solitary lesion.[10-13] Some patients may present with symptoms of peripheral neuropathy. These patients need careful evaluation to exclude POEMS syndrome, especially if there is a sclerotic element within the plasmacytoma.[14] SBP patients have no systemic manifestations (anemia, renal impairment, hypercalcemia), and if such findings exist, one should rule out MM or an unrelated condition (e.g. primary hyperparathyroidism).[2]

As in myeloma, SBP has a lytic appearance on plain radiographs. In most patients, the lesion is purely lytic and has a clear margin and a narrow zone of transition to normal surrounding bone. Computed tomography

TABLE 12.2. Characteristics of patients with SBP among various series					
Series	No. of patients	Median age	Males (%)	Spine disease (% of patients)	Monoclonal protein (% of patients)
Knowling et al.[36]	25	50	68	32	24
Brinch et al.[94]	25	56	72	68	61
Bolek et al.[32]	27	55	70	33	52
Jackson and Scarffe[95]	32	62	59	72	54
Galieni et al.[46]	32	52	81	40	47
Holland et al.[30]	32	60	70	34	NA
Frassica et al.[28]	46	56	65	54	54
Liebross et al.[18]	57	53	69	40	72
Tsang et al.[34]	32	63	65	38	41
Knobel et al. (Rare Cancer Network)[24]	206	60	65	50	NA

NA, not available

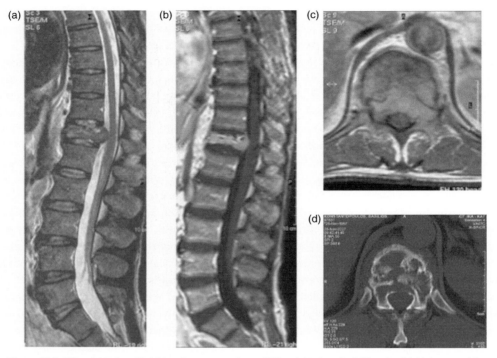

Figure 12.1. T2-weighted sagittal (a) and contrast-enhanced T1-weighted sagittal (b) and axial (c) images of the lumbosacral and lower thoracic spine shows fracture and abnormal intensity of the body of T12 vertebra. Note mass protruding in anterior epidural space (arrow). Axial CT images (d) depict bone destruction of T12.

(CT) and, particularly, MRI depict the extent of SBP more clearly and allow for more accurate treatment planning. An extraosseous soft-tissue component is often present and may impinge on the spinal cord or spinal nerve roots.[15] MRI of the spine and pelvis may show unsuspected foci of disease or diffuse involvement of the bone marrow, thus leading to the diagnosis of MM instead of SBP. One-fourth of patients thought to have SBP by conventional radiographs reveal abnormal lesions and are considered as having MM.[15,16] MRI studies (Figure 12.1) usually include T1-weighted, T2-weighted and contrast-enhanced T1-weighted sequences, depending on the circumstances. The primary tumor is imaged initially with sagittal and axial images of the involved bone, while a search for additional lesions can include coronal short-inversion time inversion recovery (STIR) images of the spine and pelvis and sagittal T1-weighted and STIR or T2-weighted fast spin echo with fat saturation images of the spine. A T1-weighted spin echo sequence remains the most important sequence for depiction of bone marrow replacement, with signal intensity lower than that of yellow bone marrow, slightly lower than

or similar to that of red bone marrow, and similar to muscle. For T2-imaging either a fast spin echo T2-weighted image with fat saturation or a short STIR can be used. For image of a large area of the skeleton (such as the entire spine) STIR images are preferred because they are less prone to artifacts due to field heterogeneity. T1-weighted contrast-enhanced images can be used to better demonstrate any associated epidural or paraspinal soft-tissue component and in cases of questionable bone marrow involvement on T1 and T2-weighted images. Lesions will enhance to a variable degree depending on tumor vascularity. In adults, normal red marrow enhances minimally. Contrast-enhanced T1-weighted images with fat saturation provide excellent contrast between the enhancing areas of bone marrow infiltration and the dark signal of the saturated bone marrow.[17] The utility of MRI in the staging of SBP is further supported by the higher rate of relapse in patients who showed unsuspected and asymptomatic lesions. In a group of 23 patients with SBP of the thoracolumbar spine, MM developed in seven of eight patients with a solitary lesion on plain radiography alone but with additional MRI lesions

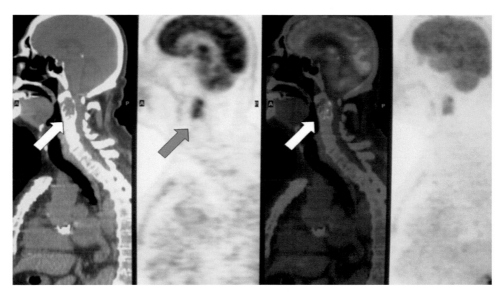

Figure 12.2. 18-FDG-PET scans showing increased uptake in a patient with SBP of the cervical spine

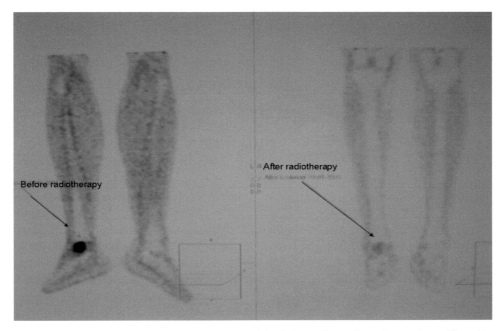

Figure 12.3. 18-FDG-PET scans before (left) and after (right) radiotherapy for a solitary plasmacytoma of the ankle

and in only one of seven who also had negative results on MRI.[15,18] PET has probably increased sensitivity over MRI mainly because of a more extensive field of view (Figures 12.2 and 12.3), as it includes more bone regions, such as the ribs, skull, and long bones. PET/CT may also allow for a more precise anatomic localization. However, MRI has increased sensitivity in the imaging of diffuse or limited bone marrow infiltration, small myelomatous bone lesions, and areas of local osteoporosis and pathological fractures. In some small series of patients with myeloma or SBP,[3,4,19]

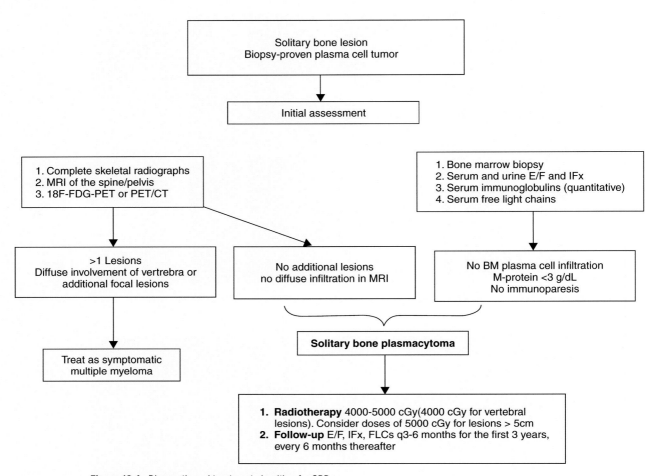

Figure 12.4. Diagnostic and treatment algorithm for SBP

PET/CT scanning resulted in the diagnosis of myeloma in some patients who were previously diagnosed as having a SBP by whole-body conventional X-rays and MRI of the spine and pelvis, as it revealed areas of involvement in the ribs or in soft tissues. However, PET/CT imaging could not detect small areas of diffuse vertebrae or marrow involvement, detected by MRI[3,4] while false negative or indeterminate results are not rare.[19]

Bone marrow studies usually show no evidence of monoclonal plasma cells; however, more sensitive techniques may show the presence of a small population of monoclonal plasma cells.[2] Patients with more than one foci of disease may still not have evidence of BM involvement, and these patients may comprise a specific subcategory of macrofocal MM.[20]

All patients with an SBP should undergo electrophoresis and immunofixation of serum and urine samples before any treatment is administered, since serial assessment of monoclonal protein after treatment has significant prognostic significance. A small monoclonal protein may be found in many patients with SBP, most commonly IgG (54%), followed by light chain only (15%) and IgA (7%), while 24% have nonsecretory disease. Median serum M-protein levels are about 0.5 g/dL, and the amount of the M-component should be less than 3 g/dL. In a series of 60 patients, a monoclonal protein was present in 37 (62%); in 26 of 37 (70%) the protein levels were ≤1 g/dL and in 30% they were 1.1 to 2.2 g/dL. In additional 8 of 60 (13%) only Bence Jones protein was present in the urine (range, 0.02-0.70 g/dL).[16] In a larger series from the Mayo Clinic a monoclonal protein was found in the serum or urine of 74 of 116 (64%) of patients, while median M-protein was 0.5 g/dL.[21] The introduction of the more sensitive free light chain assay has increased the sensitivity of the detection

TABLE 12.3. Outcome of SBP patients treated with radiotherapy alone

Series	No. of patients	Local recurrence (% of patients)	10-year DFS (% of patients)	Median survival
Knowling et al.[36]	25	0	16	7.5
Brinch et al. [94]	25	0	NA	12
Bolek et al.[32]	27	4	46	10
Frassica et al.[28]	46	11	25	9.3
Liebross et al.[18]	57	4	42	11
Knobel et al. (Rare Cancer Network)[24]	148	14	NA	NA

NA, not available

of monoclonal paraprotein, and 40% of patients with negative serum or urine immunofixation may have an abnormal FLC ratio.[21] The uninvolved immunoglobulins are preserved in the overwhelming majority of SBP patients, with less than 5% having suppressed any uninvolved immunoglobulin.[16] The low levels of monoclonal protein, the significant fraction of patients with nonsecretory disease, and the preservation of uninvolved immunoglobulins are all features consistent with the very low tumor burden of patients with SBP. Serum monoclonal protein above 3 g/dL and depressed uninvolved immunoglobulins are consistent with occult but disseminated myeloma and should trigger extensive work up to confirm this suspicion.

DIAGNOSTIC WORKUP

Histological confirmation is required for the diagnosis of SBP (Figure 12.4). Either a biopsy or fine needle aspiration is generally used. Percutaneously guided biopsy of the spine is usually feasible with CT guidance. An experienced pathologist should review the specimen, as these tumors are rare and occasional misinterpretations may lead to false diagnosis. Plasma cells are identical to those found in MM. Monoclonality of cytoplasmic light chains can be demonstrated by flow cytomtery, immunohistology, or in situ hybridization. Differential diagnosis includes reactive plasmacytosis, MM, plasmablastic lymphoma, ALK positive large B cell lymphoma, and primary effusion lymphoma. Whole-body skeletal X-rays and MRI of the spine and the pelvis are required in order to exclude the presence of other bone lesions. Although 18F-FDG PET or PET/CT increase the field of view over MRI, they do not substitute for spine and pelvis MRI. Bone marrow biopsy is needed to exclude plasmacytosis, which would place the patient in

the category of MM. Flow cytometry studies increase the sensitivity of plasma cell detection[5] but have not been validated, and light microscopy and immunohistochemistry are currently recommended for the exclusion of bone marrow involvement. All patients should have serum and urine electrophoresis and immunofixation at diagnosis and during follow-up. Free light chain assay is now widely available and should be incorporated in the initial assessment and follow-up of all SBP patients.[21] A complete workup is needed to exclude end-organ damage; thus, complete blood counts, assessment of renal function, serum calcium, serum lactate dehydrogenase, erythrocyte sedimentation rate, and β_2-microglobulin should be assessed.

TREATMENT

Definitive local radiotherapy is the treatment of choice for SBP.[22,23] Data on treatment of SBP usually derive from retrospective series, extending over prolonged periods, but no randomized trials have been conducted in the field owing to the rarity of the disease. Furthermore, in most series the majority of patients had not had MRI assessment.[24] Thus, several patients had MM rather than SBP.[15,18]

Local control, defined as long-term clinical and radiographic stability, is achieved in 83% to 96% of cases[18,25-36] (Table 12.3). After adequate radiotherapy, virtually all patients have relief of symptoms. The radiological response to radiation therapy may include sclerosis and bone remineralization in up to 50% of patients followed up with plain radiographs.[18,32] On MRI images, abnormalities of the bone marrow and an accompanying soft-tissue mass may persist even after successful treatment.[18]

A definite dose-response relationship has not been established for local radiotherapy. Mendenhall et al.[37]

reported a 6% incidence of local failure, with doses of at least 4000 cGy and a 31% incidence with lower doses. Other series used higher doses of 4500-5000 cGy,[18,29] but they did not find a dose-response curve for doses over 4000 cGy while others did not find any dose-response relationship for doses as low as 3500 cGy.[34] Frassica et al.[28] did not observe local failure when the radiotherapy dose was 4500 cGy or higher. However, relapses have been reported even with doses greater than 5000-6000 cGy.[18,24,29] Tumor bulk, defined by the size of the SBP, is considered as a risk factor for local recurrence among different series: tumors greater than 5 cm have higher rates of recurrence[24,34] compared to smaller tumors. A clear benefit from larger doses for larger tumors, however, has not been clearly established[24,34] although some reports suggest this possibility.[29,30] In some series a higher proportion of local failures was also observed in patients with spinal lesions,[28,38] but this observation was not confirmed in other series.[24]

Although the optimal dose of radiotherapy has not been established by prospective studies, most agree that a dose of approximately 4000-5000 cGy[2,22,23,39] (4000 cGy for vertebral lesions) provides the best local control without producing serious toxicity. For lesions greater than 5 cm, some suggest that perhaps doses of 5000 cGy or combined-modality approaches should be considered.[22] In the absence of large prospective studies or the convincing proof of a dose-response relationship, we recommend a radiotherapy dose of 4500 cGy in 25 fractions over 5 weeks.

The optimal clinical target volume for radiotherapy has not been clearly established and some recommend that the entire bone involved should be included in the field;[29] however, this was suggested before the advent of CT and MRI. It is now recommended that treatment fields should be designed to encompass all disease shown by MRI or CT scanning and should include a margin of normal tissue of at least 2 cm.[18,33,34] For spinal lesions, the margin should include at least one uninvolved vertebra above and below the affected vertebra.

Following radiotherapy, the monoclonal protein is reduced markedly in most patients. Serial and frequent measurements of monoclonal protein for at least 6 months after treatment are crucial and are required to confirm disease radiosensitivity. The rate of reduction may be slow, and a continuous decrease in the protein may be observed for several years.[40] The monoclonal protein disappears in a minority of patients (20%-50%), suggesting that all disease was included within the radiotherapy field.[33,41] The likelihood of disappearance of monoclonal protein is higher in patients in whom the pretreatment value is low: M-protein disappeared in 41% of patients with a pretreatment M-protein of 0.1-1 g/dL compared to none among patients with pretreatment M-protein $\geq$ 1.1 g/dL, while there was no dose-response relation between radiation dose and disappearance of monoclonal protein.[18] In most patients the monoclonal protein persists despite adequate radiotherapy,[16,18] indicating the presence of tumor beyond the field of radiation. The condition of these patients may remain stable for a long time, and further treatment should be deferred until there is clear progression of the plasma cell disorder.[2] However, patients in whom M-protein levels remain higher than 0.5 g/dL one to two years after radiotherapy have a higher risk for progression compared to those who achieve a level ≤0.5 g/dL (50% vs 13% at 5 years, p < 0.001).[21]

Although most patients with SBP of the spine can be treated with radiotherapy alone, some patients in whom the diagnosis of SBP has not yet been made present with or have rapid development of neurological dysfunction that requires laminectomy before radiotherapy. An anterior approach may be preferred because posterior procedures do not address the source of the impingement and may not reliably relieve neurological compromise.[24,27,42] Surgical intervention may also be necessary in patients with vertebral instability.[6,27] Surgical fixation of a pathological fracture of a long bone may also be required. The role of bisphosphonates in the management of SBP patients has not been defined and generally are not recommended.[22]

THE ROLE OF ADJUVANT CHEMOTHERAPY

The role for chemotherapy as an adjuvant to local radiotherapy has not been clearly defined.[2] In some series, chemotherapy was administered after completion of local radiation treatment. Mayr et al.[29] found that adjuvant chemotherapy may prevent progression to MM. Holland et al.[30] found that chemotherapy did not affect the overall rate of progression to myeloma but that adjuvant treatment changed the median time to progression from 29 to 59 months. In most other series, adjuvant chemotherapy had no beneficial effect.[32,43-46] In a small prospective trial, however, adjuvant melphalan and prednisone were given for 3 years in 53 SBP patients after radiotherapy, resulting in improved disease-free and overall survival in patients who were treated with combined therapy (p < 0.01). However, the group was too small to draw definitive conclusions, and none of the patients had been staged with MRI.[31] Thus, on the basis of the available data, we believe that adjuvant chemotherapy should not be administered to patients with SBP. Use of systemic chemotherapy or corticosteroids may obscure recognition of patients with disappearance of myeloma protein after radiotherapy who may be cured. Furthermore, early exposure to systemic treatment may hasten the evolution of resistant subclones and thereby restrict later therapeutic options, when they may be more useful. Moreover, in one series,[27] secondary leukemia developed in 4 of 7 patients with SBP who received adjuvant melphalan-based chemotherapy after completion of radiotherapy.

PROGNOSTIC FACTORS AND OUTCOME

Almost 50% of patients with solitary plasmacytoma are alive at 10 years; 25%-40% are surviving disease free at 10 years. Overt MM occurs in almost 50% of patients with solitary plasmacytoma of bone.[2] The median time to systemic progression is 2 to 4 years but myeloma may develop in occasional patients 10 or more years after the original diagnosis of SBP. The median overall survival of patients with SBP averages 10 years, and up to 20% of patients die of unrelated causes.[47] This long survival is partly due to prolonged stability of several patients who may be cured with local radiotherapy and partly due to the relatively long survival of patients who develop MM. Liebross[18] reported that their patients who developed myeloma had features of low tumor mass disease, a 77% response rate to chemotherapy and a subsequent median survival of 5.3 years.

There are two main patterns of disease progression after local treatment in patients with SBP: local relapse and development of systemic disease. As previously mentioned local control defined as long-term clinical and radiological stability is achieved in at least 90% of patients. With modern imaging techniques, MRI and PET/CT, fewer patients will have truly solitary plasmacytomas. For these patients we believe that with modern radiotherapy planning and techniques and with doses exceeding 4000 cGy local failure rates should be negligible.

The outcome of patients with SBP who received local radiotherapy without systemic adjuvant treatment is shown in Table 12.3. The majority of patients with SBP develop distant recurrence, and the most common pattern of progression consists of new bone lesions, diffuse marrow plasmacytosis, and rising of monoclonal protein. In several patients, however, new bone lesions develop without involvement of the intervening bone marrow, consistent with a pattern of multiple plasmacytomas or macrofocal myeloma. Multiple solitary plasmacytomas without evidence of MM occur in up to 5% of patients.[20,27,28,30] In some patients recurrent isolated plasmacytomas develop several months or years after treatment of the original lesion, and careful evaluation with plain radiography, MRI, and BM biopsies shows no systemic disease.[2]

Many clinical and laboratory parameters have been assessed for their possible correlation with disease outcome, either local or distant failure or survival. The dose–response relationship for local radiotherapy does not seem to affect the probability of distant relapse.[47] Clinical characteristics associated with progression to MM include impaired performance status, older age, and vertebral involvement in one series[38] but have not been confirmed by other series.[18,24,27,28,30,32,48] Only older age has been found as an independent risk factor for inferior disease-free survival in some series in which multivariate analyses were performed.[24,34]

The two main parameters that have been associated with a higher risk of progression are the depression of uninvolved immunoglobulins and the persistence of monoclonal protein after radiotherapy.[2,18,21] The MD Anderson group was the first to show that disappearance of monoclonal protein after radiotherapy was associated with prolonged stability and even cure.[49] An update of the MD Anderson series that included 61 patients with carefully staged SBP indicated that among 11 patients with disappearance of monoclonal protein myeloma developed in only 2 patients after 4 and 12 years respectively. Myeloma developed in 57% of patients with persistent monoclonal protein and in 63% of those with nonsecretory plasmacytoma (p = 0.02).[18] Patients with nonsecretory tumors appear to have a worse outcome than patients with secretory tumors, with 10-year myeloma-free survival rates of 16% and 46% respectively.[16] In multivariate analysis only persistence of monoclonal protein one year or more after radiotherapy was the only independent adverse prognostic factor for myeloma free and cause specific survival.

In a retrospective study of 116 patients with SBP the FLC ratio at the time of diagnosis was determined and was abnormal in 47% of patients. An abnormal ratio was associated with a higher risk of progression to MM, with a 44% risk of progression at 5 years in patients with abnormal FLC ratio compared to 26% of those with normal FLC ratio. Persistence of monoclonal protein level greater than 0.5 g/dL at one or two years after local treatment was also associated with increased risk of progression (p < 0.001). Abnormal FLC ratio one or two years after diagnosis was also associated with an inferior outcome (HR 3.5, 95% CI1.3-8.9; p = 0.01) in a proportion of patients who had measured FLCs. A prognostic model including FLC ratio at the time of diagnosis and M-protein levels (≤0.5 g/dL vs >0.5 g/dL) was constructed with low, intermediate, and high risk groups having 5-year progression rates of 13%, 26%, and 62% respectively (p < 0.001). Similar results were obtained when the FLC ratio at one or two years after diagnosis was used instead of the FLC ratio at the time of diagnosis.[21] In another retrospective study of 25 patients with SBP,[50] the role of angiogenesis was examined. Patients with lower MVD were less likely to progress to MM than patients with increased MVD (p = 0.02); however, this variable did not show independent significance probably due to small number of patients. Low expression of CD27 surface antigen by SBP plasma cells has also been correlated with decreased progression-free survival in another small series.[51] The presence of clonal plasma cells in the bone marrow indentified by a multiparameter flow cytometry assay has also shown prognostic significance. In a series of 52 patients with SBP the presence of neoplastic plasma cells among the bone marrow plasma cells was associated with increased rates of progression (51% vs 18%, p = 0.04).[5]

MANAGEMENT OF PROGRESSIVE DISEASE

Most patients with early disease progression presumably had occult generalized disease at diagnosis, whereas some patients with an apparent late recurrence may have had indolent growth for many years or, possibly, developed a second primary plasma cell neoplasm. The lower median age of patients with SBP compared with those with MM and the later development of MM in most patients with SBP suggest that SBP represents an early manifestation of MM in some cases. On the other hand, the condition of some patients has remained stable for more than a decade despite persistence of low-level monoclonal protein. Such patients may have had reversion to stable monoclonal gammopathy of undetermined significance (MGUS) that may have preceded the SBP. When MM evolves, most patients have features of low-tumor mass disease and a high rate of response to chemotherapy; patients with SBP average 10 years, and 10% to 20% of patients die of unrelated causes. When isolated lesions develop at long intervals (i.e., more than 2 years), radiotherapy alone may be followed by prolonged

clinical stability. When new lesions develop at shorter intervals and are accompanied by other signs that suggest MM (falling levels of uninvolved serum immunoglobulins and new abnormalities on MRI studies), systemic treatment for MM may be justified. If there is doubt, longer follow-up without chemotherapy should clarify the clinical course.

SOLITARY EXTRAMEDULLARY PLASMACYTOMA

SEP is a plasma cell tumor that arises outside the bone marrow. Similar to solitary bone plasmacytoma, the diagnosis of SEP requires a single lesion consisting of monoclonal plasma cells in the absence of MM (Table 12.1). These criteria were also defined by the International Myeloma Working Group in 2003.[1]

CLINICAL PRESENTATION

SEP is rare and less common than SBP. Often an otolaryngologist is the first physician to recognize the lesion, as approximately 85% of SEP occur in the head and neck, including the nasal cavity and sinuses, nasopharynx, and larynx (Figure 12.5).[36,52] They usually present as submucosal lesions but bone involvement in the sinuses may be noted. Regional node involvement may also occur.[53] Involvement of the tonsil has been reported.[52,54-58] Gastrointestinal involvement is the next most frequent site.[59-61] Other areas of involvement include lung,[62-65] bladder,[66,67] thyroid,[52,68-70] testis,[71] breast,[72-76] parotid,[77-82] lymph nodes,[52,83,84] and central nervous system.[52,85]

Symptoms and signs depend on the site of involvement. Epistaxis, rhinorrhoea, and nasal discharge or obstruction are the most frequent symptoms in upper airway tract involvement. Other symptoms include dysphonia, dysphagia, dyspnea, cough, epigastric pain, and headache, depending on tumor localization. Physical examination usually reveals a pedunculated or slightly raised submucosal dark-red to grayish-red swelling that bleeds easily with manipulation. The mucosa is typically intact, but ulceration and necrosis may occur in advanced cases. Patients are almost a decade younger than patients with multiple myeloma, and males predominate in a 2:1 to 5:1 ratio[36,52] to females.

Serum and urine electrophoresis and immunofixation studies may reveal a monoclonal protein, at low levels, in less than a quarter of patients.[52,80] There are no data regarding serum-free light chains in patients with SEP. IgA monoclonal protein predominates in some studies but IgG predominates in other studies.[52]

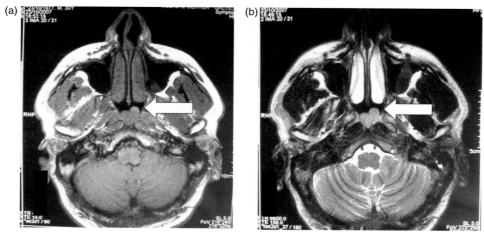

Figure 12.5. T1-weighted (a) and T2-weighted (b) axial MR images of the brain shows mass at the roof of the nasopharynx

The diagnosis of SEP is made when a monoclonal plasma cell tumour is found in an extramedullary site in the absence of multiple myeloma. Tissue is obtained with needle aspiration or surgery, depending on the site of involvement. Deep biopsies must be taken since the tumor is submucosal and the mucosa may be thickened from an inflammatory reaction. Microscopically, extramedullary plasmacytomas appear as a monocellular proliferation of plasma cells set in a sparse matrix. Nuclear and cellular atypia may be minimal or prominent. The plasma cells have round eccentric nuclei with dense nuclear chromatin clumps arranged along the nuclear membrane in a cartwheel fashion. Cytoplasm is abundant and slightly basophilic, and a perinuclear halo typically appears and corresponds to the Golgi apparatus. EMP must be distinguished from reactive plasmacytosis, plasma cell granuloma, and lymphoma (MALT, marginal zone, and immunoblastic).[22,86] Amyloid deposition may be observed within or outside the tumor. A three-grade classification has been proposed (low, intermediate, and high grade, analogous to lymphoma); however it is not widely used.[87] Plasma cells are usually of nonplasmablastic morphology and most are rated as low/ intermediate grade. Plasma cells in SEP stain positive with CD38 and show monoclonal cytoplasmic light chain expression. Negative CD20 and positive CD79 staining may further strengthen the diagnosis. Some differences between extramedullary and classical myeloma may also exist, with absence of cyclin D1 and infrequent expression of CD56, weaker staining for Bcl-2 and rare overexpression of p21 and p53. In comparison to extramedullary multiple myeloma, extramedullary plasmacytoma also shows a more mature morphology and lower proliferation indices.[88] Data on recurrent chromosome translocation typically found in myeloma and extramedullary myeloma are lacking. An experienced pathologist is needed for the correct diagnosis and in order to avoid misinterpretation of the findings. In a report from Hotz et al.[89] only 14 of 24 patients had monoclonal lesions when immunohistochemistry for light chains was applied in patients who had morphologically been diagnosed as having a SEP. The predilection of SEP for mucosal surfaces, spreading to other soft tissues, the infrequent evolution to myeloma and microscopic finding beyond plasma cells such as reactive follicles, lymphoepithelial lesions, centrocyte-like cells, and monocytoid cells suggest that SEP may actually represent a form of extranodal marginal zone lymphoma that has undergone extensive plasmacytic differentiation.[90,91]

The radiologic appearance of SEP is nonspecific. In contrast to SBP, data on the staging of SEP are limited. Thus there are no data about the diagnostic performance of spine/ pelvis MRI at diagnosis. PET and PET/CT may detect extramedullary lesions outside the field of view of the MRI or even small lesions not depicted in common CTs. Since the risk of progression to myeloma is low, most do not recommend routine MRI of the spine and pelvis during initial evaluation of a patient with SEP.[22] However, MRI is very useful in the accurate imaging of SEP lesions especially in the head and neck area and allows for more accurate treatment planning.

A bone survey with X-rays should reveal no abnormalities attributable to plasma cell dyscrasia. Initial assessment of patients diagnosed with SEP should also include complete blood counts, ESR, β_2-microglobulin, serum and urine electrophoresis and immunofixation, serum liver and renal chemistries, and serum calcium. As is the case in SBP, uninvolved immunoglobulins are normal in almost all patients with SEP.[52] Although current experience is minimal, free light chain assays may also prove useful in monitoring such patients, particularly those with normal electrophoretic and immunofixation studies.

TREATMENT

Like SBP, EMP is highly sensitive to radiation therapy and, in nearly all, local control can be achieved (80%-100%).[34,35,52,80] Approximately 50%-65% of patients remain free of disease for 10 years or longer. Because SEP is a rare tumor, data on the treatment come from small retrospective series. There are no firmly established treatment criteria; however, treatment recommendations have been published.[22] Radiation therapy usually follows guidelines applied in other more common tumors; for example, guidelines for squamous cell carcinomas of head and neck are followed for patients with SEP located in this area.[80] The entire tumor with generous margins is encompassed within the radiation field. For patients with SEP located in the nasal cavity and maxillary sinus, a three-field technique (one anterior and two lateral wedged fields) in portal arrangements are used.[80] If lymphatic tissue is involved, including Waldeyer's ring structures such as nasopharynx and tonsils, regional lymph node coverage is important to avoid a higher risk of local recurrence.[29,36,92] In patients with tumors of the oral cavity, nasopharynx, oropharynx, and larynx, standard opposed lateral fields are used. In patients with nonhead and neck tumors standard anterior-posterior and posterior-anterior fields are used.[80,86]

Optimal radiation doses are still debated. In the 1980s, Harwood[92] had recommended a dose of 3500 cGy in 15 fractions. Liebros used a median dose of 5000 cGy (range 4000-6000 cGy) with a median fraction size of 200 cGy, and no local failures were observed.[80] Tsang et al.[34] used ≥3500 cGy in 14 patients with SEP with only 1 local relapse (in a patient with disease > 5 cm). In a relatively large series, Galieni et al.[52] reported local relapse in two patients treated with low-dose radiotherapy (3000 and 3600 cGy, respectively) after surgery. In another retrospective analysis a dose response, even for larger tumors, was not found.[35] On the basis of these retrospective data and in agreement with others,[22] we

recommend a dose of 4000 cGy in 20 fractions of 200 cGy, for tumors less than 5 cm. For larger tumors, a dose of 5000 cGy in 25 fractions should be considered. Cervical nodes should be included in the radiation field whenever they are involved, and if SEP is located in Waldeyer's ring (which is considered at high risk for local recurrence) then first echelon cervical nodes should also be included. Prophylactic neck radiotherapy is not recommended for patients with SEP of the nasal cavity or the paranasal sinuses.[39,80,86]

Since SEP is a highly radiosensitive tumor, surgical procedures of the head and neck are not recommended; however, surgery may be considered for other sites of disease, such as the gastrointestinal tract. Furthermore, SEP has no specific imaging features; thus in many patients a primary surgical approach is followed before establishing the diagnosis of SEP. In a retrospective literature review[41] patients with SEP located in sites other than the head and neck who received surgery, radiation, or a combined-modality treatment had similar outcome, suggesting that either surgery or radiotherapy is reasonable for such patients. These authors suggested that surgery, when clear surgical margins are achieved, is also an option for tumors in the aerodigestive tract; however, we believe that since current experience shows a high rate of local control with radiotherapy, this should remain the treatment of choice. Adjuvant radiotherapy after complete tumor excision cannot be recommended in the absence of any data. No data support primary or adjuvant systemic chemotherapy or administration of glucocorticoids in the management of SEP.[52]

Local recurrence rates for patients with SEP treated with local radiotherapy are low and do not exceed 10% in almost all series.[34-36,80,92] In some series[34,52] these local relapses are seen in patients with bulky tumors or in those treated with lower doses of radiation; however, this has not been constant across series.[35,80] Most patients with SEP remain disease free for long periods and perhaps more than two-thirds survive more than 10 years. Progression to MM is less frequent than in SBP,[34,35] ranging from 11% to 36%,[35,52,80] with most of these progressions occurring during the first 3 years after diagnosis. Other patterns of progression include distant relapses of SEP, with lymph nodes, skin, and subcutaneous tissues most frequently involved, bone localization leading to an SBP or multiple bone lytic lesions without or with low levels of monoclonal paraprotein, and absence of marrow plasmacytosis.[52] Patients relapsing at distant sites either with an SEP or with an SBP may be treated with local radiotherapy; however, patients with multiple sites of relapse or marrow plasmacytosis should be treated for myeloma. Patients developing myeloma usually have a protracted course and generally respond to therapy[52,80] although rare cases with rapid dissemination in multiple organs, resistance to alkylating therapy, and short survival are reported.[52]

Owing to the small numbers of patients enrolled in these retrospective studies and the low rates of relapse, it has been difficult to establish prognostic factors for local relapse or evolution to myeloma. No difference has been observed in outcome if destruction of adjacent bone has been observed in most[29,53,80] but not all series.[92] The localization of SEP may influence dissemination, with worse outcome for tumors located outside head and neck.[52] In a small published series with literature review, patients with pulmonary SEP had a relatively poor 5-year survival of 40%, although some patients may survive for more than 20 years.[93] The presence of monoclonal paraprotein at diagnosis has been associated by some with higher risk for dissemination but not its persistence;[52] however, given the low rates of monoclonal paraprotein in patients with SEP, it is difficult to draw firm conclusions. Patients having plasmablastic-type tumors developed local recurrences in a significantly higher rate than those with low grade tumors.[53]

FUTURE DIRECTIONS

SBR and SEP are rare tumors with a generally favorable outcome when treated with local radiotherapy. This will probably remain the treatment of choice at least in the near future. The introduction of novel agents, with enhanced antimyeloma activity, such as thalidomide, lenalidomide, and bortezomib, may partly change the management of these tumors, since these drugs may be incorporated in an adjuvant or neoadjuvant setting. Until then, adequate radiation doses and accurate field design are the most important parameters for the management of SBP and SEP. New technology provides new tools for more accurate 3D-conformal design of radiation fields and dose delivery. The introduction of whole-body MRI, PET, and PET/CT may also reduce the incidence of true SBPs and SEPs since many patients will be diagnosed with disseminated disease and managed for myeloma. In any case, treating physicians should always investigate thoroughly all patients for the presence of more extensive disease than a solitary focus.

REFERENCES

1. International Myeloma Working Group. Criteria for the classification of monoclonal gammopathies, multiple myeloma and related disorders.. *Br J Haematol* 2003;121(5):749-57.
2. Dimopoulos MA, Moulopoulos LA, Maniatis A, Alexanian R. Solitary plasmacytoma of bone and asymptomatic multiple myeloma. *Blood* 2000;96(6):2037-44.
3. Nanni C, Zamagni E, Farsad M, Franchi R, Franti S. Role of 18F-FDG PET/CT in the assessment of bone involvement in newly diagnosed multiple myeloma: preliminary results. *Eur J Nucl Med Mol Imaging* 2006;33(5):525-31.
4. Zamagni E, Nanni C, Patriarca F, et al. A prospective comparison of 18F-fluorodeoxyglucose positron emission tomography-computed tomography, magnetic resonance imaging and whole-body planar radiographs in the assessment of bone disease in newly diagnosed multiple myeloma. *Haematologica* 2007;92(1):50-5.
5. Hill QA, de Tute RM, Child JA, De Tute RM, Owen RG. Neoplastic plasma cells are demonstrable at bone marrow sites distant to solitary plasmacytoma of bone and predict for progression to multiple myeloma. ASH Annual Meeting Abstracts 2006;108(11):3512-.
6. McLain RF, Weinstein JN. Solitary plasmacytomas of the spine: a review of 84 cases. *J Spinal Disord* 1989;2(2):69-74.
7. Alexander MP, Goodkin DE, Poser CM. Solitary plasmacytoma producing cranial neuropathy. *Arch Neurol* 1975;32(11):777-8.
8. Prasad ML, Mahapatra AK, Kumar L, et al. Solitary intracranial plasmacytoma of the skull base. *Indian J Cancer* 1994;31(3):174-9.
9. Higurashi M, Yagishita S, Fujitsu K, Kitsuta Y, Yakemoto Y, Osano S. Plasma cell myeloma of the skull base: report of two cases. *Brain Tumor Pathol* 2004;21(3):135-41.
10. Pambuccian SE, Horyd ID, Cawte T, Huvos AG. Amyloidoma of bone, a plasma cell/plasmacytoid neoplasm. Report of three cases and review of the literature. *Am J Surg Pathol* 1997;21(2):179-86.
11. Rawlings NG, Brownstein S, Robinson JW, Jordan DR. Solitary osseous plasmacytoma of the orbit with amyloidosis. *Ophthal Plast Reconstr Surg* 2007;23(1):79-80.
12. Cooper JH, Rootman J, Ramsey MS. Extramedullary plasmacytoma (amyloid tumour) of the caruncle. *Can J Ophthalmol* 1989;24(4):166-8.
13. Nagasaka T, Lai R, Kuno K, Nakashima T, Nakashima N. Localized amyloidosis and extramedullary plasmacytoma involving the larynx of a child. *Hum Pathol* 2001;32(1):132-4.
14. Dispenzieri A, Kyle RA, Lacy MQ, et al. POEMS syndrome: definitions and long-term outcome. *Blood* 2003;101(7):2496-506.
15. Moulopoulos LA, Dimopoulos MA, Weber D, Fuller L, Libshitz HI, Alexanian R. Magnetic resonance imaging in the staging of solitary plasmacytoma of bone. *J Clin Oncol* 1993;11(7):1311-5.
16. Wilder RB, Ha CS, Cox JD, Weber D, Delasalle K, Alexanian R. Persistence of myeloma protein for more than one year after radiotherapy is an adverse prognostic factor in solitary plasmacytoma of bone. *Cancer* 2002;94(5):1532-7.
17. Moulopoulos LA, Dimopoulos MA. Magnetic resonance imaging of the bone marrow in hematologic malignancies. *Blood* 1997;90(6):2127-47.
18. Liebross RH, Ha CS, Cox JD, Weber D, Delasalle K, Alexanian R. Solitary bone plasmacytoma: outcome and prognostic

factors following radiotherapy. *Int J Radiat Oncol Biol Phys* 1998;41(5):1063-7.

19. Schirrmeister H, Buck AK, Bergmann L, et al. Positron emission tomography (PET) for staging of solitary plasmacytoma. *Cancer Biother Radiopharm* 2003;18(5):841-5.

20. Dimopoulos MA, Pouli A, Anagnostopoulos A, et al. Macrofocal multiple myeloma in young patients: a distinct entity with favorable prognosis. *Leuk Lymphoma* 2006;47(8):1553-6.

21. Dingli D, Kyle RA, Rajkumar SV, et al. Immunoglobulin free light chains and solitary plasmacytoma of bone. *Blood* 2006;108(6):1979-83.

22. Soutar R, Lucraft H, Jackson G, et al. Guidelines on the diagnosis and management of solitary plasmacytoma of bone and solitary extramedullary plasmacytoma. *Br J Haematol* 2004;124(6):717-26.

23. Barosi G, Boccadoro M, Cavo M, et al. Management of multiple myeloma and related-disorders: guidelines from the Italian Society of Hematology (SIE), Italian Society of Experimental Hematology (SIES) and Italian Group for Bone Marrow Transplantation (GITMO). *Haematologica* 2004;89(6):717-41.

24. Knobel D, Zouhair A, Tsang RW, et al. Prognostic factors in solitary plasmacytoma of the bone: a multicenter Rare Cancer Network study. *BMC Cancer* 2006;6:118.

25. Mill WB, Griffith R. The role of radiation therapy in the management of plasma cell tumors. *Cancer* 1980;45(4):647-52.

26. Chak LY, Cox RS, Bostwick DG, et al. Solitary plasmacytoma of bone: treatment, progression, and survival. *J Clin Oncol* 1987;5(11):1811-5.

27. Delauche-Cavallier MC, Laredo JD, Wybier M, et al. Solitary plasmacytoma of the spine. Long-term clinical course. *Cancer* 1988;61(8):1707-14.

28. Frassica DA, Frassica FJ, Schray MF, et al. Solitary plasmacytoma of bone: Mayo Clinic experience. *Int J Radiat Oncol Biol Phys* 1989;16(1):43-8.

29. Mayr NA, Wen BC, Hussey DH, et al. The role of radiation therapy in the treatment of solitary plasmacytomas. *Radiother Oncol* 1990;17(4):293-303.

30. Holland J, Trenkner DA, Wasserman TH, et al. Plasmacytoma. Treatment results and conversion to myeloma. *Cancer* 1992;69(6):1513-7.

31. Aviles A, Huerta-Guzman J, Delgado S, et al. Improved outcome in solitary bone plasmacytomata with combined therapy. *Hematol Oncol* 1996;14(3):111-7.

32. Bolek TW, Marcus RB, Mendenhall NP. Solitary plasmacytoma of bone and soft tissue. *Int J Radiat Oncol Biol Phys* 1996;36(2):329-33.

33. Jyothirmayi R, Gangadharan VP, Nair MK, et al. Radiotherapy in the treatment of solitary plasmacytoma. *Br J Radiol* 1997;70(833):511-6.

34. Tsang RW, Gospodarowicz MK, Pintilie M, et al. Solitary plasmacytoma treated with radiotherapy: impact of tumorsize on outcome. *Int J Radiat Oncol Biol Phys* 2001;50(1):113-20.

35. Ozsahin M, Tsang RW, Poortmans P, et al. Outcomes and patterns of failure in solitary plasmacytoma: a multicenter Rare

Cancer Network study of 258 patients. *Int J Radiat Oncol Biol Phys* 2006;64(1):210-7.

36. Knowling MA, Harwood AR, Bergsagel DE. Comparison of extramedullary plasmacytomas with solitary and multiple plasma cell tumors of bone. *J Clin Oncol* 1983;1(4):255-62.

37. Mendenhall CM, Thar TL, Million RR. Solitary plasmacytoma of bone and soft tissue. *Int J Radiat Oncol Biol Phys* 1980;6(11):1497-501.

38. Bataille R, Sany J. Solitary myeloma: clinical and prognostic features of a review of 114 cases. *Cancer* 1981;48(3):845-51.

39. Weber DM. Solitary bone and extramedullary plasmacytoma. *Hematology Am Soc Hematol Educ Program* 2005;373-6.

40. Alexanian R. Localized and indolent myeloma. *Blood* 1980;56(3):521-5.

41. Alexiou C, Kau RJ, Dietzfelbinger H, et al. Extramedullary plasmacytoma: tumor occurrence and therapeutic concepts. *Cancer* 1999;85(11):2305-14.

42. Durr HR, Kuhne JH, Hagena FW, et al. Surgical treatment for myeloma of the bone. A retrospective analysis of 22 cases. *Arch Orthop Trauma Surg* 1997;116(8):463-9.

43. Burt M, Karpeh M, Ukoha O, et al. Medical tumors of the chest wall. Solitary plasmacytoma and Ewing's sarcoma. *J Thorac Cardiovasc Surg* 1993;105(1):89-96.

44. Chang MY, Shih LY, Dunn P, et al. Solitary plasmacytoma of bone. *J Formos Med Assoc* 1994;93(5):397-402.

45. Shih LY, Dunn P, Leung WM, et al. Localised plasmacytomas in Taiwan: comparison between extramedullary plasmacytoma and solitary plasmacytoma of bone. *Br J Cancer* 1995;71(1):128-33.

46. Galieni P, Cavo M, Avvisati G, et al. Solitary plasmacytoma of bone and extramedullary plasmacytoma: two different entities? *Ann Oncol* 1995;6(7):687-91.

47. Dimopoulos MA, Kiamouris C, Moulopoulos LA. Solitary plasmacytoma of bone and extramedullary plasmacytoma. *Hematol Oncol Clin North Am* 1999;13(6):1249-57.

48. Dimopoulos MA, Moulopoulos A, Delasalle K, et al. Solitary plasmacytoma of bone and asymptomatic multiple myeloma. *Hematol Oncol Clin North Am* 1992;6(2):359-69.

49. Dimopoulos MA, Goldstein J, Fuller L, et al. Curability of solitary bone plasmacytoma. *J Clin Oncol* 1992;10(4):587-90.

50. Kumar S, Fonseca R, Dispenzieri A, et al. Prognostic value of angiogenesis in solitary bone plasmacytoma. *Blood* 2003;101(5):1715-7.

51. Morgan TK, Zhao S, Chang KL, et al. Low CD27 expression in plasma cell dyscrasias correlates with high-risk disease: an immunohistochemical analysis. *Am J Clin Pathol* 2006;126(4):545-51.

52. Galieni P, Cavo M, Pulsoni A, et al. Clinical outcome of extramedullary plasmacytoma. *Haematologica* 2000;85(1):47-51.

53. Susnerwala SS, Shanks JH, Banerjee SS, et al. Extramedullary plasmacytoma of the head and neck region: clinicopathological correlation in 25 cases. *Br J Cancer* 1997;75(6):921-7.

54. Webb HE, Harrison EG, Masson JK, et al. Solitary extramedullary myeloma (plasmacytoma) of the upper part of the respiratory tract and oropharynx. *Cancer* 1962;15:1142-55.

55. Helmus C. Extramedullary plasmacytoma of the head and neck. *Laryngoscope* 1964;74:553-9.

56. Kotner LM, Wang CC. Plasmacytoma of the upper air and food passages. *Cancer* 1972;30(2):414-8.

57. Medini E, Rao Y, Levitt SH. Solitary extramedullary plasmacytoma of the upper respiratory and digestive tracts. *Cancer* 1980;45(11):2893-6.

58. Segas J, Skoulakis H, Katrinakis G, et al. Solitary extramedullary plasmacytoma of the oropharynx: a rare location. *Ear Nose Throat J* 1993;72(11):743-5.

59. Remigio PA, Klaum A. Extramedullary plasmacytoma of stomach. *Cancer* 1971;27(3):562-8.

60. Preud'homme JL, Galian A, Danon F, et al. Extramedullary plasmacytoma with gastric and lymph node involvement: an immunological study. *Cancer* 1980;46(8):1753-8.

61. Chim CS, Wong WM, Nicholls J, et al. Extramedullary sites of involvement in hematologic malignancies: case 3. Hemorrhagic gastric plasmacytoma as the primary presentation in multiple myeloma. *J Clin Oncol* 2002;20(1):344-7.

62. Amin R. Extramedullary plasmacytoma of the lung. *Cancer* 1985;56(1):152-6.

63. Chen KY, Wu HD, Chang YL, et al. Primary pulmonary plasmacytoma with lobar consolidation: an unusual presentation. *J Formos Med Assoc* 1998;97(7):507-10.

64. Joseph G, Pandit M, Korfhage L. Primary pulmonary plasmacytoma. *Cancer* 1993;71(3):721-4.

65. Shin MS, Carcelen MF, Ho KJ. Diverse roentgenographic manifestations of the rare pulmonary involvement in myeloma. *Chest* 1992;102(3):946-8.

66. Takahashi R, Nakano S, Namura K, et al. Plasmacytoma of the urinary bladder in a renal transplant recipient. *Int J Hematol* 2005;81(3):255-7.

67. Yang C, Motteram R, Sandeman TF. Extramedullary plasmacytoma of the bladder: a case report and review of literature. *Cancer* 1982;50(1):146-9.

68. More JR, Dawson DW, Ralston AJ, et al. Plasmacytoma of the thyroid. *J Clin Pathol* 1968;21(5):661-7.

69. Salazar JE, Nelson JF, Winer-Muram HT. Extramedullary plasmacytoma of the thyroid. *Can Assoc Radiol J* 1987;38(2):136-8.

70. Bourtsos EP, Bedrossian CW, De Frias DV, et al. Thyroid plasmacytoma mimicking medullary carcinoma: a potential pitfall in aspiration cytology. *Diagn Cytopathol* 2000;23(5):354-8.

71. Iizumi T, Shinohara S, Amemiya H, et al. Plasmacytoma of the testis. *Urol Int* 1995;55(4):218-21.

72. Proctor NS, Rippey JJ, Shulman G, et al. Extramedullary plasmacytoma of the breast. *J Pathol* 1975;116(2):97-100.

73. Kirshenbaum G, Rhone DP. Solitary extramedullary plasmacytoma of the breast with serum monoclonal protein: a case report and review of the literature. *Am J Clin Pathol* 1985;83(2):230-2.

74. Alhan E, Calik A, Kucuktulu U, et al. Solitary extramedullary plasmocytoma of the breast with kappa monoclonal gammopathy. *Pathologica* 1995;87(1):71-3.

75. Cangiarella J, Waisman J, Cohen JM, et al. Plasmacytoma of the breast. A report of two cases diagnosed by aspiration biopsy. *Acta Cytol* 2000;44(1):91-4.

76. De Chiara A, Losito S, Terracciano L, et al. Primary plasmacytoma of the breast. *Arch Pathol Lab Med* 2001;125(8):1078-80.

77. Ferlito A, Polidoro F, Recher G. Extramedullary plasmacytoma of the parotid gland. *Laryngoscope* 1980;90(3):486-93.

78. Simi U, Marchetti G, Bruno R, et al. Plasmacytoma of the parotid gland. Report of a case and review of the world literature. *Acta Otorhinolaryngol Belg* 1988;42(1):93-6.

79. Gonzalez-Garcia J, Ghufoor K, Sandhu G, et al. Primary extramedullary plasmacytoma of the parotid gland: a case report and review of the literature. *J Laryngol Otol* 1998;112(2):179-81.

80. Liebross RH, Ha CS, Cox JD, et al. Clinical course of solitary extramedullary plasmacytoma. *Radiother Oncol* 1999;52(3):245-9.

81. Hari CK, Roblin DG. Solitary plasmacytoma of the parotid gland. *Int J Clin Pract* 2000;54(3):197-8.

82. Kanthan R, Torkian B. Solitary plasmacytoma of the parotid gGland with crystalline inclusions: a case report. *World J Surg Oncol* 2003;1(1):12.

83. Lin BT, Weiss LM. Primary plasmacytoma of lymph nodes. *Hum Pathol* 1997;28(9):1083-90.

84. Lim YH, Park SK, Oh HS, et al. A case of primary plasmacytoma of lymph nodes. *Korean J Intern Med* 2005;20(2):183-6.

85. Inbasekaran V, Vijayarathinam P, Arumugam S. Solitary intracerebral plasmacytoma. *J Indian Med Assoc* 1991;89(1):16-7.

86. Dimopoulos MA, Hamilos G. Solitary bone plasmacytoma and extramedullary plasmacytoma. *Curr Treat Options Oncol* 2002;3(3):255-9.

87. Bartl R, Frisch B, Fateh-Moghadam A, et al. Histologic classification and staging of multiple myeloma. A retrospectiveand prospective study of 674 cases. *Am J Clin Pathol* 1987;87(3):342-55.

88. Kremer M, Ott G, Nathrath M, et al. Primary extramedullary plasmacytoma and multiple myeloma: phenotypic differences revealed by immunohistochemical analysis. *J Pathol* 2005;205(1):92-101.

89. Hotz MA, Schwaab G, Bosq J, et al. Extramedullary solitary plasmacytoma of the head and neck. A clinicopathological study. *Ann Otol Rhinol Laryngol* 1999;108(5):495-500.

90. Hussong JW, Perkins SL, Schnitzer B, et al. Extramedullary plasmacytoma. A form of marginal zone cell lymphoma? *Am J Clin Pathol* 1999;111(1):111-6.

91. Wiltshaw E. The natural history of extramedullary plasmacytoma and its relation to solitary myeloma of bone and myelomatosis. *Medicine (Baltimore)* 1976;55(3):217-38.

92. Harwood AR, Knowling MA, Bergsagel DE. Radiotherapy of extramedullary plasmacytoma of the head and neck. *Clin Radiol* 1981;32(1):31-6.

93. Koss MN, Hochholzer L, Moran CA, et al. Pulmonary plasmacytomas: a clinicopathologic and immunohistochemical study of five cases. *Ann Diagn Pathol* 1998;2(1):1-11.

94. Brinch L, Hannisdal E, Abrahamsen AF, et al. Extramedullary plasmacytomas and solitary plasma cell tumours of bone. *Eur J Haematol* 1990;44(2):132-5.

95. Jackson A, Scarffe JH. Prognostic significance of osteopenia and immunoparesis at presentation in patients with solitary myeloma of bone. *Eur J Cancer* 1990;26(3):363-71

13 Monoclonal Gammopathy of Undetermined Significance and Smoldering Multiple Myeloma

Robert A. Kyle and S. Vincent Rajkumar

INTRODUCTION

In 1952, Jan Waldenström introduced the term "essential hyperglobulinemia" to describe patients with a small spike in the electrophoretic pattern but no evidence of multiple myeloma (MM), Waldenström macroglobulinemia (WM), amyloidosis (AL), or related disorders. Benign, idiopathic, asymptomatic, nonmyelomatous, cryptogenic, lanthanic, and rudimentary monoclonalgammopathy; dysimmunoglobulinemia; idiopathic paraproteinemia; and asymptomatic paraimmunoglobulinemia have been used to describe the entity. According to Waldenström,[1] the protein spike remained constant in size in contrast to the increasing protein spike of the protein in MM. The entity became known as "benign monoclonal gammopathy," but this is misleading because a monoclonal (M) protein may remain stable or it may increase and develop into symptomatic MM, WM, AL, or a related disorder. Because of this, the term "monoclonal gammopathy of undetermined significance" is a more appropriate term.

Monoclonal gammopathy of undetermined significance (MGUS) is characterized by the proliferation of a single clone of plasma cells that produces a homogeneous monoclonal (M) protein. Each M protein consists of two heavy polypeptide chains of the same class and subclass and two light chain polypeptide chains of the same type. In contrast, polyclonal immunoglobulins are produced by many clones of plasma cells. They contain all heavy chain classes and both light chain types. Each M protein consists of two heavy polypeptide chains of the same class: gamma (γ) constitutes immunoglobulin G (IgG), alpha (α) is found in IgA, mu (μ) is present in IgM, delta (δ) occurs in IgD, and epsilon (ε) is present in IgE. Two light polypeptide chains (kappa [κ] and lambda [λ]) of the

This study was supported by grant CA 62242 and CR107476 from the National Cancer Institute.

same type are found in each M protein. A monoclonal increase in immunoglobulins results from a clonal process that is malignant or potentially malignant, whereas a polyclonal increase in immunoglobulins is caused by a reactive or inflammatory process.

In 1978, the term "monoclonal gammopathy of undetermined significance" was introduced.[2] MGUS is defined as a serum M protein < 3 g/dL, <10% plasma cells in the bone marrow, and no evidence of end-organ damage (CRAB: hyperCalcemia, Renal insufficiency, Anemia, Bone lesions) related to the plasma cell proliferative disorder.[3]

LABORATORY APPROACH TO MGUS

Serum protein electrophoresis should be performed whenever MM, WM, or AL is suspected.[4] Unexplained weakness or fatigue, anemia, unexplained back pain, osteoporosis,osteolytic lesions or fractures, hypercalcemia, renal insufficiency, or recurrent infections are indications for serum protein electrophoresis. It should also be performed in adults with unexplained sensorimotor peripheral neuropathy, carpal tunnel syndrome, refractory congestive heart failure, orthostatic hypotension, nephrotic syndrome, or malabsorbtion because an M protien suggests AL. All patients with a spike or a localized band on agarose gel electrophoresis or a localized spike on the densitometer tracing require immunofixation to confirm the presence of an M protein and determine its type. In addition, immunofixation should be carried out whenever MM, AL, or a related disorder is suspected clinically.

Quantitation of immunoglobulins should be performed with a rate nephelometer. Levels of IgM obtained by nephelometry may be at least 1000 mg/dL higher than that expected on the basis of the serum protein electrophoretic tracing. The nephelometric IgG and IgA levels may also be increased.

The serum free light chain (FLC) assay is an automated nephelometric test that measures the level of free kappa and free lambda light chains in the serum. The normal ratio for FLC (κ/λ) is 0.26-1.65.[5] The FLC assay is useful for monitoring patients with nonsecretory MM and is of prognostic value in MGUS,[6] solitary plasmacytoma of bone,[7] smoldering multiple myeloma (SMM),[8] and MM (CLH Snozek, JA Katzmann et al., accepted for publication). In short, it is also helpful for following patients with plasma cell disorders who do not have a measurable M spike in the serum or urine.

Screening for the presence of an M protein in a patient with a suspected monoclonal gammopathy does not require the collection of a 24-h urine specimen. In a group of 428 patients with a serum M protein and a urine M protein, serum immunofixation was abnormal in 93.5%, serum protein electrophoresis was abnormal in 81%, and serum FLC assay was abnormal in 86%. All three serum tests were normal in only 2 out of 428 patients. Consequently, a 24-h urine study is not required for screening of a monoclonal gammopathy. However, a 24-h urine specimen must be collected for electrophoresis and immunofixation if a serum M protein is found.[9]

In addition, all patients with a serum M protein of >1.5 g/dL should have electrophoresis and immunofixation of an aliquot from a 24-h urine specimen. The size of the urinary M protein provides an indirect measurement of the patient's tumor mass and is useful for monitoring the course of the disease.

In 2007, 1,770 persons with an M protein in the serum or urine were identified at Mayo Clinic: MGUS, 1,005 (57%); MM, 272 (15%); AL, 189 (10.5%); lymphoproliferative disorder, 71 (4%); SMM, 69 (4%); solitary or extramedullary plasmacytoma, 12 (1%); WM, 37 (2%); and other, 115 (6.5%) (see Figure 13.1).

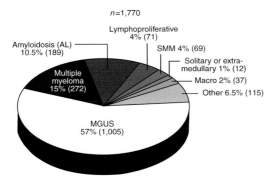

Figure 13.1. Monoclonal gammopathies seen at Mayo clinic during 2007.

PREVALENCE OF MGUS

The presence of an M protein without evidence of MM or a related disorder (MGUS) has been reported in approximately 3% of persons older than 70 years in Sweden,[10] the United States,[11] and France.[12] MGUS occurs more often among older patients. The prevalence in African Americans is two- to threefold greater than that in Caucasians.[13,14] In contrast, the prevalence of MGUS in Japanese patients is less than that in Caucasians.[15]

The first population-based study that used sensitive laboratory techniques to detect M proteins was performed in Olmsted County, Minnesota. Serum samples were obtained from 21 463 of the 28 038 enumerated residents (77%) who were 50 years of age or older. MGUS was identified in 694 (3.2%) of these subjects. Age-adjusted rates were greater in men than in women (4.0% vs. 2.7%) (p < 0.001) (Table 13.1, Figure 13.2). The prevalence increased with advancing age and was almost four times as high among persons aged 80 years or older than among those 50-59 years of age. The prevalence of MGUS was 5.3% among patients 70 years or older and 7.5% among those 85 years or older. The prevalence of MGUS was 8.9% in men older than 85 years, while in women it was 7.0%. The concentration of the M protein was <1 g/dL in 63.5% and more than 2 g/dL in 4.5% of the 694 patients. The M protein was too small to measure in 13.1%. The median size was 0.5 g/dL and 0.7 g/dL if the unmeasurable M proteins were excluded. The isotype of the M protein was IgG in 69% of the 694 patients with MGUS, IgM in 17%, IgA in 11%, and biclonal in 3%. The light chain type was κ in 62% and λ in 38%. The concentration of uninvolved immunoglobulins was reduced in 28% of 447 patients tested. Of the 79 patients tested, 21% had a monoclonal light chain in the urine.

Percentage detected clinically and duration

The prevalence of MGUS in Olmsted County, Minnesota, in a population-based screening study found that MGUS was present in 1.3% of persons 50 years of age and 3.8% of those 70 years of age. In contrast, 0.1% of patients at age 50 had an MGUS discovered on the basis of clinical practice and only 0.8% of patients at age 70. Thus, only 21% of patients with MGUS at age 70 had been recognized on the basis of clinical practice. This is probably higher in Olmsted County than elsewhere because serum protein electrophoresis is

TABLE 13.1. Prevalence of MGUS according to age group and sex among residents of Olmsted County, Minnesota

Age (years)	Number/total number (%)*		
	Men	Women	Total
50-59	82/4038 (2.0)	59/4335 (1.4)	141/8373 (1.7)
60-69	105/2864 (3.7)	73/3155 (2.3)	178/6019 (3.0)
70-79	104/1858 (5.6)	101/2650 (3.8)	205/4508 (4.6)
≥80	59/709 (8.3)	110/1854 (6.0)	170/2563 (6.6)
Total	350/9469 (3.7)[†]	343/11 994 (2.9)[†]	694/21 463 (3.2)[†,‡]

*The percentage was calculated as the number of patients with MGUS divided by the number who were tested.
[†]Prevalence was age-adjusted to the 2000 US total population as follows: men, 4.0% (95% confidence interval, 3.5-4.4); women, 2.7% (95% confidence interval, 2.4-3.0); and total, 3.2% (95% confidence interval, 3.0-3.5).
[‡]Prevalence was age- and sex-adjusted to the 2000 US total population.
Source: From Kyle et al., Prognosis in monoclonal gammopathy of undetermined significance. *N Engl J Med* 2006;354:13. © 2006 Massachusetts Medical Society. All rights reserved.

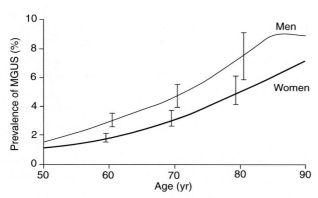

Figure 13.2. Prevalence of monoclonal gammopathy of undetermined significance (MGUS) according to age. The I bars represent 95% confidence intervals. Years of age greater than 90 have been collapsed to 90 years of age.
Source: From Kyle et al., Prognosis in monoclonal gammopathy of undetermined significance. *N Engl J Med* 2006;354:1362-9. © 2006 Massachusetts Medical Society. All rights reserved.

frequently ordered on Mayo Clinic patients given our long-standing interest in monoclonal gammopathies. The duration of MGUS before detection at age 70 can be calculated if one knows the prevalence of MGUS, the risk of progression (1% per year), and the differential difference in the death rate of MGUS patients compared with non-MGUS patients. By calculating the incidence from the known prevalence and the differential survival, one can determine the duration of MGUS before its recognition. MGUS discovered at age 70 has been present for 0-5 years in 27%, 6-10 years in

20%, 11-15 years in 15%, 16-20 years in 11%, and for more than 20 years in 27%. Thus, 30% of patients recognized to have MGUS at age 70 probably had MGUS at age 50. The median duration of MGUS before its recognition on the basis of clinical practice is 11 years.[16]

NATURAL HISTORY OF MGUS

MGUS is asymptomatic and may be found unexpectedly during laboratory testing of an apparently normal person or may be found during evaluation of an unrelated disorder. MGUS is a common finding in the medical practice of all physicians. It is important for both patient and physician to determine whether the monoclonal protein remains benign or progresses to MM or a related disorder.

Mayo Clinic referral population of 241 patients

The medical records of all patients with a monoclonal gammopathy who were seen at Mayo Clinic from 1956 through 1970 were reviewed.[2,17] Patients with MM, WM, AL, lymphoma, or a related condition were excluded. A total of 241 patients remained for long-term study. After 3579 patient-years of follow-up (median, 13.7 years; range, 0-39 years), the number of patients who were alive and whose M-protein level had remained stable and thus could be classified as having benign monoclonal gammopathy had decreased to 14 (6%). The serum M-protein value increased to 3 g/dL or more in 25 patients (10%) but did not require chemotherapy for symptomatic MM, WM, or AL.

TABLE 13.2. Development of multiple myeloma or related disorder in 64 patients with MGUS*

	No. (%) of patients	Interval to disease (years)	
		Median	Range
Multiple myeloma	44 (69)	10.6	1-32
Macroglobulinemia	7 (11)	10.3	4-16
Amyloidosis	8 (12)	9.0	6-19
Lymphoproliferative disease	5 (8)	8.0	4-19
Total	64 (100)	10.4	1-32

*MGUS = monoclonal gammopathy of undetermined significance.
Source: Used with permission from Kyle RA, Therneau TA, Rajkumar SV, et al. Long-tern follow-up of 241 patients with monoclonal gammopathy of undetermined significance: the original Mayo Clinic Series 25 years later. Mayo Clinic Proc 2004;79:859-66.

A total of 138 patients (57%) died without evidence of symptomatic MM, WM, AL, lymphoma, or a related disorder. Cardiac disease, cerebrovascular disease, or a nonplasma cell malignancy accounted for the majority of deaths. MM, WM, AL, or a lymphoproliferative disorder developed in 64 patients (27%). The actuarial risk of progression was 17% at 10 years, 34% at 20 years, and 39% at 25 years; the rate was approximately 1.5% per year. Sixty-nine percent of the 64 patients who progressed developed MM. The interval from recognition of MGUS to the diagnosis of MM ranged from 1 to 32 years (median 10.6 years) (Table 13.2). In 10 patients, the diagnosis of MM was made 20 years after recognition of MGUS. WM developed in seven patients. All had serum IgM κ-protein levels ranging from 3.1 g/dL to 8.5 g/dL at diagnosis. Systemic AL amyloidosis was found in eight patients of 6-19 years (median 9 years) after the recognition of an M protein in the serum. A malignant lymphoproliferative disorder (malignant lymphoma, 3; chronic lymphocytic leukemia, 1; and an atypical malignant lymphoproliferative disorder, 1) developed in five patients of 4-19 years (median 8 years) after the detection of the M protein.

Because the 241 Mayo Clinic patients came from all parts of the United States and other countries and may be subject to referral bias, we conducted a population-based study to confirm the findings of the Mayo Clinic study. A total of 1384 patients who resided in the 11 counties of southeastern Minnesota were identified as having MGUS. The patients were evaluated at Mayo Clinic from January 1, 1960, through December 31, 1964.[18] The median age at diagnosis of MGUS

was 72 years, in contrast to 64 years for the 241 cohort. This suggests that older patients are less likely to visit referral centers. Fifty-four percent were male. Only 2% (24 patients) were younger than 40 years at diagnosis, whereas 810 (59%) were aged 70 years or older. The M-protein value at diagnosis ranged from unmeasurable to 3.0 g/dL. Seventy percent of the M proteins were IgG, 12% IgA, and 15% IgM. Three percent (45 patients) had a biclonal gammopathy. The light chain type was κ in 61% and λ in 39%. A reduction of uninvolved (normal or background) immunoglobulins was found in 38% of 840 patients in whom quantitation of immunoglobulins was determined. Thirty-one percent of the 418 patients who had immunofixation of urine had a monoclonal light chain. Only 17% had an M-protein value >150 mg per 24 h.

The bone marrow contained 0%-10% plasma cells (median, 3%) in the 160 patients who underwent the procedure. The hemoglobin value was <10 g/dL in 7% and 12.0 g/dL or less in 23%. However, the anemia was related to causes other than the plasma cell proliferative process and was due to iron deficiency, renal insufficiency, myelodysplasia, and so forth in each instance. The serum creatinine level was >2 mg/dL in 6% but was attributable to unrelated causes such as hypertension, diabetes, or glomerulonephritis.

After a follow-up of 11 009 person-years (median, 15.4 years; range, 0-35 years), 70% had died, indicating a robust follow-up. MM, AL, lymphoma with an IgM serum protein, WM, plasmacytoma, or chronic lymphocytic leukemia developed in 8% (115 patients) during follow-up. Progression to one of these disorders occurred in 1% of patients each year. At 10 years, 10% had progressed; at 20 years, 21% had progressed; and at 25 years, 26% had progressed (Figure 13.3). Patients were at risk for progression even after more than 25 years of follow-up. In addition, 32 patients were identified in whom the M-protein value was >3 g/dL or the percentage of bone marrow plasma cells increased to more than 10% but in whom symptomatic MM did not develop. The number of patients with progression to a plasma cell disorder (115 patients) was 7.3 times the number expected on the basis of the incidence rates for those conditions in the general population[19] (Table 13.3). The risk of development of MM was increased 25-fold; WM, 46-fold; and AL, 8.4-fold. The risk of development of lymphoma was only modestly increased at 2.4-fold, but this risk was underestimated because only lymphomas associated with an IgM protein were

Type of progression	Observed no. of patients	Expected no. of patients[†]	Relative Risk (95% CI)
Multiple myeloma	75	3.0	25.0 (20-32)
Lymphoma	19[‡]	7.8	2.4 (2-4)
Primary amyloidosis	10	1.2	8.4 (4-16)
Macroglobulinemia	7	0.2	46.0 (19-95)
Chronic lymphocytic leukemia	3[§]	3.5	0.9 (0.2-3)
Plasmacytoma	1	0.1	8.5 (0.2-47)
Total	115	15.8	7.3 (6-9)

*CI denotes confidence interval.

[†]Expected numbers of cases were derived from the age- and sex-matched white population of the Surveillance, Epidemiology, and End Results program in Iowa[19], except for primary amyloidosis.

[‡]All 19 patients had serum IgM monoclonal protein. If the 30 patients with IgM, IgA, or IgG monoclonal protein and lymphoma were included, the relative risk would be 3-9 (95% confidence interval, 2.6-5.5).

[§]All three patients had serum IgM monoclonal protein. If all six patients with IgM, IgA, or IgG monoclonal protein and chronic lymphocytic leukemia were included, the relative risk would be 1.7 (95% confidence interval, 0.6-3.7).

Source: This table is reprinted with permissions from Kyle et al., A long-term study of prognosis in monoclonal gammopathy of undetermined significance. *N Engl J Med* 2002;346:564-9. © 2002 Massachusetts Medical Society. All rights reserved.

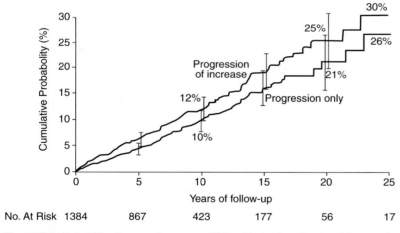

Figure 13.3. Probability of progression among 1384 residents of southeastern Minnesota in whom MGUS was diagnosed from 1960 through 1994. The top curve shows the probability of progression to a plasma cell cancer (115 patients) or of an increase in the monoclonal protein concentration to more than 30 g/L or the proportion of plasma cells in bone marrow to more than 10% (32 patients). The bottom curve shows only the probability of progression of MGUS to multiple myeloma, IgM lymphoma, primary amyloidosis, macroglobulinemia, chronic lymphocytic leukemia, or plasmacytoma (115 patients). The bars show 95% confidence intervals.
Source: From Kyle et al., A long-term study of prognosis in monoclonal gammopathy of undetermined significance. *N Engl J Med* 2002;346(8):564-9. © 2002 Massachusetts Medical Society. All rights reserved.

counted in the observed number, while the incidence rates for lymphoma associated with IgG, IgA, and IgM proteins were used to calculate the expected number. Sixty-five percent (*n* = 75) of the 115 patients who progressed developed MM. The characteristics of these 75 patients were comparable with those of 1027 patients with newly diagnosed myeloma who were referred to Mayo Clinic between 1985 and 1998[20] except that the southeastern Minnesota patients were older (median, 72 vs. 66 years) and less likely to be male (45% vs. 60%).

The mode of development of MM among the patients with MGUS was variable. The M-protein level increased within 2 years of the recognition of MGUS in 11 patients, whereas the serum M-protein level was stable for more than 10 years and then increased within 2 years in 19 patients; in 9 others, the M protein increased gradually after having been stable for at least 2 years. In nine patients, the M-protein level increased gradually during follow-up until the diagnosis of symptomatic MM was made. In 10 patients, the serum M-protein level remained essentially stable; the diagnosis of MM was unequivocal in these 10 patients because of an increase in bone marrow plasma cells, development of lytic lesions, or occurrence of anemia, renal insufficiency, or an increased level of urine M protein. Seventeen patients had an insufficient number of serum M-protein measurements to determine the pattern of increase. In patients with WM, the M-protein level showed a gradual increase in three, stable levels were followed by a sudden increase in two, and data were insufficient in two.

During follow-up, the M protein disappeared in 66 patients (5%). All had low initial values of an M protein; only 17 had a value higher than 0.5 g/dL at diagnosis. Disappearance of the M protein occurred in 39 patients because of therapy for MM or lymphoma or other disorders such as idiopathic thrombocytopenic purpura or vasculitis unrelated to the monoclonal gammopathy. The M protein disappeared without an apparent cause in 27 patients (2%). Only 6 of these 27 patients (0.4% of all patients) had a discrete spike on the densitometer tracing of the initial electrophoretic pattern (median 1.2 g/dL). Thus, spontaneous disappearance of an M protein after diagnosis of MGUS was rare.

FOLLOW-UP IN OTHER SERIES

Similar findings have been reported in several other series. In one group, 13 out of 128 patients with MGUS developed a malignant disease during a median follow-up of 56 months.[21] In another study, 6.6% of 334 patients with MGUS had progression after a median follow-up of 8.4 years.[22] During a median follow-up of 70 months, 6.8% of 335 persons with MGUS progressed.[23] The actuarial probability of development of malignancy was 31% at 20 years in a series of 263 patients with MGUS.[24] Malignant transformation was the cause of death in 97 of 1324 patients with MGUS in North Jutland, Denmark, while only 4.9 deaths were expected.[25] Sixty-four new cases of malignancy (5 expected; relative risk 12.9) were found among 1229 patients with MGUS.[26] The risk of developing MM, WM, or lymphoma was 34.3-fold, 63.8-fold, and 5.9-fold, respectively. In a series of 504 patients with MGUS from Iceland, malignancy developed in 10% after a median follow-up of 6 years.[27] Thus, these series confirm a risk of progression from MGUS to MM or a related disorder of approximately 1% per year. It must be emphasized that this risk of progression does not disappear even after long-term follow-up.

PATHOGENESIS OF PROGRESSION OF MGUS

Genetic changes, bone marrow angiogenesis, cytokines related to myeloma bone disease, and possibly infectious agents may all play a role in the progression of MGUS to MM or a related disorder. However, the events responsible for malignant transformation are poorly understood.[28]

Genetic changes

Approximately 60% of patients with MM have IgH (14q32) translocations.[29] These same translocations are also present in MGUS.[30] Forty-six percent of patients with MGUS studied with fluorescence in situ hybridization (FISH) had IgH

translocations consisting of t(11;14)(q13;q32) in 25%, t(4;14) (p16.3;q32) in 9%, and t(14;16)(q32;q23) in 5%. These translocations resulted in dysregulation of oncogenes such as cyclin D1 (11q13), c-*maf* (16q23), and FGFR3/MMSET (fibroblastic growth factor receptor 3/MM SET domain) (4p16.3) and cyclin D3 (6p21) and may be playing a role in the initiation of MGUS rather than progression of MGUS to MM. Most of the patients with MGUS who lack evidence of IgH translocations have hyperdiploidy. Hyperdiploidy was reported in 11 out of 28 patients (40%) with SMM or MGUS.[31] The frequency is similar to that of hyperdiploid MM reported in the literature. It suggests that hyperdiploid MM originates early during disease evolution. Thus, almost all cases of MGUS are associated with genomic instability that is manifested as primary IgH translocations in approximately one-half and hyperdiploidy in most of the remaining patients.

Deletions of chromosome 13 have been found in both MGUS and MM.[32] However, it is not clear whether the rate of progression from MGUS to MM is increased because the frequency of deletion of chromosome 13 is similar in both MGUS and MM.

K- or N-*ras* mutations were reported in 5% of 20 patients with MGUS in contrast to 31% of 58 patients with MM. The authors postulated that *ras* mutations are often a genetic marker if not a causal event in the progression of MGUS to MM.[33] Aberrant methylation of the 5′ gene-promoter regions of tumor suppressor genes has been found in MGUS, but aberrant methylation is lower in frequency compared with MM. The possible role of these changes in the progression of MGUS is not clear.

Angiogenesis

Increased angiogenesis was first reported in MM by Vacca et al. in 1994.[34] Angiogenesis was studied in 400 patients with MGUS, SMM, newly diagnosed active MM, relapsed MM, and AL. The median microvessel density (in vessels per high-power field) was 1.3 in 42 normal controls, 1.7 in AL, 3 in MGUS, 4 in SMM, 11 in MM, and 20 in relapsed MM. It is evident that bone marrow angiogenesis increases progressively from MGUS to MM.[35] Vacca et al.,[36] using a chick embryo chorioallantoic membrane angiogenesis assay, reported that 76% of MM bone marrow samples had increased angiogenic potential compared to 20% of MGUS samples.

An alteration in the balance between pro- and antiangiogenic facts appears responsible for progression rather than overexpression of a single pro-angiogenic cytokine. In addition, there may be a loss of angiogenesis inhibitory activity with disease progression from MGUS to MM. In one study, 63% of MGUS sera inhibited angiogenesis, whereas 43% of SMM and 4% of MM serum samples did so. Vascular endothelial growth factor (VEGF) did not eliminate the inhibitory effect.[37] Thus, loss of an endogenous angiogenesis inhibitor may play a role in the increased angiogenesis that occurs with disease progression.

Myeloma bone disease–associated cytokines

The presence of lytic bone lesions, osteopenia, hypercalcemia, and pathological fractures differentiate MM from MGUS. Nevertheless, we found a 2.7-fold increase in axial fractures in 488 Olmsted County residents with MGUS.[38]

Osteoclastic activation and inhibition of osteoblast differentiation are responsible for bone lesions in MM. Osteoclastic activation is caused by overexpression of various cytokines including receptor activator of nuclear factor κ-β ligand (RANKL) and macrophage inflammatory protein 1-α (MIP-1α).[39] Consequently, myeloma bone disease may occur from excess RANKL or reduced levels of osteoprotegerin.[40] Interleukin-1β (IL-1β) induces osteoclast formation and may play a role in the transformation of MGUS to myeloma.[41] IL-6 and tumor necrosis factor-α may also play a role.

Helicobacter pylori

It was reported that eradication of *H. pylori* led to the resolution of MGUS in 11 out of 39 patients who had a *H. pylori* infection.[42] In contrast, we found that 30% of 93 patients with MGUS who were residents of Olmsted County, Minnesota, had *H. pylori*, as did 32% of 98 control patients from the same population. In addition, 51 out of 154 patients (33%) from Mayo Clinic with MGUS were positive for *H. pylori* as were 365 out of 1103 (33%) without MGUS. Thus, the role of *H. pylori* infection in MGUS is controversial.[43]

RISK FACTORS FOR MALIGNANT TRANSFORMATION IN MGUS

Prediction of MGUS patients who remain stable and those in whom progression develops is very difficult at the time of recognition of MGUS.[44]

Size of M protein

The size of the M protein at the time of recognition of MGUS is the most important predictor of progression.[18] Twenty years after recognition of MGUS, the risk of progression to MM or a related disorder was 14% for patients with an initial M-protein value of 0.5 g/dL or less, 25% for 1.5 g/dL, 41% for 2.0 g/dL, and 49% in those with an M spike of 2.5 g/dL. The risk of progression of an M protein of 1.5 g/dL was almost double that of a patient with an M-protein value of 0.5 g/dL. The risk of progression with an M protein of 2.5 g/dL was 4.6 times that of a patient with a 0.5 g/dL M protein. Rosinol et al.[45] reported that a progressive increase in the size of the M protein during the first year of follow-up was the most important risk factor for progression.

Type of immunoglobulin

In the southeastern Minnesota population, patients with IgM or IgA monoclonal protein had an increased risk of progression compared to those with an IgG monoclonal protein (p = 0.001). Blade et al.[21] also noted that patients with an IgA MGUS had a greater probability for progression to MM.

Bone marrow plasma cells

Cesana et al.[46] reported that the presence of more than 5% bone marrow plasma cells was an independent risk factor for progression. Baldini et al.[23] found a malignant transformation of 6.8% when the bone marrow plasma cell content was <10% and 37% for those with bone marrow plasma cell of 10%-30%.

Serum FLC ratio

Thirty-three percent of 1148 patients with MGUS from southeastern Minnesota had an abnormal FLC ratio. The risk of progression in patients with an abnormal FLC ratio was significantly greater than that in patients with a normal ratio (hazard ratio 3.5; p < 0.001) and was independent of the size and type of the serum M protein.[6]

Risk-stratification model for MGUS

Patients with risk factors consisting of an abnormal serum FLC, non-IgG MGUS, and an elevated serum M-protein value ≥1.5 g/dL had a risk of progression at 20 years of 58%

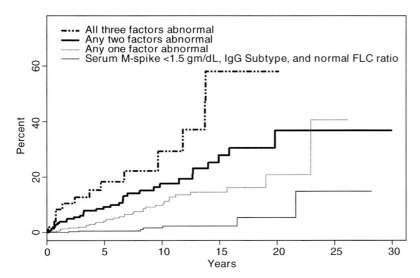

Figure 13.4. Risk of progression of MGUS to myeloma or related disorder using a risk-stratification model that incorporates the free light chain ratio and the size and type of the serum monoclonal protein. The top curve illustrates risk of progression with time in patients with all three risk factors, namely an abnormal serum kappa/lambda free light chain ratio (<0.26 or >1.65), a high serum monoclonal protein level (>15 g/L), and non-IgG MGUS; the second gives the risk of progression in patients with any two of these risk factors; the third curve illustrates the risk of progression with one of these risk factors; the bottom curve is the risk of progression for patients with none of the risk factors.

Source: This research was originally published in Rajkumar et al., Serum free light chain ratio is an independent risk factor for progression in monoclonal gammopathy of undetermined significance (MGUS). *Blood* 2005;106:812-17. © The American Society of Hematology.

compared with 37% for only two risk factors present, 21% with one risk factor present, and 5% when none of the risk factors was present (Figure 13.4). When competing causes of death were taken into account, the risk of progression was only 2% at 20 years in those with no risk factors.

LIFE EXPECTANCY AND CAUSE OF DEATH IN MGUS

In our experience, survival was significantly shorter among 241 patients with MGUS diagnosed before 1971, compared with an age- and sex-adjusted 1980 US population (13.7 vs. 15.7 years). Median duration of survival was 8.1 years for the 1384 patients with MGUS in southeastern Minnesota, compared to an expected 11.8 years (p < 0.001) for Minnesota residents of matched age and sex. Rates of death at 10 years were 6% from plasma cell disorders and 53% from nonplasma cell disorders such as cardiovascular and cerebrovascular diseases and nonplasma cell malignancies (Figure 13.5). After 20 years' follow-up, the rates were 10% from plasma cell disorders and 72% from nonplasma cell disorders.

DIFFERENTIAL DIAGNOSIS

Differentiation of a patient with MGUS from one with MM may be difficult at the time of presentation and is based on the clinical and laboratory features. A radiographic bone survey and a bone marrow aspirate and biopsy are indicated in all patients with an M-protein value of 1.5 g/dL or more, and all patients who have an abnormality in the complete blood count, creatinine, or calcium values consistent with MM. Additional risk factors are the presence of an IgA or IgM MGUS and patients with an abnormal FLC ratio. The size of the serum M protein is useful because higher levels are associated with a greater likelihood of MM or WM. The reduction of uninvolved immunoglobulins or the presence of an M protein in the urine (Bence Jones proteinuria) are of little help in differentiation because they may be present in both MGUS and MM. Patients with a serum M protein ≥3 g/dL or bone marrow plasma cells ≥10% without other manifestations of MM are considered to have SMM.[47] The presence of osteolytic lesions strongly suggests MM, but metastatic carcinoma may produce lytic lesions and be associated with an unrelated serum M protein and plasmacytosis. Magnetic resonance imaging may be useful in that 24 patients with MGUS had normal images, but abnormalities were found in 86% of 44 patients with MM.[48] An elevated plasma cell labeling index usually indicates symptomatic MM, but one-third of patients with symptomatic MM have a normal labeling index. The presence of circulating plasma cells in the peripheral blood is suggestive of symptomatic MM.[49] Conventional cytogenetic studies are not useful because an abnormal karyotype is rare in MGUS because of the low proliferative rate and the small number of plasma cells. Furthermore, FISH is not helpful because abnormalities are found in both MGUS and MM.

In summary, the differentiation of symptomatic MM from MGUS or SMM depends mainly on the presence or absence of end-organ damage (CRAB) that is due to the underlying plasma cell proliferative disorder. MGUS and SMM are distinguished from each other by the size of the serum M protein and the number of bone marrow plasma cells.

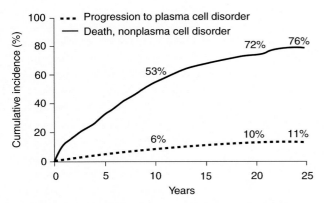

Figure 13.5. Rate of death from non-plasma cell disorders compared with progression to plasma cell disorders in 1384 patients with MGUS from southeastern Minnesota.
Source: From Kyle and Rajkumar, Monoclonal gammopathies of undetermined significance. *Immunol Rev* 2003;194:125. © Wiley-Blackwell, UK.

MANAGEMENT

Serum protein electrophoresis should be repeated 3-6 months after recognition of MGUS; if the results are stable and the patient has no clinical features of MM, WM, or AL and a serum M-protein value < 1.5 g/dL, IgG type, and normal FLC ratio, serum protein electrophoresis may be repeated every 2-3 years. In this setting, skeletal radiography or bone marrow examination are rarely necessary.

In an MGUS patient with a serum M-protein value >1.5 g/dL, a metastatic bone survey and a bone marrow aspirate and biopsy should be performed. The presence of an IgA or an IgM protein type or an abnormal FLC ratio are additional reasons to consider bone marrow evaluation. Bone marrow examination is also indicated in patients who have unexplained anemia, renal insufficiency, hypercalcemia, or bone lesions. Cytogenetic studies (both conventional and FISH), determination of the plasma cell labeling index, and a search for circulating plasma cells in the peripheral blood should be performed.[50] Computed tomographic scan of the abdomen may be helpful in patients with an IgM monoclonal protein because asymptomatic retroperitoneal lymphadenopathy may be present. If MM or WM is present, serum lactate dehydrogenase, β_2-microglobulin, and C-reactive protein should be determined.

If the results of the above tests are satisfactory, serum protein electrophoresis and a complete blood count should be repeated at 6-month intervals for a year and then

annually. Patients must contact their physicians immediately if there is any change in their clinical condition.

VARIANTS OF MGUS

Biclonal gammopathy

Biclonal gammopathies are characterized by the presence of two different M proteins and occur in 3%-6% of patients with monoclonal gammopathies. Two M proteins may be due to the proliferation of two different clones of plasma cells, each producing an unrelated M protein, or by the production of two M proteins by a single clone of plasma cells. Biclonal gammopathy of undetermined significance was found in 37 out of 57 patients with a biclonal gammopathy.[51] The age range was 39-93 years (median, 67 years). Localized bands were found in only 18 patients with electrophoresis on cellulose acetate; in the others, a second M protein was not recognized until immunoelectrophoresis or immunofixation was performed. The clinical findings of biclonal gammopathies are similar to those of monoclonal gammopathies. Thirty-five percent of the 57 patients had MM, WM, or another malignant lymphoproliferative disorder.

Triclonal gammopathy

In a review of 24 patients with triclonal gammopathy, 16 were associated with a malignant lymphoproliferative disorder, 5 occurred in nonhematologic diseases, and 3 were of undetermined significance.[52] In another case report of a patient with non-Hodgkin lymphoma, IgG kappa, IgG lambda, and IgM lambda monoclonal proteins were described. Three separate populations of M-component producing cells were identified.[53]

Idiopathic Bence Jones proteinuria

Two patients with a stable serum M protein excreted 0.8 g/day or more of Bence Jones protein for more than 17 years without developing MM or a related disorder.[54] Seven additional patients have been described who presented with Bence Jones proteinuria with >1.0 g per 24 h, but in whom no M protein was found in the serum and no evidence of MM or a related disorder was found.[55] Multiple myeloma developed in two of the seven patients, SMM in one, and AL in one. Two patients died of unrelated causes. One out of the seven patients had excreted up to 1.8 g κ-light chain/24 h for 37 years without the development of symptomatic MM or renal insufficiency. He died of a sudden cardiac arrhythmia and no evidence of systemic AL or MM was found at autopsy. Although idiopathic Bence Jones proteinuria may remain stable for years, MM or AL often develops, so the patients must be followed up indefinitely.

IgM MGUS

IgM MGUS is defined as a serum IgM monoclonal protein <3 g/dL, bone marrow lymphoplasmacytic infiltration <10%, and no evidence of anemia, constitutional symptoms, hyperviscosity, lymphadenopathy, or hepatosplenomegaly.[56] Of 430 patients in whom an IgM serum clonal protein was detected on laboratory testing at Mayo Clinic between 1956 and 1978, 56% had MGUS.[57]

IgM MGUS was diagnosed in 213 Mayo Clinic patients who resided in the 11 counties of southeastern Minnesota.[58] Twenty-nine (14%) of these 213 patients developed non-Hodgkin lymphoma ($n = 17$), WM ($n = 6$), chronic lymphocytic leukemia ($n = 3$), or AL ($n = 3$) with relative risks of 15-, 262-, 6-, and 16-fold, respectively. The risk of progression was 1.5% per year. This rate persisted even after 20 years of follow-up. The initial levels of serum M protein and a lower serum albumin level at diagnosis were independent predictors of progression.

Morra et al.[59] reported that 14 (10%) out of 138 patients with IgM MGUS progressed after having remained stable for 12 months. Another group of 83 patients with an IgM-related disorder consisting of type 1 cryoglobulinemia in 19, type 2 cryoglobulinemia in 56, peripheral neuropathy in 5, and idiopathic thrombocytopenic purpura in 3 overt WM or a related disorder developed in 8 out of the 83 patients.[60] In another report, 15 out of 217 patients with IgM MGUS and 45 out of 201 patients with indolent WM progressed to symptomatic WM.[61] The size of the initial M-protein value, hemoglobin level, and gender are important variables relating to progression.

IgD MGUS

The presence of an IgD monoclonal protein almost always indicates MM, AL, or plasma cell leukemia. However, IgD MGUS has been reported in two patients.

IgE MGUS

Only two patients have been reported with IgE MGUS.[62]

ASSOCIATION OF MGUS WITH OTHER DISEASES

Many diseases are associated with MGUS, as would be expected in an older population. The association of any two diseases depends on the frequency with which each occurs independently. In addition, an apparent association may occur because of differences in the referral pattern or in other selected patient groups. Valid epidemiological and statistical methods are essential for evaluating these associations. The need for appropriate control populations cannot be overemphasized.[63,64]

Lymphoproliferative disorders

Azar et al.[65] reported that malignant lymphoma and lymphatic leukemia were associated with a myeloma-type serum protein. Kyle et al.[66] described six patients with lymphoma who had serum electrophoretic patterns similar to those of MM. In a group of 640 patients with diffuse NHL or CLL, an M protein was found in 44 (7%), but only 4 out of 292 (1.4%) patients with nodular lymphoma and 1 out of 218 (0.5%) patients with Hodgkin lymphoma had an M protein.[67] In a cohort of 430 patients with a serum IgM monoclonal gammopathy seen at Mayo Clinic between 1956 and 1978, the following diseases were found: MGUS (56%), WM (17%), malignant lymphoproliferative disease (14%), NHL (7%), CLL (5%), and AL (1%).[57] In another series of 382 patients with a lymphoid neoplasm and an associated IgM monoclonal protein, 59% had lymphoplasmacytic lymphoma/WM. Chronic lymphocytic leukemia/small lymphocytic lymphoma accounted for 20%; marginal zone lymphoma, 7%; follicular lymphoma, 5%; mantle cell lymphoma, 3%; diffuse large B-cell lymphoma, 2%; and miscellaneous, 4%.[68] In a series of 26 patients with extranodal marginal zone lymphoma, 7 (27%) had an M protein.[69]

Leukemia

We described 100 patients with chronic lymphocytic leukemia and an M protein in the serum or urine.[70] IgM accounted for 38%, while IgG was found in 51%. No major differences were apparent in patients whether they had an IgG or an IgM monoclonal protein. M proteins have also been recognized in hairy cell leukemia, adult T-cell leukemia, chronic myelocytic leukemia, acute lymphoblastic leukemia, chronic neutrophilic leukemia, acute leukemia, Sézary syndrome, mycosis fungoides, Kaposi sarcoma, and erythema elevatum diutinum.

Other hematologic disorders

Acquired von Willebrand disease has been reported with MGUS.[71] On the other hand, thromboembolic events were found in 19 (6.1%) out of 310 patients with MGUS.[72] Monoclonal proteins have also been reported in myelodysplastic syndrome, idiopathic myelofibrosis, polycythemia vera, paroxysmal nocturnal hemoglobinuria, lupus anticoagulant activity, pernicious anemia, and red cell aplasia.

Connective tissue disorders

Rheumatoid arthritis, lupus erythematosus, scleroderma, polymyositis, and inclusion body myositis have been noted with a monoclonal gammopathy. Polymyalgia rheumatica has been reported with monoclonal gammopathy, but both conditions occur more commonly in an older population, so the relationship is questionable.

Neurological disorders

In 279 patients with a sensorimotor peripheral neuropathy of unknown cause, we found 16 cases (6%) with MGUS.[73] An association exists between MGUS and peripheral neuropathy. The incidence is variable and depends on patient selection bias, vigor with which the presence of an M protein is sought, and whether the diagnosis of peripheral neuropathy is made on clinical or electrophysiological grounds.

IgM is the most common monoclonal protein associated with peripheral neuropathy. The M protein binds to myelin-associated glycoprotein (MAG) in about one-half of patients with an IgM monoclonal gammopathy and peripheral neuropathy. The role of antibodies and peripheral neuropathy has been reviewed.[74] Gosselin et al.[75] reported a series of 65 patients with MGUS and sensorimotor peripheral neuropathy; IgM was present in 31, IgG in 24, and IgA in 10. The size of the M protein and the presence

of anti-MAG activity apparently do not influence the type and severity of the neuropathy. MGUS neuropathies differ from those associated with AL in the following manner: (1) the lower extremities are more often involved in MGUS, but both upper and lower extremities may be involved in AL; (2) the course of neuropathy in AL is almost always slowly progressive; and (3) autonomic features such as orthostatic hypotension, anhidrosis, and bowel habit changes, and heart or kidney failure often occur in AL.

Treatment of peripheral neuropathy and monoclonal gammopathy is unsatisfactory. Plasmapheresis has been of benefit to some patients, while chlorambucil has been useful to some with IgM MGUS. Melphalan and prednisone can be helpful for IgG and IgA gammopathies. Both fludarabine and rituximab have been reported as producing some benefit, but the results are disappointing. Intravenous immunoglobulin infusions have been of occasional benefit. Therapy of neuropathy associated with monoclonal gammopathies has been reviewed.[76] MGUS has been reported with myasthenia gravis, ataxia telangectasia, motor neuron disease, and nemaline myopathy.

POEMS syndrome (osteosclerotic myeloma)

POEMS syndrome is characterized by Polyneuropathy, Organomegaly, Endocrinopathy, Monoclonal protein, and Skin changes. It is defined by the presence of a monoclonal plasma cell disorder, sensorimotor peripheral neuropathy, and at least one of the following seven features: osteosclerotic bone lesions, Castleman disease, organomegaly, endocrinopathy (excluding diabetes mellitus or hypothyroidism), edema, typical skin changes, and papilledema.[56,77] Actually, the absence of osteosclerotic lesions should make the diagnosis suspect. Hypertrichosis, hyperpigmentation, gynecomastia, and testicular atrophy may be present. Thrombocytosis or erythrocytosis are not uncommon. Almost all patients have a monoclonal protein of the λ light chain type. The serum M protein is modest in size, while Bence Jones proteinuria, renal insufficiency, hypercalcemia, and skeletal fractures, all of which are common in MM, are rarely seen. The bone marrow usually contains <5% plasma cells. Elevated levels of IL-1β, TNF-α, IL-6, and VEGF are seen frequently. If the patient has single or multiple sclerotic lesions, a limited area of tumoricidal radiation therapy is the treatment of choice. If the lesions are widespread, autologous stem cell transplantation or alkylating agent therapy is indicated.[78] The median survival was 13.8 years in a 99-patient cohort.[77]

Endocrine disorders

The association of hyperparathyroidism and MGUS is controversial. We reported that 9 (1%) out of 911 patients >50 years of age with hyperparathyroidism at Mayo Clinic had MGUS, which is similar to that in a normal population.[79] In contrast, 20 out of 101 patients with hyperparathyroidism had an M protein compared to only 2 out of 127 controls.[80]

Dermatologic diseases

Lichen myxedematosus (papular mucinosis, scleromyxedema) is a rare dermatologic condition frequently associated with a cathodal IgG λ protein. Necrobiotic xanthogranuloma and pyoderma gangrenosum are frequently associated with a monoclonal protein. Schnitzler syndrome is characterized by the presence of chronic urticaria and an IgM monoclonal protein. A review of dermatologic disorders associated with an M protein has been published.[81]

Immunosuppression

Monoclonal proteins are frequently seen after kidney, liver, heart, or autologous bone marrow transplantation. In five patients with MGUS undergoing organ transplantation, SMM developed in two and an increase in the M protein was found in one.[82]

Miscellaneous conditions

Capillary leak syndrome[83] and acquired C1q inhibitor deficiency[84] have been reported with monoclonal gammopathies. Idiopathic focal and segmental glomerulosclerosis may be associated with an M protein.[85] Although MGUS has been reported following silicone breast implants, the frequency does not appear to be increased.[86] Monoclonal proteins may be bound to calcium, copper, transferrin, or serum phosphorus. Monoclonal proteins may also have apparent antibody activity.[87]

SMOLDERING MULTIPLE MYELOMA

Smoldering multiple myeloma is defined as having an IgG or an IgA monoclonal protein of 3 g/dL or higher and/or 10% or more plasma cells in the bone marrow but no evidence of end-organ damage (hypercalcemia, renal insufficiency, anemia, or skeletal lesions).[3,56] Previous reports have used a variety of definitions of the entity, and this has resulted in important differences in its clinical course.[46,47,88-92] SMM should be differentiated from MGUS because it is associated with a significantly higher risk of progression. Similarly, it should be differentiated from symptomatic myeloma because observation alone is the standard of care and chemotherapy is not required.

We reported a cohort of 276 patients with SMM.[93] The median age at diagnosis was 64 years (range, 26-90 years). Only 3% were younger than 40 years of age at diagnosis. Males accounted for 62%. Eleven percent had an M protein ≥4 g/dL. IgG accounted for 74% of the M proteins, while 22.5% were IgA, 0.5% were IgD, and 3% were biclonal. The light chain was κ in 67% and λ in 33%. The levels of uninvolved or normal immunoglobulins were reduced in 83% of 230 patients in whom the immunoglobulins were measured. Ninety-two (36%) out of 259 patients had a monoclonal κ light chain in the urine, while 43 (17%) had a λ light chain and 123 (47%) had no monoclonal light chain. Only four patients (1.5%) excreted more than 1 g of light chain per 24 h.

During 2131 cumulative person-years of follow-up (range, 0-29 years; median, 6.1 years), 85% of the patients with SMM died (median follow-up of those still living was 11.6 years). Active MM developed in 158 patients (57%), while AL amyloidosis developed in 5 (2%) (Table 13.4). The cumulative probability of progression to active MM or AL was 51% at 5 years, 66% at 10 years, and 73% at 15 years. Median time to progression was 4.8 years (Figure 13.6). The overall risk of progression was 10% per year for the first 5 years, approximately 3% per year for the next 5 years, and 1% per year for the next 10 years.

The number of patients with progression to active MM was 522 times the number of persons without SMM who would be expected to have active disease, while the risk of AL amyloidosis was increased by a factor of 50. Rates of death owing to other diseases, including cardiovascular and cerebrovascular disease and nonplasma cell cancers were 18% at 5 years, 26% at 10 years, 30% at 15 years, and 35%

TABLE 13.4. Relative risk of progression in 276 patients with smoldering multiple myeloma, according to prognostic group*

Progression	No. of patients	Expected rate of disease[†]	Relative risk (95% CI)[‡]
Multiple myeloma			
All patients	157[§]	0.301	522 (443-610)
Group 1	75	0.072	1038 (817-1302)
Group 2	72	0.174	413 (323-520)
Group 3	10	0.054	184 (88-338)
Amyloidosis			
All patients	5	0.100	50 (16-117)
Group 1	3	0.022	136 (28-402)
Group 2	2	0.060	33 (4-121)
Group 3	0	0.019	0 (0-198)
Total	162	0.401	404 (344-471)

*Patients were divided into three prognostic groups: Group 1 (bone marrow plasma cells, ≥10%; monoclonal protein level, ≥3 g/dL), Group 2 (plasma cells, ≥10%; monoclonal protein level, <3 g/dL), and Group 3 (plasma cells, <10%; monoclonal protein level, ≥3 g/dL). The 162 patients with disease progression were followed for a total of 641 person-years. CI denotes confidence interval.

[†]The expected rate of multiple myeloma obtained from Iowa Surveillance, Epidemiology, and End Results program (1973-2002).[19] The expected rate of amyloidosis was calculated from data for patients in Olmsted County, Minnesota.

[‡]Expected rate of amyloidosis based on the data from Olmsted County, Minnesota.

[§]One patient had progression, but the date of progression was not available; therefore, this patient was excluded from the analysis of progression.

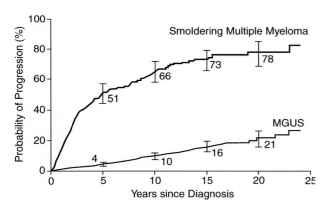

Figure 13.6. Probability of progression to multiple myeloma or primary amyloidosis in smoldering multiple myeloma (SMM) and MGUS. Vertical bars denote 95% confidence limits.

at 20 years. The overall rate of survival was 60% at 5 years, 34% at 10 years, and 20% at 15 years (median, 6.3 years).

The study cohort was stratified into three groups at initial diagnosis: Group 1, bone marrow plasma cells of ≥10% and a serum M-protein level of 3 g/dL or more; Group 2, bone marrow plasma cells of 10% or more and a serum M protein <3 g/dL; and Group 3, bone marrow plasma cells of <10% and a serum M-protein level of 3 g/dL or more.

Risk factors for progression

Significant baseline risk factors for the progression of SMM to active MM or AL in the univariate and multivariate analyses are shown in Table 13.5. Significant baseline risk factors for progression of SMM to MM or AL in the univariate analysis included the level of serum M protein (p < 0.001), presence of IgA monoclonal protein (p = 0.004), presence of urinary light chain (p = 0.04), extent of bone marrow involvement (plasma cells ≥20%; p = 0.001), reduction in levels of uninvolved immunoglobulins (p = 0.001), and the pattern of plasma cell involvement in bone marrow (sheets of cells spanning the interfatty marrow space) (p < 0.001).

On the basis of a fitted model containing the proportion of plasma cells in the bone marrow and serum monoclonal protein level, the risk of progression to MM or AL at 10 years was 55% for patients with an initial plasma cell level of 10%-14%; progression occurred in 70% of the

TABLE 13.5. Risk factors for disease progression among 276 patients with smoldering multiple myeloma (1970-1995)*

Variable	Patients (no.)	Events (no.)	Median time to progression (months)	Univariate analysis	Multivariate analysis[†]	5 years	10 years	15 years
Prognostic groups				<0.001	<0.001			
Group 1	106	78	27			69	77	87
Group 2	143[‡]	74	93			43	64	70
Group 3	27	10	228			15	33	39
Serum heavy chain				0.004	0.01			
IgA	62	46	27			66	77	80
IgG	205	112	75			46	62	71
Bone marrow plasma cells (%)				<0.001	0.005			
<20	164	78	117			36	53	61
20–50	84	65	26			68	82	92
>50	27	19	21			85	93	NA
Serum monoclonal protein (g/dL)				<0.001	0.04			
<4	244	138	75			47	64	71
≥4	31	24	18			80	80	90
Urinary light chain				0.04	0.09			
Negative	123	71	89			46	62	68
κ or λ	135	84	49			56	70	80
Type of urinary light chain				0.08	0.12			
Negative	123	71	89			46	62	68
κ	92	57	60			51	67	82
λ	43	27	32			68	77	77
Reduction of uninvolved immunoglobulins				<0.001	0.003			
0	40	16	159			24	33	59
1	71	35	89			38	59	62
2	119	85	32			68	81	84
Pattern of bone marrow plasma cell involvement				<0.001	0.02			
Interfat space or sheets	103	77	28			68	79	88
Singly distributed or small clusters	160	78	103			40	57	63
Overall	276[§]	162	58			51	66	73

*Patients were divided into three prognostic groups: Group 1 (bone marrow plasma cells, ≥10%; monoclonal protein level, ≥3 g/dL), Group 2 (plasma cells, ≥10%; monoclonal protein level, <3 g/dL), and Group 3 (plasma cells, <10%; monoclonal protein level, ≥3 g/dL). NA denotes not applicable.
†The multivariate p values for the type of heavy chain represent the test for an additional significant contribution to the predictive ability of a model already containing the prognostic groups; the multivariate p values for the remaining variables represent the test for an additional significant contribution when added individually to a model already containing prognostic groups and the type of heavy chain. Expected rate of multiple myeloma obtained from Iowa Surveillance, Epidemiology, and End Results program (1973-2002).[19] The expected rate of amyloidosis was calculated from data for patients in Olmsted County, Minnesota.
‡One patient had progression, but the date of progression was not available; therefore, this patient was excluded from the analysis of progression.

27 patients with more than 50% plasma cells in the bone marrow (median time to progression, 21 months). The risk of progression to active MM or AL at 10 years was 57% in patients with an initial M-protein level of 2 g/dL and 70% in those whose initial level was 5.0 g/dL. Hemoglobin, gender, serum albumin level, proportion of normal hematopoietic elements, and expression of cyclin D1 were not significantly associated with progression.

On multivariate analysis, the serum M-protein level and the number of plasma cells in the bone marrow emerged as significant, independent risk factors for progression. On the basis of these findings and the fact that these two variables were also the main components of the definition of SMM, we constructed a risk-stratification model containing three risk groups. The cumulative probability of progression at 15 years was 87% for the 106 patients in Group 1 (≥10% plasma cells and ≥3 g/dL of monoclonal protein), 70% for the 142 patients in Group 2 (≥10% plasma cells and <3 g/dL of M protein), and 39% for the 27 patients in Group 3 (<10% plasma cells and ≥3 g/dL of M protein). The median time to progression was 2 years in Group 1, 8 years in Group 2, and 19 years in Group 3 (p < 0.001). The type of serum heavy chain (IgA) added significantly to the multivariate model containing the three prognostic risk groups (p = 0.01).

Incorporating the FLC ratio into the risk model, the 5-year progression rates in high-, intermediate-, and low-risk groups were 76%, 51%, and 25%, respectively. Thus, the serum immunoglobulin FLC ratio is an important additional determinant of clinical outcome in patients with SMM.[8]

REFERENCES

1. Waldenström J. Studies on conditions associated with disturbed gamma globulin formation (gammopathies). *Harvey Lectures* 1960-1961;56:211-31.
2. Kyle RA. Monoclonal gammopathy of undetermined significance. Natural history in 241 cases. *Am J Med* 1978;64(5):814-26.
3. Criteria for the classification of monoclonal gammopathies, multiple myeloma and related disorders: a report of the international myeloma working group. *Br J Haematol* 2003;121(5):749-57.
4. Katzmann JA, Kyle RA. Immunochemical characterization of immunoglobulins in serum, urine, and cerebrospinal fluid. In: B. Detrick, R. Hamilton, J. Folds, eds. Manual of molecular and clinical laboratory immunology. 7th ed. Washington DC, ASM Press;2006:88-100.
5. Katzmann JA, Clark RJ, Abraham RS, et al. Serum reference intervals and diagnostic ranges for free kappa and free lambda immunoglobulin light chains: relative sensitivity for detection of monoclonal light chains. *Clinical Chemistry* 2002;48(9):1437-44.

6. Rajkumar SV, Kyle RA, Therneau TM, et al. Serum free light chain ratio is an independent risk factor for progression in monoclonal gammopathy of undetermined significance. *Blood* 2005;106(3):812-17.
7. Dingli D, Kyle RA, Rajkumar SV, et al. Immunoglobulin free light chains and solitary plasmacytoma of bone. *Blood* 2006;108(6):1979-83.
8. Dispenzieri A, Kyle RA, Katzmann JA, et al. Immunoglobulin free light chain ratio is an independent risk factor for progression of smoldering (asymptomatic) multiple myeloma. *Blood* 2008;111(2):785-9.
9. Katzmann JA, Dispenzieri A, Kyle RA, et al. Elimination of the need for urine studies in the screening algorithm for monoclonal gammopathies by using serum immunofixation and free light chain assays. *Mayo Clin Proc* 2006;81(12):1575-8.
10. Axelsson U, Bachmann R, Hallen J. Frequency of pathological proteins (m-components) om 6,995 sera from an adult population. *Acta Medica Scandinavica* 1966;179(2):235-47.
11. Kyle RA, Finkelstein S, Elveback LR, Kurland LT. Incidence of monoclonal proteins in a Minnesota community with a cluster of multiple myeloma. *Blood* 1972;40(5):719-24.
12. Saleun JP, Vicariot M, Deroff P, Morin JF. Monoclonal gammopathies in the adult population of finistere, France. *J Clin Pathol* 1982;35(1):63-8.
13. Landgren O, Gridley G, Turesson I, et al. Risk of monoclonal gammopathy of undetermined significance (MGUS) and subsequent multiple myeloma among African American and white veterans in the United States. *Blood* 2006;107(3):904-6.
14. Landgren O, Katzmann JA, Hsing AW, et al. Prevalence of monoclonal gammopathy of undetermined significance among men in Ghana. *Mayo Clin Proc* 2007;82(12):1468-73.
15. Iwanaga M, Tagawa M, Tsukasaki K, Kamihira S, Tomonaga M. Prevalence of monoclonal gammopathy of undetermined significance: study of 52,802 persons in Nagasaki city, Japan. *Mayo Clin Proc* 2007;82(12):1474-9.
16. Kyle RA, Therneau TM, Melton Iii LJ, et al. Monoclonal gammopathy of undetermined significance: estimated incidence and duration prior to recognition. *Blood* 2007;10(11):79a (Abstract #246).
17. Kyle RA, Therneau TM, Rajkumar SV, Larson DR, Plevak MF, Melton LJ III. Long-term follow-up of 241 patients with monoclonal gammopathy of undetermined significance: The original Mayo Clinic series 25 years later [see comment]. *Mayo Clin Proc* 2004;79(7):859-66.
18. Kyle RA, Therneau TM, Rajkumar SV, et al. A long-term study of prognosis in monoclonal gammopathy of undetermined significance [see comment]. *N Engl J Med* 2002;346(8):564-9.
19. Surveillance, Epidemiology, and End Results (SEER) Program public-use data CD ROM (1973-1998). Bethesda, MD, National Cancer Institute, Cancer Statistics Branch, 2001.
20. Kyle RA, Gertz MA, Witzig TE, et al. Review of 1027 patients with newly diagnosed multiple myeloma [see comment]. *Mayo Clin Proc* 2003;78(1):21-33.
21. Blade J, Lopez-Guillermo A, Rozman C, et al. Malignant transformation and life expectancy in monoclonal gammopathy

of undetermined significance. *Br J Haematol* 1992;81(3): 391-4.

22. Van De Poel MH, Coebergh JW, Hillen HF. Malignant transformation of monoclonal gammopathy of undetermined significance among out-patients of a community hospital in southeastern Netherlands. *Br J Haematol* 1995;91(1):121-5.

23. Baldini L, Guffanti A, Cesana BM, et al. Role of different hematologic variables in defining the risk of malignant transformation in monoclonal gammopathy. *Blood* 1996;87(3):912-18.

24. Pasqualetti P, Festuccia V, Collacciani A, Casale R. The natural history of monoclonal gammopathy of undetermined significance. A 5- to 20-year follow-up of 263 cases. *Acta Haematol* 1997;97(3):174-9.

25. Gregersen H, Ibsen J, Mellemkjoer L, Dahlerup J, Olsen J, Sorensen H. Mortality and causes of death in patients with monoclonal gammopathy of undetermined significance. *Br J Haematol* 2001;112(2):353-7.

26. Gregersen H, Mellemkjaer L, Salling Ibsen J, et al. Cancer risk in patients with monoclonal gammopathy of undetermined significance. *Am J Hematol* 2000;63(1):1-6.

27. Ogmundsdottir HM, Haraldsdottir V, G MJ, et al. Monoclonal gammopathy in Iceland: a population-based registry and follow-up. *Br J Haematol* 2002;118(1):166-73.

28. Kyle RA, Rajkumar SV. Monoclonal gammopathy of undetermined significance and smouldering multiple myeloma: emphasis on risk factors for progression. *Br J Haematol* 2007;139(5):730-43.

29. Avet-Loiseau H, Li JY, Facon T, et al. High incidence of translocations t(11;14)(q13;q32) and t(4;14)(p16;q32) in patients with plasma cell malignancies. *Cancer Res* 1998;58(24):5640-5.

30. Fonseca R, Bailey RJ, Ahmann GJ, et al. Genomic abnormalities in monoclonal gammopathy of undetermined significance. *Blood* 2002;100(4):1417-24.

31. Chng WJ, Van Wier SA, Ahmann GJ, et al. A validated fish trisomy index demonstrates the hyperdiploid and nonhyperdiploid dichotomy in MGUS. *Blood* 2005;106(6):2156-61.

32. Avet-Loiseau H, Li JY, Morineau N, et al. Monosomy 13 is associated with the transition of monoclonal gammopathy of undetermined significance to multiple myeloma. Intergroupe francophone du myelome. *Blood* 1999;94(8):2583-9.

33. Rasmussen T, Kuehl M, Lodahl M, Johnsen HE, Dahl I, MS. Possible roles for activating ras mutations in the MGUS to MM transition and in the intramedullary to extramedullary transition in some plasma cell tumors. *Blood* 2005;105(1)317-23.

34. Vacca A, Ribatti D, Roncali L, et al. Bone marrow angiogenesis and progression in multiple myeloma. *Br J Haematol* 1994;87(3):503-8.

35. Rajkumar SV, Mesa RA, Fonseca R. Bone marrow angiogenesis in 400 patients with monoclonal gammopathy of undetermined significance, multiple myeloma, and primary amyloidosis. *Clin Cancer Res* 2002;8(7):2210-16.

36. Vacca A, Ribatti D, Presta M, et al. Bone marrow neovascularization, plasma cell angiogenic potential, and matrix metalloproteinase-2 secretion parallel progression of human multiple myeloma. *Blood* 1999;93(9):3064-73.

37. Kumar S, Witzig TE, Timm M, et al. Bone marrow angiogenic ability and expression of angiogenic cytokines in myeloma: evidence favoring loss of marrow angiogenesis inhibitory activity with disease progression. *Blood* 2004;104(4):1159-65.

38. Melton LJ III, Rajkumar SV, Khosla S, et al. Fracture risk in monoclonal gammopathy of undetermined significance. *J Bone Miner Res* 2004;19(1):25-30.

39. Roodman GD, Biology of myeloma bone disease. In: VC Broudy, JL. Abkowitz, JM Vose, eds. *Hematology 2002: American society of hematology education program book.* Washington, DC:2002; 227-32.

40. Croucher PI, Shipman CM, Lippitt J, et al. Osteoprotegerin inhibits the development of osteolytic bone disease in multiple myeloma. *Blood* 2001;98(13):3534-40.

41. Lust JA, Donovan KA. Biology of the transition of monoclonal gammopathy of undetermined significance (MGUS) to multiple myeloma. *Cancer Control* 1998;5(3):209-17.

42. Malik AA, Ganti AK, Potti A, Levitt R, Hanley JF. Role of *Helicobacter pylori* infection in the incidence and clinical course of monoclonal gammopathy of undetermined significance. *Am J Gastroenterol* 2002;97(6):1371-4.

43. Rajkumar SV, Kyle RA, Plevak MF, Murray JA, Therneau TM. *Helicobacter pylori* infection and monoclonal gammopathy of undetermined significance. *Br J Haematol* 2002;119(3):706-8.

44. Kyle RA. "Benign" monoclonal gammopathy–after 20 to 35 years of follow-up. *Mayo Clin Proc* 1993;68(1):26-36.

45. Rosinol L, Cibeira MT, Montoto S, et al. Monoclonal gammopathy of undetermined significance: predictors of malignant transformation and recognition of an evolving type characterized by a progressive increase in M protein size. *Mayo Clin Proc* 2007;82(4):428-34.

46. Cesana C, Klersy C, Barbarano L, et al. Prognostic factors for malignant transformation in monoclonal gammopathy of undetermined significance and smoldering multiple myeloma. *J Clin Oncol* 2002;20(6):1625-34.

47. Kyle RA, Greipp PR. Smoldering multiple myeloma. *N Engl J Med* 1980;302(24):1347-9.

48. Bellaiche L, Laredo JD, Liote F, et al. Magnetic resonance appearance of monoclonal gammopathies of unknown significance and multiple myeloma. The GRI study group. *Spine* 1997;22(21):2551-7.

49. Kumar S, Rajkumar SV, Kyle RA, et al. Prognostic value of circulating plasma cells in monoclonal gammopathy of undetermined significance. *J Clin Oncol* 2005;23(24):5668-74.

50. Nowakowski GS, Witzig TE, Dingli D, et al. Circulating plasma cells detected by flow cytometry as a predictor of survival in 302 patients with newly diagnosed multiple myeloma. *Blood* 2005;106(7):2276-9.

51. Kyle RA, Robinson RA, Katzmann JA. The clinical aspects of biclonal gammopathies. Review of 57 cases. *Am J Med* 1981;71(6):999-1008.

52. Grosbois B, Jego P, De Rosa H, et al. [Triclonal gammopathy and malignant immunoproliferative syndrome]. [review] [25 refs] [in French]. *Revue de Medecine Interne* 1997;18(6):470-3.

53. Tirelli A, Guastafierro S, Cava B, Lucivero G. Triclonal gammopathy in an extranodal non-Hodgkin lymphoma patient. *Am J Hematol* 2003;73(4):273-5.

54. Kyle RA, Maldonado JE, Bayrd ED. Idiopathic Bence Jones proteinuria–a distinct entity? *Am J Med* 1973;55(2):222-6.

55. Kyle RA, Greipp PR. "Idiopathic" Bence Jones proteinuria: long-term follow-up in seven patients. *N Engl J Med* 1982; 306(10):564-7.

56. Rajkumar SV, Dispenzieri A, Kyle RA. Monoclonal gammopathy of undetermined significance, Waldenstrom macroglobulinemia, AL amyloidosis, and related plasma cell disorders: diagnosis and treatment. *Mayo Clin Proc* 2006;81(5):693-703.

57. Kyle RA, Garton JP. The spectrum of IgM monoclonal gammopathy in 430 cases. *Mayo Clin Proc* 1987;62(8):719-31.

58. Kyle RA, Therneau TM, Rajkumar SV, et al. Long-term follow-up of IgM monoclonal gammopathy of undetermined significance. *Blood* 2003;102(10):3759-64.

59. Morra E, Cesana C, Klersy C, et al. Prognostic factors for transformation in asymptomatic immunoglobulin M monoclonal gammopathies. *Clin Lymphoma* 2005;5(4):265-9.

60. Cesana C, Barbarano L, Miqueleiz S, et al. Clinical characteristics and outcome of immunoglobulin M-related disorders. *Clin Lymphoma* 2005;5(4):261-4.

61. Baldini L, Goldaniga M, Guffanti A, et al. Immunoglobulin M monoclonal gammopathies of undetermined significance and indolent Waldenstrom's macroglobulinemia recognize the same determinants of evolution into symptomatic lymphoid disorders: proposal for a common prognostic scoring system. *J Clin Oncol* 2005;23(21):4662-8.

62. Ayto RM, Lambert C, Lampert I, Salooja, N. Monoclonal gammopathy of undetermined significance with an IgE paraprotein. *Blood* 2007;110(11):259b (Abstract #4744).

63. Kyle RA, Rajkumar SV. Monoclonal gammopathies of undetermined significance. In: J. Malpas and E. Al, eds. *Myeloma: biology and management.* 3rd ed. Philadelphia, PS: Saunders, 2004:315-52.

64. Kyle RA, Rajkumar SV. Monoclonal gammopathy of undetermined significance. *Br J Haematol* 2006;134(6):573-89.

65. Azar HA, Hill WT, Osserman EF. Malignant lymphoma and lymphatic leukemia. *Am J Med* 1957;23:239-49.

66. Kyle RA, Bayrd ED, Mckenzie BF, Heck FJ. Diagnostic criteria for electrophoretic patterns of serum and urinary proteins in multiple myeloma: study of one hundred and sixty-five multiple myeloma patients with similar electrophoretic patterns. *J Am Med Assoc* 1960;174:245-51.

67. Alexanian R. Monoclonal gammopathy in lymphoma. *Arch Intern Med* 1975;135(1):62-6.

68. Lin P, Hao S, Handy BC, Bueso-Ramos CE, Medeiros LJ. Lymphoid neoplasms associated with IgM paraprotein: a study of 382 patients. *Am J Clin Pathol* 2005;123(2):200-5.

69. Asatiani E, Cohen P, Ozdemirli M, Kessler CM, Mavromatis B, Cheson, BD. Monoclonal gammopathy in extranodal marginal zone lymphoma (ENMZL) correlates with advanced disease and bone marrow involvement. *Am J Hematol* 2004;77(2): 144-6.

70. Noel P, Kyle RA. Monoclonal proteins in chronic lymphocytic leukemia. *Am J Clin Pathol* 1987;87(3):385-8.

71. Lamboley V, Zabraniecki L, Sie P, Pourrat J, Fournie B. Myeloma and monoclonal gammopathy of uncertain significance associated with acquired von Willebrand's syndrome. Seven new cases with a literature review. *Joint, Bone, Spine: Revue du Rhumatisme* 2002;69(1):62-7.

72. Sallah S, Husain A, Wan J, Vos P, Nguyen NP. The risk of venous thromboembolic disease in patients with monoclonal gammopathy of undetermined significance. *Ann Oncol* 2004;15(10):1490-4.

73. Kelly JJ Jr, Kyle RA, O'brien PC, Dyck PJ. Prevalence of monoclonal protein in peripheral neuropathy. *Neurology* 1981; 31(11):1480-3.

74. Quarles RH, Weiss MD. Autoantibodies associated with peripheral neuropathy. [review] [197 refs]. *Muscle Nerve* 1999;22(7):800-22.

75. Gosselin S, Kyle RA, Dyck PJ. Neuropathy associated with monoclonal gammopathies of undetermined significance [see comment]. *Ann Neurol* 1991;30(1):54-61.

76. Nobile-Orazio E. Treatment of dys-immune neuropathies. *J Neurol* 2005;252(4):385-95.

77. Dispenzieri A, Kyle RA, Lacy MQ, et al. Poems syndrome: definitions and long-term outcome. *Blood* 2003;101(7):2496-506.

78. Dispenzieri A, Moreno-Aspitia A, Suarez GA, et al. Peripheral blood stem cell transplantation in 16 patients with POEMS syndrome, and a review of the literature. *Blood* 2004;104(10):3400-7.

79. Mundis RJ, Kyle RA. Primary hyperparathyroidism and monoclonal gammopathy of undetermined significance. *Am J Clin Pathol* 1982;77(5):619-21.

80. Arnulf B, Bengoufa D, Sarfati E, et al. Prevalence of monoclonal gammopathy in patients with primary hyperparathyroidism: a prospective study. *Arch Intern Med* 2002;162(4):464-7.

81. Daoud MS, Lust JA, Kyle RA, Pittelkow MR. Monoclonal gammopathies and associated skin disorders. [review] [214 refs]. *J Am Acad Dermatol* 1999;40(4):507-35; quiz 536-8.

82. Rostaing L, Modesto A, Abbal M, Durand D. Long-term follow-up of monoclonal gammopathy of undetermined significance in transplant patients. *Am J Nephrol* 1994;14(3):187-91.

83. Droder RM, Kyle RA, Greipp PR. Control of systemic capillary leak syndrome with aminophylline and terbutaline. *Am J Med* 1992;92(5):523-6.

84. Pascual M, Widmann JJ, Schifferli JA. Recurrent febrile panniculitis and hepatitis in two patients with acquired complement deficiency and paraproteinemia. *Am J Med* 1987;83(5):959-62.

85. Dingli D, Larson DR, Plevak MF, Grande JP, Kyle RA. Focal and segmental glomerulosclerosis and plasma cell proliferative disorders. *Am J Kidney Dis* 2005;46(2):278-82.

86. Karlson EW, Tanasijevic M, Hankinson SE, et al. Monoclonal gammopathy of undetermined significance and exposure to breast implants. *Arch Intern Med* 2001;161(6):864-7.

87. Merlini G, Farhangi M, Osserman EF. Monoclonal immuno-globulins with antibody activity in myeloma, macroglobuline-mia and related plasma cell dyscrasias. [review] [202 refs]. *Semin Oncol* 1986;13(3):350-65.

88. Alexanian R, Barlogie B, Dixon D. Prognosis of asymptomatic multiple myeloma. *Arch Intern Med* 1988;148(9):1963-5.

89. Dimopoulos MA, Moulopoulos A, Smith T, Delasalle KB, Alexanian R. Risk of disease progression in asymptomatic multiple myeloma. *Am J Med* 1993;94(1):57-61.

90. Facon T, Menard JF, Michaux JL, et al. Prognostic factors in low tumour mass asymptomatic multiple myeloma: a report on 91 patients. The groupe d'etudes et de recherche sur le myelome (germ). *Am J Hematol* 1995;48(2):71-5.

91. Rosinol L, Blade J, Esteve J, et al. Smoldering multiple myeloma: natural history and recognition of an evolving type. *Br J Haematol* 2003;123(4):631-6.

92. Weber DM, Dimopoulos MA, Moulopoulos LA, Delasalle KB, Smith T, Alexanian R. Prognostic features of asymptomatic multiple myeloma. *Br J Haematol* 1997;97(4):810-14.

93. Kyle RA, Remstein ED, Therneau TM, et al. Clinical course and prognosis of smoldering (asymptomatic) multiple myeloma. *N Engl J Med* 2007;356(25):2582-90.

14 Diagnosis and Treatment of POEMS Syndrome

Angela Dispenzieri

INTRODUCTION

POEMS syndrome is a paraneoplastic disorder associated with an underlying plasma cell dyscrasia. The major clinical feature of the syndrome is a chronic progressive polyneuropathy with a predominant motor disability.[1,2] The acronym POEMS (Polyneuropathy, Organomegaly, Endocrinopathy, M protein, and Skin changes) captures several dominant features of the syndrome. Important traits not included in the acronym include elevated levels of vascular endothelial growth factor (VEGF), sclerotic bone lesions, Castleman disease, papilledema, peripheral edema, ascites, effusions, thrombocytosis, polycythemia, fatigue, clubbing, and abnormal pulmonary function test. Other names for the syndrome include osteosclerotic myeloma, Crow-Fukase syndrome, and Takatsuki syndrome.[3,4] Although the vast majority of patients have osteosclerotic myeloma, these same patients usually have only 5% bone marrow plasma cells or less (almost always monoclonal λ), and rarely have anemia, hypercalcemia, or renal insufficiency. These characteristics and the superior median survival differentiate POEMS syndrome from multiple myeloma.

The complexity of the interaction of plasma cell dyscrasia and peripheral neuropathy (PN) became increasingly evident in 1956 with Crow's description of two patients with osteosclerotic plasmacytomas with neuropathy, and other "striking features," which included clubbing, skin pigmentation, dusky discoloration of skin, white finger nails, mild lymphadenopathy, and ankle edema.[5] As many as 50% of patients with osteosclerotic myeloma were noted to have PN[6-8] in contrast to 1%-8% of multiple myeloma patients.[9,10]

Support in part by the Robert A. Kyle Hematologic Malignancies Fund, Mayo Clinic.

A syndrome distinct from multiple myeloma–associated neuropathy became to be recognized. In Iwashita's 1977 review of the literature, the 30 patients with osteosclerotic myeloma and PN, as compared to the 29 patients without PN, more commonly had hyperpigmentation, edema, skin thickening, hepatomegaly, hypertrichosis, and clubbing.[7] In 1980, Bardswick described two patients and coined the acronym POEMS.[1] In 1981, Kelly et al. reported on 16 cases seen at Mayo,[11] and in 1983[3] and 1984[4] two large series of cases collected from Japan were reported solidifying the existence of a distinct pathological entity. Another series from France further bolstered these concepts in the early 1990s with a report of 25 patients.[12]

PATHOGENESIS

The pathogenesis of this multisystem disease is complex. Elevations of VEGF,[13-15] proangiogenic,[14-23] and proinflammatory[14,17,18,23] cytokines are the hallmark of this disorder. Little is known about the plasma cells except that more than 95% of the time they are λ light chain restricted with restricted Vλ1 germline gene usage.[24,25] Aneuploidy[18] and deletion of chromosome 13[26] have been described. POEMS is not a deposition disease like primary systemic amyloidosis.[4,27] Nerve biopsies do not have deposition of monoclonal proteins[4,27,28] nor are auto-antibodies against peripheral nerve antigens (SGPG and SGLPG glycolipids, GM1, GD1a, GD1b, GT1b gangliosides) found.[18] Prior hypotheses have included implication of hyperestrogenemia[12] and HHV-8.[29-31] The coagulation pathway and its relationship to VEGF has also been proposed,[32] but more data will be required to solidify this hypothesis.

Although the cytokine network is highly complex and interrelated, VEGF appears to be the dominant driving cytokine in this disorder. VEGF normally targets endothelial cells and induces a rapid and reversible increase in vascular permeability. It is important in angiogenesis, and osteogenesis is strongly dependent on angiogenesis. VEGF is expressed by osteoblasts in bone tissue, macrophages, tumor cells[14] (including plasma cells),[33,34] and megakaryocytes/platelets.[35] Both interleukin-1β (IL-1β) and IL-6 have been shown to stimulate VEGF production.[14] Plasma and serum levels of VEGF are markedly elevated in patients with POEMS[13-15] and correlate with the activity of the disease.[14,36,37] The principal isoform of VEGF expressed is VEGF165.[36] VEGF levels are independent of M-protein size.[36] Increased VEGF has been found in ascitic fluid[38] and the cerebrospinal fluid (CSF).[37] Arimura et al. studied the direct effects of VEGF on blood nerve barrier function using an animal model and found that VEGF increased the microvascular permeability inducing endoneurial edema.[39] The authors postulate that this increased permeability could allow serum components toxic to nerves, such as complement and thrombin, to induce further damage.

Although POEMS patients have higher levels of IL-1β, tumor necrosis factor-α (TNF-α), and IL-6 than classic multiple myeloma patients[14,40] and controls[17,18,23,40] this relationship appears to be less consistent.[17-22] For some patients levels of IL-6 correlate with disease activity,[17] especially those with co-existent Castleman disease, and increased levels have been found in the CSF,[19] pericardium,[41] and ascites.[20] Elevated levels of matrix metalloproteinases and tissue inhibitor of metalloproteinases (TIMP) have been observed in patients with POEMS. Serum levels of VEGF and TIMP-1 were strongly correlated with each other.[42] The significance of these findings is not yet fully understood. Finally, aberrations in the coagulation cascade have been implicated. Circulating coagulation factors such as fibrinopeptide A and thrombin-antithrombin complex are increased during the active phase of illness, but other factors relating to fibrinolysis, plasminogen, a2 plasmin inhibitor plasmin complex, and FDP did not increase.[43]

DIAGNOSTIC CRITERIA

Establishing diagnostic criteria for any syndrome is fraught with difficulty, POEMS notwithstanding. They must be broad enough to diagnose patients early to avoid cumulative morbidity, but narrow enough that patients without the syndrome are not mislabeled as having the syndrome. Soubrier et al.[12] demonstrated that prognosis was not dependent on the number of features present in these patients. We confirmed that in our series of 99 patients and proposed criteria, which were later criticized for being too broad.[44] With increasing information about the role of cytokines in this disorder, Arimura et al. have suggested including elevated levels of VEGF as one of the diagnostic criteria.[45] Table 14.1 includes revised criteria for a diagnosis of POEMS syndrome, based on our experience and that of the literature.[2,3,12,16,36,45]

CLINICAL FEATURES

Figure 14.1 demonstrates the most common features and their frequencies. The peak incidence of the POEMS syndrome is in the fifth and sixth decades of life, unlike multiple myeloma, which has a peak incidence in the seventh and eighth decades. Symptoms of PN usually dominate the clinical picture.[11] Symptoms begin in the feet and consist of tingling, paresthesias, and coldness. Motor involvement follows the sensory symptoms. Both are distal, symmetric, and progressive with a gradual proximal spread. Severe weakness occurs in more than one-half of patients and results in inability to climb stairs, arise from a chair, or grip objects firmly with their hands. The course is usually progressive and patients may be confined to a wheelchair. Impotence occurs, but autonomic symptoms are not a feature. Bone pain and fractures rarely occur. Patients gradually lose weight to muscular atrophy. They report fatigue, which may be cytokine mediated or due to associated respiratory disease. Because patients become so restricted in their movement owing to their neuropathy, it is rare for them to report dyspnea despite markedly abnormal pulmonary testing.

As time progresses, muscle weakness is more marked than sensory loss. Touch, pressure, vibratory, and joint position senses are usually involved. Loss of temperature discrimination and nociception is less frequent. The cranial nerves are not involved except for papilledema. Hyperpigmentation is common. Coarse black hair may appear on the extremities. Other skin changes include skin thickening, rapid accumulation of glomeruloid angiomata, flushing, dependent rubor or acrocyanosis, white nails, and clubbing. Testicular atrophy and gynecomastia may be present in men and galactorrhea may be present in women. Pitting edema of the lower extremities is common. Ascites and pleural effusion occur in approximately one-third of patients. The liver is palpable in almost one-half

TABLE 14.1. Criteria for the diagnosis of POEMS syndrome*

Major criteria	1. Polyneuropathy (typically demyelinating)
	2. Monoclonal plasma cell proliferative disorder (almost always λ)
	3. Castleman disease
	4. Sclerotic bone lesions
	5. Vascular endothelial growth factor elevation
Minor criteria	6. Organomegaly (splenomegaly, hepatomegaly, or lymphadenopathy)
	7. Extravascular volume overload (edema, pleural effusion, or ascites)
	8. Endocrinopathy (adrenal, thyroid,[†] pituitary, gonadal, parathyroid, pancreatic[†])
	9. Skin changes (hyperpigmentation, hypertrichosis, glomeruloid hemangiomata, plethora, acrocyanosis, flushing, white nails)
	10. Papilledema
	11. Thrombocytosis/polycythemia[‡]
Other symptoms and signs	Clubbing, weight loss, hyperhidrosis, pulmonary hypertension/restrictive lung disease, thrombotic diatheses, diarrhea, low vitamin B_{12} values
Possible associations	Arthralgias, cardiomyopathy (systolic dysfunction), and fever

POEMS, Polyneuropathy, Organomegaly, Endocrinopathy, M protein, Skin changes.
*Polyneuropathy and monoclonal plasma cell disorder or Castleman disease present in all patients; to make diagnosis *at least* one other major criterion and one minor criterion is required to make diagnosis.
[†]Because of the high prevalence of diabetes mellitus and thyroid abnormalities, this diagnosis alone is not sufficient to meet this minor criterion.
[‡]Anemia and/or thrombocytopenia are distinctively unusual in this syndrome unless Castleman disease is present.

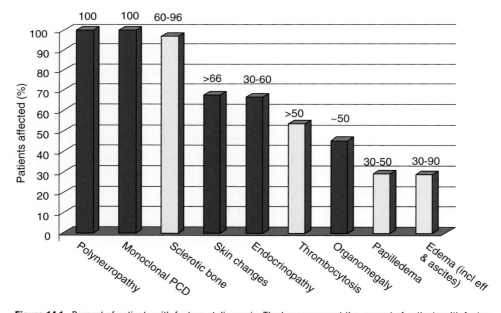

Figure 14.1. Percent of patients with feature at diagnosis. The bars represent the percent of patients with feature in the Mayo series;[2] the numbers over the bars represent the percent of patients with feature in three other large series.[3,4,12] The dark blue bars represent the features in acronym and the light blue bars refer to other features that are a part of the syndrome.

of patients, but splenomegaly and lymphadenopathy is found in fewer patients. On lymph node biopsy, in 11%-30% the histology is angiofollicular lymph node hyperplasia (Castleman disease) or Castleman disease-like.[1,2,4,12] This estimate may be conservative since most patients do not undergo lymph node biopsies. The neuropathy in Castleman disease patients tends to be more subtle than that of POEMS patients with osteosclerotic myeloma and is more often sensory. At its worst, however, it is a mixture of demyelination and axonal degeneration with normal myelin spacing on electron microscopy,[46] and abnormal capillary proliferation, similar to what is seen in the affected lymph nodes, has been described.[46]

Patients may develop arterial and/or venous thromboses during their course. Lesprit et al. observed 4 out of 20 patients to have arterial occlusion.[47] In the Mayo series, there were 18 patients suffering serious events such as stroke, myocardial infarction, and Budd-Chiari syndrome.[2] Affected vessels include carotid, iliac, celiac, subclavian, mesenteric, and femoral.[48-51] The POEMS-associated strokes tend to be end artery border-zone infarctions.[51] Gangrene of lower extremities can occur.[50] Whether the thromboses are due to the use of corticosteroids, chemotherapy, and/or elevations of proinflammatory cytokines[47,50] or VEGF is unknown.[49] It seems likely that VEGF and platelets play a role in arterial occlusion because when vascular injury occurs to endothelial cells, platelets aggregate to repair damaged vascular intima and release VEGF.[35]

LABORATORY INVESTIGATIONS

Thrombocytosis is common, and polycythemia may be seen.[2,11] Anemia and thrombocytopenia are not characteristic unless there is co-existing Castleman disease. Hypercalcemia and renal insufficiency are rarely present. The size of the M-protein on electrophoresis is small (median 1.1 g/dL) and is rarely more than 3.0 g/dL. The M protein is usually IgG or IgA and almost always of the λ type.[2,3] Levels of serum erythropoietin are low and are inversely correlated with VEGF levels.[37]

Bence Jones proteinuria is uncommon. Protein levels in the CSF are elevated in virtually all patients. Plasma cells are not present in the CSF, but increased levels of IL-6 receptor[52] and VEGF[37] have been described. Bone marrow usually contains <5% plasma cells, and when clonal cells are found they are almost always monoclonal λ. Osteosclerotic lesions occur in approximately 95% of patients, and can be confused with benign bone islands, aneurysmal bone cysts, nonossifying fibromas, and fibrous dysplasia. Some lesions are densely sclerotic, while others are lytic with a sclerotic rim, while still others have a mixed soap-bubble appearance (Figure 14.2). Bone windows of computed tomography (CT) body images are often very informative. FDG avidity is variable.

Endocrinopathy is a central but poorly understood feature of POEMS. In a recent large series from the Mayo Clinic,[53] approximately 84% of patients have a recognized endocrinopathy, with hypogonadism as the most common, followed by thyroid abnormalities, glucose metabolism abnormalities, and finally by adrenal insufficiency.

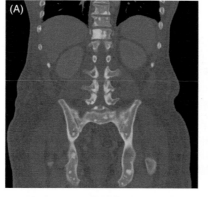
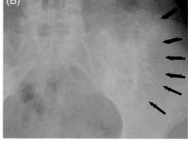
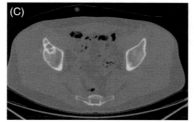
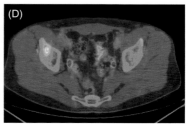

Figure 14.2. Bone lesions in POEMS syndrome. (A) Diffuse sclerotic lesions seen on bone windows of CT scan. (B) Mixed lytic and sclerotic lesions, "soap-bubble lesion." (C) Lytic lesion with sclerotic rim right ischium. (D) FDG avidity of lesion seen in (C).
Source: Printed with permission form Elsevier Press from Dispenzieri A. POEMS syndrome. *Blood Rev* 2007;21:285-99.

The majority of patients have evidence of multiple endocrinopathies in the four major endocrine axes (gonadal, thyroid, glucose, and adrenal).

Nerve conduction studies and electromyelography demonstrate a polyneuropathy with prominent demyelination as well as features of axonal degeneration, which are similar to the findings of patients with chronic inflammatory demyelinating polyradiculoneuropathy (CIDP).[11,54,55] Biopsy of the sural nerve usually shows both axonal degeneration and demyelination. VEGF is highly expressed in blood vessels and some nonmyelin-forming Schwann cells.[37] In most cases of POEMS syndrome, the nerve biopsy shows typical features of uncompacted myelin lamellae. At ultrastructural examination there are no features of macrophage-associated demyelination, which are seen in some cases of chronic inflammatory demyelinating polyneuropathy.[19,27,56,57]

Renal dysfunction is usually not a dominant feature of this syndrome. A slight excess in urinary protein is not unusual. In our experience, approximately 9% of patients have proteinuria exceeding 0.5 g/24 h and only 6% have a serum creatinine greater than or equal to 1.5 mg/dL. A total of four patients in our series developed renal failure as preterminal events.[2] Renal disease is more likely to occur in patients who have co-existing Castleman disease. The renal histology is diverse, with membranoproliferative features and evidence of endothelial injury being most common.[58] On both light and electron microscopy, mesangial expansion, narrowing of capillary lumina, basement membrane thickening, subendothelial deposits, widening of the subendothelial space, swelling and vacuolization of endothelial cells, and mesangiolysis predominate.[28,59-64] Standard immunofluorescence is negative,[28,65] and this differentiates it from primary membranoproliferative glomerulitis.[58] Rarely, infiltration by plasma cells nests or Castleman-like lymphoma can be seen.[64]

The pulmonary manifestations are protean, including pulmonary hypertension,[2,18,28,66-75] restrictive lung disease, impaired neuromuscular respiratory function, and impaired diffusion capacity of carbon monoxide,[74] but improve with effective therapy (Figure 14.3).[67,70,74] In a series of 20 patients with POEMS, followed over a 10-year period, 25% manifested pulmonary hypertension.[70] Findings on autopsy[70] or biopsy[76] are those of classic pulmonary hypertension, including eccentric intimal fibrosis, medial hypertrophy, and marked dilatation of arteries and arterioles. Whether the digital clubbing seen in POEMS is a reflection of underlying pulmonary hypertension and/or parenchymal disease is yet to be determined. Parallels between hypertrophic osteoarthropathy and POEMS, including digital clubbing, periostosis of tubular bones, pachydermia, hyperhydrosis, and acro-osteolysis, have been drawn.[77]

DIFFERENTIAL DIAGNOSIS

The dominant feature of this syndrome is PN, and not infrequently patients are initially diagnosed with CIDP or, less frequently, Guillan-Barre. An algorithm for making the diagnosis is shown in Figure 14.4. If a monoclonal protein is detected, monoclonal gammopathy–associated PN and AL amyloidosis enter the differential diagnosis. The two best ways to distinguish POEMS from these entities is to measure a plasma or serum VEGF level and to determine whether there are other POEMS syndrome symptoms or signs. Watanabe et al. studied serum levels of VEGF in 10 POEMS patients and compared them with measurements from normal controls ($n = 25$), CIDP ($n = 7$), Guillain-Barre ($n = 12$), and other neurological disorders ($n = 20$).[36] Seventy percent of POEMS patients had elevated levels while all other patients had normal levels. VEGF levels are higher in POEMS patients than in patients with monoclonal gammopathy of undetermined significance[14] and multiple myeloma.[14,16]

PROGNOSIS

The course of POEMS syndrome is chronic, and patients typically survive for more than a decade in contrast to multiple myeloma. In our experience, the median survival was 13.8 years.[2] Individual reports of patients with the disease for more than 5 years are not unusual, and in one French study, at least 7 out of 15 patients were alive for more than 5 years.[12] In Nakanishi's series of 102 patients, the median survival was 33 months[4] although in Takatsuki's study of 109 patients, the authors stated that the "clinical course is very chronic … some patients survived greater than 10 years."[3] The number of POEMS features does not affect survival.[2,12] In our experience, only fingernail clubbing and extravascular volume overload, that is, effusions, edema, and ascites, were significantly associated with a shorter overall survival. Other variables such as the number

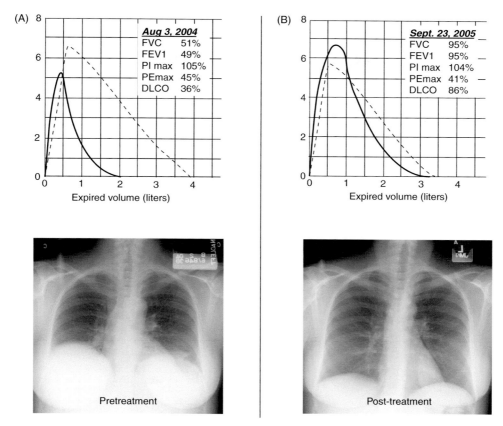

Figure 14.3. Pulmonary findings of pre- and post-therapy. (A) Pretreatment pulmonary function tests and CXR. (B) Post-treatment pulmonary function tests and CXR.
Source: Printed with permission form Elsevier Press from Dispenzieri A. POEMS syndrome. *Blood Rev* 2007;21:285-99.

of POEMS features, age, alkylator use, number of bone lesions, endocrine involvement, weight loss, lymphadenopathy, Castleman disease, organomegaly, papilledema, skin, gender, serum M-protein, urine M-protein, thrombocytosis, or hemoglobin had no predictive value for overall survival in the Mayo series.[2] More recently, we have identified respiratory symptoms to be predictive of adverse outcome.[75] In the French series, patients without plasmocytoma or bone lesions had a worse prognosis than those with other types of plasma cell dyscrasia in the absence of bone lesions.[12]

Additional features typically arise over time if treatment is unsuccessful or if the diagnosis is delayed.[2] The most common causes of death are cardiorespiratory failure, progressive inanition, infection, capillary-leak-like syndrome, and renal failure. Even those patients with multiple bone lesions or more than 10% plasma cells do not progress to classic multiple myeloma. The renal pathology in the occasional patient who develops renal failure is different from that of patients with classic myeloma. Stroke and myocardial infarction are also observed causes of death.

THERAPY

Our treatment approach is outlined in Figure 14.5, but there are no randomized, controlled trials in patients with POEMS. Information about benefits of therapy is

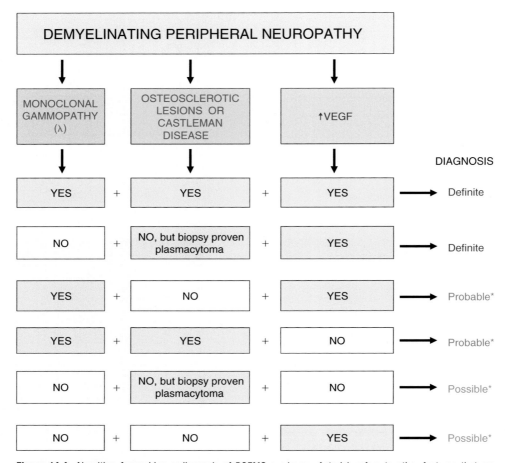

Figure 14.4. Algorithm for making a diagnosis of POEMS syndrome. Asterisk refers to other features that are defined in Table 14.1 to make diagnosis.

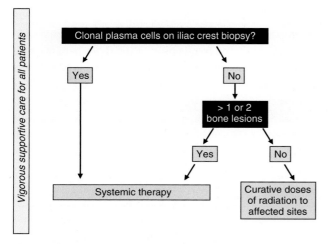

Figure 14.5. Treatment approach for POEMS syndrome.

most typically derived retrospectively (Table 14.2). Given these limitations, however, there are therapies that benefit patients with POEMS syndrome, including radiation therapy,[2,7,78-81] alkylator-based therapies,[2,4,10,63,82,83] and corticosteroids.[2] Intensive supportive care measures must also be instituted. Single or multiple osteosclerotic lesions in a limited area should be treated with radiation. If a patient has widespread osteosclerotic lesions or diffuse bone marrow plasmacytosis, systemic therapy is warranted. In contrast to CIDP, plasmapheresis and intravenous immunoglobulin do not produce clinical benefit. High-dose chemotherapy with peripheral blood transplant is yielding very promising results.[58,84-97] When the selected therapy is effective, response of systemic symptoms and skin changes typically precede those of the neuropathy, with the former

References	Treatment	Improvement rates (%)
2,7,10,78,79	Radiation	$\geq$50
2,10,82,119,120	Standard dose alkylator-based therapy	$\geq$40
2,4,19,60,121	Corticosteroids	$\geq$15
58,84-98	High-dose chemotherapy with PBSCT	$\geq$90

TABLE 14.2. Response to standard therapies

beginning to respond within a month, and the latter within 3-6 months, with maximum benefit frequently not seen before 2 to 3 years. Clinical response to therapy correlates better with VEGF level than M-protein level,[34,45] and complete hematological response is not required to derive substantial clinical benefit.[98]

Melphalan is among the most effective agents against plasmaproliferative disorders. On the basis of retrospective data, approximately 40% of patients with POEMS syndrome will respond to melphalan and prednisone.[2] The optimal duration of therapy has not been established, but borrowing from the experience of multiple myeloma, 12-24 months of treatment is reasonable.[99] Limiting the melphalan exposure is important because secondary myelodysplastic syndrome or acute leukemia can occur.[100] Cyclophosphamide is another alkylator that can control the disease in a limited number of patients. If the patient is considered to be a candidate for peripheral blood stem cell transplantation, melphalan-containing regimens should be avoided until after stem cell harvest.

High-dose chemotherapy with peripheral blood stem cell transplant is an emerging therapy for patients with POEMS. The first report was that of a 25-year-old female who was treated with high-dose chemotherapy followed by bone marrow transplantation; she died of multiorgan failure 63 days after her stem cell transplant.[84] Subsequently, there have been an additional 38 transplanted patients who have been reported.[58,85-98] All patients have improvement of their neuropathy over time; as in the case with radiation therapy and other chemotherapy, improvement of the PN takes months to years. Other clinical features improve after stem cell transplant, including levels of VEGF in several of the patients studied.[87,89]

Among the first 16 patients we transplanted, the treatment-related morbidity was higher than expected.[91]

Thirty-seven percent of our patients spent time in the intensive care unit and 37% required mechanical ventilation. Though only one of our patients died (6.2% mortality rate), if the published experience of transplanted POEMS patients is pooled, the mortality figure is 2 out of 27 or 7.4%. These numbers appear higher than the 2% transplant-related mortality observed in patients with multiple myeloma[101] but lower than the 14% transplant-related mortality observed in patients with primary systemic amyloidosis.[102]

We subsequently looked at our experience with 30 patients undergoing stem cell transplant and found that from day 8-16 patients with POEMS had higher than expected rates of fever, diarrhea, weight gain, and rash (93%, 77%, 53%, and 43%, respectively), and up to 50% had engraftment-like syndrome that appeared to be corticosteroid responsive.[98] Splenomegaly was the baseline factor that best predicted for a complicated peritransplant course. Patients had a higher than expected transfusion need, with median numbers of platelet and erythrocyte transfusions being five aphesis units (IQR, 2.0-10) and 6 units (IQR, 2.5-8.5), respectively. POEMS patients had delayed engraftment with a median time to absolute neutrophil count 0.5×10^9/L of 16 days (interquartile range [IQR] 15-18), with only 10% reaching an ANC of 0.5×10^9/L by day 13. Their times to platelets 20×10^9/L and 50×10^9/L were 14.5 days (IQR 11-22) and 19.5 days (IQR 15-39), respectively.

Other treatments that have been reported are shown in Table 14.3, and include plasmapheresis,[52,82,103] intravenous immunoglobulin,[104] interferon-α,[43,105] tamoxifen,[106,107] trans-retinoic acid,[108] thalidomide,[109] ticlopidine,[110] argatroban,[32,43] strontium-89,[111] bevacizumab,[112,113] and lenalidomide.[114] Plasmapheresis is not an effective treatment in this disorder.[103] Those reports purporting efficacy of plasma exchange combine the treatment with corticosteroids and/or other therapies confounding interpretation.[52,82] Intravenous immunoglobulin also cannot be recommended on the basis of our experience or on a review of the literature.[104] Once again the few reports claiming effectiveness simultaneously use other immunosuppressants or treatments.[115-118] Although there is a theoretical rationale (anti-VEGF and anti-TNF effects) for using thalidomide in POEMS patients, enthusiasm for its use should be tempered by the high rate of PN induced by the drug. In contrast, the next-generation immune

TABLE 14.3. Experience with experimental therapies

References	Treatment	N	Outcomes
106	Tamoxifen	1	Disappearance of edema, effusions, and regression of PN
110	Ticlopidine	1	Improved edema, ascites, effusions, and VEGF for "several months;" no improvement in PN, other labs, or thyroid function
32	Argatroban	2	Improvement in 1; no response in 1
43	Interferon + argatroban	2	Improvement in paraprotein, neuropathy, and coagulation parameters—doing well at 2 years
105	Interferon-α	1	POEMS + CD: Begun after radiation. Remarkable improvement of PN and organomegaly and lymphadenopathy after 3 months
108	*Trans* retinoic acid	1	Improved cytokines, platelet count, but worsening PN
111	Strontium-89	1	Improvement of LA, hepatomegaly, PN, platelets
122	Thalidomide + dexamethasone	1	POEMS + CD: improved PN, ascites, pleural effusion, dyspnea, creatinine, CBC, IL-6 w/in 2 months
109	Thalidomide	1*	Improved ascites, anemia, leukopenia, thrombocytopenia, ESR, and sense of well-being
112	Bevacizumab	1	Patient also receiving melphalan + dexamethasone; improved edema, pain, weakness, VEGF
113	Bevacizumab	1	Worsening PN, anasarca, MOF; died of pneumonia 5 weeks after treatment
113	Bevacizumab	1	Initial worsening; dose repeated with cyclophosphamide resulted in improvement of pulmonary HTN, anasarca, skin changes
114	Lenaldiomide + low-dose dexamethasone	1	Improvement in ascites, performance status, PN, VEGF levels, testosterone levels, pulmonary function tests

CD, Castleman disease; HTN, hypertension; IL-6, interleukin-6; LA, lymphadenopathy; MOF, multi-organ failure; PN, peripheral neuropathy; VEGF, vascular endothelial growth factor.
*POEMS (w/ normal IL-6 and no bone lesions), but CD-like since anemia, leukopenia, thrombocytopenia, incr. ESR.

modulatory drug, lenalidomide, has a much lower risk of PN. We have observed dramatic improvements in one patient treated with this drug.[114] Bevacizumab has been tried with mixed results. Two patients who had also received alkylator during and/or predating the bevacizumab had benefit. One who received it after radiation died.[112,113]

All-*trans*-retinoic acid (ATRA) has been tried on the basis of the theory that it represses the AP-1 (a protein complex of c-jun and c-fos proto-oncogene products) mediated induction of gene expression. AP-1 responsive elements are present on the *IL-6*, *IL-1*, and *TNF*-α genes, suggesting a possible inhibition of these cytokines by ATRA.[108] A patient was treated with ATRA, and 26 days into treatment, radiation therapy was also begun. Before the radiation therapy began, there was an insignificant drop in the serum IgA λ level, a significant drop in the platelet, and lymphocyte count, and the levels of IL-1β, IL-6, and TNF-α. However, there was only worsening of the neuropathy during therapy.

The physical limitations of the patient should not be overlooked while evaluating and/or treating the underlying plasma cell disorder. As always a multidisciplinary, thoughtful treatment program will improve a complex patient's treatment outcome. A physical therapy and occupational therapy program is essential to maintain flexibility and assist in lifestyle management despite the neuropathy. In those patients with respiratory muscle weakness and/or pulmonary hypertension, overnight oxygen, or continuous positive airway pressure (CPAP) may be useful.

CONCLUSIONS

POEMS syndrome is a complex syndrome that shares elements with other diseases – most notably other plasma cell dyscrasias and Castleman disease. Significant clues to the underlying pathogenesis lies in the monoclonal lambda light chain restriction, the osteosclerotic lesions, and the cytokine profile. Unraveling the elements of this paraneoplastic syndrome has the potential to provide insight into a number of other disorders. For now, the best treatments appear to be those that are useful to treat patients with myeloma, although neurotoxic therapies should be avoided, limiting the treatment armamentarium. One of the greatest practical challenges is making the diagnosis in a timely manner to prevent severe irreversible neurological disability.

REFERENCES

1. Bardwick PA, Zvaifler NJ, Gill GN, Newman D, Greenway GD, Resnick DL. Plasma cell dyscrasia with polyneuropathy, organomegaly, endocrinopathy, M protein, and skin changes: the POEMS syndrome. Report on two cases and a review of the literature. *Medicine* 1980;59:311-22.

2. Dispenzieri A, Kyle RA, Lacy MQ, et al. POEMS syndrome: definitions and long-term outcome. *Blood* 2003;101:2496-506.

3. Takatsuki K, Sanada I. Plasma cell dyscrasia with polyneuropathy and endocrine disorder: clinical and laboratory features of 109 reported cases. *Jpn J Clin Oncol* 1983;13:543-55.

4. Nakanishi T, Sobue I, Toyokura Y, et al. The Crow-Fukase syndrome: a study of 102 cases in Japan. *Neurology* 1984;34:712-20.

5. Crow R. Peripheral neuritis in myelomatosis. *Br Med J* 1956;2:802-4.

6. Driedger H, Pruzanski W. Plasma cell neoplasia with osteosclerotic lesions. A study of five cases and a review of the literature. *Arch Intern Med* 1979;139:892-6.

7. Iwashita H, Ohnishi A, Asada M, Kanazawa Y, Kuroiwa Y. Polyneuropathy, skin hyperpigmentation, edema, and hypertrichosis in localized osteosclerotic myeloma. *Neurology* 1977;27:675-81.

8. Mangalik A, Veliath AJ. Osteosclerotic myeloma and peripheral neuropathy. A case report. *Cancer* 1971;28:1040-5.

9. Evison G, Evans KT. Sclerotic bone deposits in multiple myeloma [letter]. *Br J Radiol* 1983;56:145.

10. Reitan JB, Pape E, Fossa SD, Julsrud OJ, Slettnes ON, Solheim OP. Osteosclerotic myeloma with polyneuropathy. *Acta Med Scand* 1980;208:137-44.

11. Kelly JJ Jr., Kyle RA, Miles JM, Dyck PJ. Osteosclerotic myeloma and peripheral neuropathy. *Neurology* 1983;33:202-10.

12. Soubrier MJ, Dubost JJ, Sauvezie BJ. POEMS syndrome: a study of 25 cases and a review of the literature. French study group on POEMS syndrome. *Am J Med* 1994;97:543-53.

13. Watanabe O, Arimura K, Kitajima I, Osame M, Maruyama I. Greatly raised vascular endothelial growth factor (VEGF) in POEMS syndrome [letter]. *Lancet* 1996;347:702.

14. Soubrier M, Dubost JJ, Serre AF, et al. Growth factors in POEMS syndrome: evidence for a marked increase in circulating vascular endothelial growth factor. *Arthritis Rheum* 1997;40:786-7.

15. Hashiguchi T, Arimura K, Matsumuro K, et al. Highly concentrated vascular endothelial growth factor in platelets in Crow-Fukase syndrome. *Muscle Nerve* 2000;23:1051-6.

16. Gherardi RK, Belec L, Soubrier M, Malapert D, Zuber M, Viard JP. Overproduction of proinflammatory cytokines imbalanced by their antagonists in POEMS syndrome. *Blood* 1996;87:1458-65.

17. Hitoshi S, Suzuki K, Sakuta M. Elevated serum interleukin-6 in POEMS syndrome reflects the activity of the disease. *Intern Med* 1994;33:583-7.

18. Rose C, Zandecki M, Copin MC, et al. POEMS syndrome: report on six patients with unusual clinical signs, elevated levels of cytokines, macrophage involvement and chromosomal aberrations of bone marrow plasma cells. *Leukemia* 1997;11:1318-23.

19. Orefice G, Morra VB, De Michele G, et al. POEMS syndrome: clinical, pathological and immunological study of a case. *Neurol Res* 1994;16:477-80.

20. Nakazawa K, Itoh N, Shigematsu H, Koh CS. An autopsy case of Crow-Fukase (POEMS) syndrome with a high level of IL-6 in the ascites. Special reference to glomerular lesions. *Acta Pathol Jpn* 1992;42:651-6.

21. Emile C, Danon F, Fermand JP, Clauvel JP. Castleman disease in POEMS syndrome with elevated interleukin-6 [letter; comment]. *Cancer* 1993;71:874.

22. Saida K, Ohta M, Kawakami H, Saida T. Cytokines and myelin antibodies in Crow-Fukase syndrome. *Muscle Nerve* 1996;19:1620-2.

23. Feinberg L, Temple D, de Marchena E, Patarca R, Mitrani A. Soluble immune mediators in POEMS syndrome with pulmonary hypertension: case report and review of the literature. *Crit Rev Oncog* 1999;10:293-302.

24. Soubrier M, Labauge P, Jouanel P, Viallard JL, Piette JC, Sauvezie B. Restricted use of Vlambda genes in POEMS syndrome. *Haematologica* 2004;89:ECR02.

25. Nakaseko C, Abe D, Takeuchi M, et al. Restricted oligo-clonal usage of monoclonal immunoglobulin {lambda} light chain germline in POEMS syndrome. *ASH Annual Meeting Abstracts* 2007;110:2483.

26. Bryce AH, Ketterling RP, Gertz MA, et al. Cytogenetic analysis using multiple myeloma targets in POEMS syndrome. Proceedings of American Society of Oncology Meeting, Chicago, IL, 2007.

27. Bergouignan FX, Massonnat R, Vital C, et al. Uncompacted lamellae in three patients with POEMS syndrome. *Eur Neurol* 1987;27:173-81.

28. Viard JP, Lesavre P, Boitard C, et al. POEMS syndrome presenting as systemic sclerosis. Clinical and pathologic study of a case with microangiopathic glomerular lesions. *Am J Med* 1988;84:524-8.

29. Belec L, Mohamed AS, Authier FJ, et al. Human herpesvirus 8 infection in patients with POEMS syndrome-associated multicentric Castleman's disease. *Blood* 1999;93:3643-53.

30. Belec L, Authier FJ, Mohamed AS, Soubrier M, Gherardi RK. Antibodies to human herpesvirus 8 in POEMS (polyneuropathy, organomegaly, endocrinopathy, M protein, skin changes) syndrome with multicentric Castleman's disease. *Clin Infect Dis* 1999;28:678-9.

31. Bosch EP, Smith BE. Peripheral neuropathies associated with monoclonal proteins. [Review] [63 refs]. *Med Clin North Am* 1993;77:125-39.

32. Tokashiki T, Hashiguchi T, Arimura K, Eiraku N, Maruyama I, Osame M. Predictive value of serial platelet count and VEGF determination for the management of DIC in the Crow-Fukase (POEMS) syndrome. *Intern Med* 2003;42:1240-3.

33. Endo I, Mitsui T, Nishino M, Oshima Y, Matsumoto T. Diurnal fluctuation of edema synchronized with plasma VEGF concentration in a patient with POEMS syndrome. *Intern Med* 2002;41:1196-8.

34. Nakano A, Mitsui T, Endo I, Takeda Y, Ozaki S, Matsumoto T. Solitary plasmacytoma with VEGF overproduction: report of a patient with polyneuropathy. *Neurology* 2001;56:818-19.

35. Koga H, Tokunaga Y, Hisamoto T, et al. Ratio of serum vascular endothelial growth factor to platelet count correlates with disease activity in a patient with POEMS syndrome. *Eur J Intern Med* 2002;13:70-4.

36. Watanabe O, Maruyama I, Arimura K, et al. Overproduction of vascular endothelial growth factor/vascular permeability factor is causative in Crow-Fukase (POEMS) syndrome. *Muscle Nerve* 1998;21:1390-7.

37. Scarlato M, Previtali SC, Carpo M, et al. Polyneuropathy in POEMS syndrome: role of angiogenic factors in the pathogenesis. *Brain* 2005;128:1911-20.

38. Loeb JM, Hauger PH, Carney JD, Cooper AD. Refractory ascites due to POEMS syndrome. *Gastroenterology* 1989;96:247-9.

39. Arimura K. Increased vascular endothelial growth factor (VEGF) is causative in Crow-Fukase syndrome. [Japanese]. *Rinsho Shinkeigaku* 1999;39:84-5.

40. Gherardi RK, Belec L, Fromont G, et al. Elevated levels of interleukin-1 beta (IL-1 beta) and IL-6 in serum and increased production of IL-1 beta mRNA in lymph nodes of patients with polyneuropathy, organomegaly, endocrinopathy, M protein, and skin changes (POEMS) syndrome. *Blood* 1994;83:2587-93.

41. Shikama N, Isono A, Otsuka Y, Terano T, Hirai A. A case of POEMS syndrome with high concentrations of interleukin-6 in pericardial fluid. *J Intern Med* 2001;250:170-3.

42. Michizono K, Umehara F, Hashiguchi T, et al. Circulating levels of MMP-1, -2, -3, -9, and TIMP-1 are increased in POEMS syndrome. *Neurology* 2001;56:807-10.

43. Saida K, Kawakami H, Ohta M, Iwamura K. Coagulation and vascular abnormalities in Crow-Fukase syndrome. *Muscle Nerve* 1997;20:486-92.

44. Yishay O, Eran E. POEMS syndrome: failure of newly suggested diagnostic criteria to anticipate the development of the syndrome. *Am J Hematol* 2005;79:316-18.

45. Mineta M, Hatori M, Sano H, et al. Recurrent Crow-Fukase syndrome associated with increased serum levels of vascular endothelial growth factor: a case report and review of the literature. *Tohoku J Exp Med* 2006;210:269-77.

46. Donaghy M, Hall P, Gawler J, et al. Peripheral neuropathy associated with Castleman's disease. *J Neurol Sci* 1989;89:253-67.

47. Lesprit P, Authier FJ, Gherardi R, et al. Acute arterial obliteration: a new feature of the POEMS syndrome? *Medicine* 1996;75:226-32.

48. Zenone T, Bastion Y, Salles G, et al. POEMS syndrome, arterial thrombosis and thrombocythaemia. *J Intern Med* 1996;240:107-9.

49. Soubrier M, Guillon R, Dubost JJ, et al. Arterial obliteration in POEMS syndrome: possible role of vascular endothelial growth factor. *J Rheumatol* 1998;25:813-15.

50. Bova G, Pasqui AL, Saletti M, Bruni F, Auteri A. POEMS syndrome with vascular lesions: a role for interleukin-1beta and interleukin-6 increase—a case report. *Angiology* 1998;49:937-40.

51. Kang K, Chu K, Kim DE, Jeong SW, Lee JW, Roh JK. POEMS syndrome associated with ischemic stroke. *Arch Neurol* 2003;60:745-9.

52. Atsumi T, Kato K, Kurosawa S, Abe M, Fujisaku A. A case of Crow-Fukase syndrome with elevated soluble interleukin-6 receptor in cerebrospinal fluid. Response to double-filtration plasmapheresis and corticosteroids. *Acta Haematol* 1995;94:90-4.

53. Ghandi GY, Basu R, Dispenzieri A, Basu A, Montori V, Brennan MD. Endocrinopathy in POEMS syndrome: the Mayo clinic experience. *Mayo Clin Proc* 2007;82:836-42.

54. Sung JY, Kuwabara S, Ogawara K, Kanai K, Hattori T. Patterns of nerve conduction abnormalities in POEMS syndrome. *Muscle Nerve* 2002;26:189-93.

55. Suarez GA, Dispenzieri A, Gertz MA, Kyle RA. The electrophysiologic findings of the peripheral neuropathy associated with POEMS. *Clin Neurophysiol* 2002;113:S9.

56. Vital C, Vital A, Ferrer X, et al. Crow-Fukase (POEMS) syndrome: a study of peripheral nerve biopsy in five new cases. *J Peripher Nerv Syst* 2003;8:136-44.

57. Crisci C, Barbieri F, Parente D, Pappone N, Caruso G. POEMS syndrome: follow-up study of a case. *Clin Neurol Neurosurg* 1992;94:65-8.

58. Sanada S, Ookawara S, Karube H, et al. Marked recovery of severe renal lesions in POEMS syndrome with high-dose melphalan therapy supported by autologous blood stem cell transplantation. *Am J Kidney Dis* 2006;47:672-9.

59. Navis GJ, Dullaart RP, Vellenga E, Elema JD, de Jong PE. Renal disease in POEMS syndrome: report on a case and review of the literature. [Review] [25 refs]. *Nephrology, Dialysis, Transplantation* 1994;9:1477-81.

60. Sano M, Terasaki T, Koyama A, Narita M, Tojo S. Glomerular lesions associated with the Crow-Fukase syndrome. *Virchows Arch A Pathol Anat Histopathol* 1986;409:3-9.

61. Takazoe K, Shimada T, Kawamura T, et al. Possible mechanism of progressive renal failure in Crow-Fukase syndrome [letter]. *Clin Nephrol* 1997;47:66-7.

62. Mizuiri S, Mitsuo K, Sakai K, et al. Renal involvement in POEMS syndrome. *Nephron* 1991;59:153-6.

63. Stewart PM, McIntyre MA, Edwards CR. The endocrinopathy of POEMS syndrome. *Scott Med J* 1989;34:520-2.

64. Nakamoto Y, Imai H, Yasuda T, Wakui H, Miura AB. A spectrum of clinicopathological features of nephropathy associated with POEMS syndrome. *Nephrol Dial Transplant* 1999;14:2370-8.

65. Fukatsu A, Ito Y, Yuzawa Y, et al. A case of POEMS syndrome showing elevated serum interleukin 6 and abnormal expression of interleukin 6 in the kidney. *Nephron* 1992;62:47-51.

66. Mufti GJ, Hamblin TJ, Gordon J. Melphalan-induced pulmonary fibrosis in osteosclerotic myeloma [letter]. *Acta Haematol* 1983;69:140-1.

67. Iwasaki H, Ogawa K, Yoshida H, et al. Crow-Fukase syndrome associated with pulmonary hypertension. *Intern Med* 1993;32:556-60.

68. Ribadeau-Dumas S, Tillie-Leblond I, Rose C, et al. Pulmonary hypertension associated with POEMS syndrome. [Review] [17 refs]. *Eur Respir J* 1996;9:1760-2.

69. Okura H, Gohma I, Hatta K, Imanaka T. Thiamine deficiency and pulmonary hypertension in Crow-Fukase syndrome. *Intern Med* 1995;34:674-5.

70. Lesprit P, Godeau B, Authier FJ, et al. Pulmonary hypertension in POEMS syndrome: a new feature mediated by cytokines. *Am J Respir Crit Care Med* 1998;157:907-11.

71. Brazis PW, Liesegang TJ, Bolling JP, Kashii S, Trachtman M, Burde RM. When do optic disc edema and peripheral neuropathy constitute poetry? *Surv Ophthalmol* 1990;35:219-25.

72. Kishimoto S, Takenaka H, Shibagaki R, Noda Y, Yamamoto M, Yasuno H. Glomeruloid hemangioma in POEMS syndrome shows two different immunophenotypic endothelial cells. *J Cutan Pathol* 2000;27:87-92.

73. Paciocco G, Bossone E, Erba H, Rubenfire M. Reversible pulmonary hypertension in POEMS syndrome—another etiology of triggered pulmonary vasculopathy?. [Review] [17 refs]. *Can J Cardiol* 2000;16:1007-12.

74. Dispenzieri A, Moreno-Aspitia A, Suarez GA, et al. Peripheral blood stem cell transplantation in 16 patients with POEMS syndrome, and a review of the literature. *Blood* 2004;104:3400-7.

75. Allam JS, Kennedy CC, Aksamit TR, Dispenzieri A. Pulmonary manifestations are common and associated with shortened survival in POEMS syndrome: a retrospective review of 141 patients. 2008;133(4):969-74.

76. Lewerenz J, Gocht A, Hoeger PH, et al. Multiple vascular abnormalities and a paradoxical combination of vitamin B(12) deficiency and thrombocytosis in a case with POEMS syndrome. *J Neurol* 2003;250:1488-91.

77. Martinez-Lavin M, Vargas AS, Cabre J, et al. Features of hypertrophic osteoarthropathy in patients with POEMS syndrome: a metaanalysis [letter]. *J Rheumatol* 1997;24:2267-8.

78. Morley JB, Schwieger AC. The relation between chronic polyneuropathy and osteosclerotic myeloma. *J Neurol Neurosurg Psychiatry* 1967;30:432-42.

79. Davis L, Drachman D. Myeloma neuropathy. *Arch Neurol* 1972;27:507-11.

80. Philips ED, el-Mahdi AM, Humphrey RL, Furlong MB Jr. The effect of the radiation treatment on the polyneuropathy of multiple myeloma. *J Can Assoc Radiol* 1972;23:103-6.

81. Broussolle E, Vighetto A, Bancel B, Confavreux C, Pialat J, Aimard G. P.O.E.M.S. syndrome with complete recovery after treatment of a solitary plasmocytoma. *Clin Neurol Neurosurg* 1991;93:165-70.

82. Ku A, Lachmann E, Tunkel R, Nagler W. Severe polyneuropathy: initial manifestation of Castleman's disease associated with POEMS syndrome. *Arch Phys Med Rehabil* 1995;76:692-4.

83. Cabezas-Agricola JM, Lado-Abeal JJ, Otero-Anton E, Sanchez-Leira J, Cabezas-Cerrato J. Hypoparathyroidism in POEMS syndrome [letter]. *Lancet* 1996;347:701-2.

84. Wong VA, Wade NK. POEMS syndrome: an unusual cause of bilateral optic disk swelling. *Am J Ophthalmol* 1998;126:452-4.

85. Hogan WJ, Lacy MQ, Wiseman GA, Fealey RD, Dispenzieri A, Gertz MA. Successful treatment of POEMS syndrome with autologous hematopoietic progenitor cell transplantation. *Bone Marrow Transplant* 2001;28:305-9.

86. Rovira M, Carreras E, Blade J, et al. Dramatic improvement of POEMS syndrome following autologous haematopoietic cell transplantation. *Br J Haematol* 2001;115:373-5.

87. Jaccard A, Royer B, Bordessoule D, Brouet JC, Fermand JP. High-dose therapy and autologous blood stem cell transplantation in POEMS syndrome. *Blood* 2002;99:3057-9.

88. Peggs KS, Paneesha S, Kottaridis PD, et al. Peripheral blood stem cell transplantation for POEMS syndrome. *Bone Marrow Transplant* 2002;30:401-4.

89. Soubrier M, Ruivard M, Dubost JJ, Sauvezie B, Philippe P. Successful use of autologous bone marrow transplantation in treating a patient with POEMS syndrome. *Bone Marrow Transplant* 2002;30:61-2.

90. Wiesmann A, Weissert R, Kanz L, Einsele H. Long-term follow-up on a patient with incomplete POEMS syndrome undergoing high-dose therapy and autologous blood stem cell transplantation. *Blood* 2002;100:2679-80.

91. Dispenzieri A, Kyle RA, Lacy MQ, et al. Superior survival in primary systemic amyloidosis patients undergoing peripheral blood stem cell transplantation: a case-control study. *Blood* 2004;103:3960-3.

92. Takai K, Niikuni K, Kurasaki T. Successful treatment of POEMS syndrome with high-dose chemotherapy and autologous peripheral blood stem cell transplantation. *Rinsho Ketsueki* 2004;45:1111-14.

93. Ganti AK, Pipinos I, Culcea E, Armitage JO, Tarantolo S. Successful hematopoietic stem-cell transplantation in multicentric Castleman disease complicated by POEMS syndrome. *Am J Hematol* 2005;79:206-10.

94. Kastritis E, Terpos E, Anagnostopoulos A, Xilouri I, Dimopoulos MA. Angiogenetic factors and biochemical markers of bone metabolism in POEMS syndrome treated with high-dose therapy and autologous stem cell support. *Clin Lymphoma Myeloma* 2006;7:73-6.

95. Kuwabara S, Misawa S, Kanai K, et al. Autologous peripheral blood stem cell transplantation for POEMS syndrome. *Neurology* 2006;66:105-7.

96. Kojima H, Katsuoka Y, Katsura Y, et al. Successful treatment of a patient with POEMS syndrome by tandem high-dose chemotherapy with autologous CD34+ purged stem cell rescue. *Int J Hematol* 2006;84:182-5.

97. Imai N, Kitamura E, Tachibana T, et al. Efficacy of autologous peripheral blood stem cell transplantation in POEMS syndrome with polyneuropathy. *Intern Med* 2007;46:135-8.

98. Dispenzieri A, Lacy MQ, Hayman SR, et al. Peripheral blood stem cell transplant for POEMS syndrome is associated with high rates of engraftment syndrome. *Eur J Haematol* 2008;80:397-406.

99. Anonymous. Combination chemotherapy versus melphalan plus prednisone as treatment for multiple myeloma: an overview of 6,633 patients from 27 randomized trials. Myeloma Trialists' Collaborative Group. *J Clin Oncol* 1998;16:3832-42.

100. Satoh K, Miura I, Chubachi A, Utsumi S, Imai H, Miura AB. Development of secondary leukemia associated with (1;7) (q10;p10) in a patient with Crow-Fukase syndrome. *Intern Med* 1996;35:660-2.

101. Attal M, Harousseau JL, Stoppa AM, et al. A prospective, randomized trial of autologous bone marrow transplantation and chemotherapy in multiple myeloma. Intergroupe Francais du Myelome [see comments]. *N Engl J Med* 1996;335:91-7.

102. Gertz MA, Lacy MQ, Dispenzieri A, et al. Stem cell transplantation for the management of primary systemic amyloidosis. *Am J Med* 2002;113:549-55.

103. Silberstein LE, Duggan D, Berkman EM. Therapeutic trial of plasma exchange in osteosclerotic myeloma associated with the POEMS syndrome. *J Clin Apher* 1985;2:253-7.

104. Chang YJ, Huang CC, Chu CC. Intravenous immunoglobulin therapy in POEMS syndrome: a case report. *Chung Hua i Hsueh Tsa Chih Chinese Med J* 1996;58:366-9.

105. Coto V, Auletta M, Oliviero U, et al. POEMS syndrome: an Italian case with diagnostic and therapeutic implications. *Ann Ital Med Int* 1991;6:416-19.

106. Barrier JH, Le Noan H, Mussini JM, Brisseau JM. Stabilisation of a severe case of P.O.E.M.S. syndrome after tamoxifen administration [letter]. *J Neurol Neurosurg Psychiatry* 1989;52:286.

107. Enevoldson TP, Harding AE. Improvement in the POEMS syndrome after administration of tamoxifen [letter]. *J Neurology Neurosurg Psychiatry* 1992;55:71-2.

108. Authier FJ, Belec L, Levy Y, et al. All-trans-retinoic acid in POEMS syndrome. Therapeutic effect associated with decreased circulating levels of proinflammatory cytokines. *Arthritis Rheum* 1996;39:1423-26.

109. Sinisalo M, Hietaharju A, Sauranen J, Wirta O. Thalidomide in POEMS syndrome: case report. *Am J Hematol* 2004;76:66-8.

110. Matsui H, Udaka F, Kubori T, Oda M, Nishinaka K, Kameyama M. POEMS syndrome demonstrating VEGF decrease by ticlopidine. *Intern Med* 2004;43:1082-3.

111. Sternberg AJ, Davies P, Macmillan C, Abdul-Cader A, Swart S. Strontium-89: a novel treatment for a case of osteosclerotic myeloma associated with life-threatening neuropathy. *Br J Haematol* 2002;118:821-4.

112. Badros A, Porter N, Zimrin A. Bevacizumab therapy for POEMS syndrome. *Blood* 2005;106:1135.

113. Straume O, Bergheim J, Ernst P. Bevacizumab therapy for POEMS syndrome. *Blood* 2006;107:4972-3; author reply 4973-4.

114. Dispenzieri A, Klein CJ, Mauermann ML. Lenalidomide therapy in a patient with POEMS syndrome. *Blood* 2007;110:1075-6.

115. Benito-Leon J, Lopez-Rios F, Rodriguez-Martin FJ, Madero S, Ruiz J. Rapidly deteriorating polyneuropathy associated with osteosclerotic myeloma responsive to intravenous immunoglobulin and radiotherapy. *J Neurol Sci* 1998;158:113-17.

116. Henze T, Krieger G. Combined high-dose 7S-IgG and dexamethasone is effective in severe polyneuropathy of the POEMS syndrome [letter] [see comments]. *J Neurol* 1995;242:482-3.

117. Rotta FT, Bradley WG. Marked improvement of severe polyneuropathy associated with multifocal osteosclerotic myeloma following surgery, radiation, and chemotherapy. *Muscle Nerve* 1997;20:1035-7.

118. Huang CC, Chu CC. Poor response to intravenous immunoglobulin therapy in patients with Castleman's disease and the POEMS syndrome [letter; comment]. *J Neurol* 1996;243:726-7.

119. Judge MR, McGibbon DH, Thompson RP. Angioendotheliomatosis associated with Castleman's lymphoma and POEMS syndrome. *Clin Exp Dermatol* 1993;18:360-2.

120. Kuwabara S, Hattori T, Shimoe Y, Kamitsukasa I. Long term melphalan-prednisolone chemotherapy for POEMS syndrome. *J Neurol Neurosurg Psychiatry* 1997;63:385-7.

121. Arima F, Dohmen K, Yamano Y, et al. Five cases of Crow-Fukase syndrome [Japanese]. *Fukuoka Igaku Zasshi* 1992;83:112-20.

122. Kim SY, Lee SA, Ryoo HM, Lee KH, Hyun MS, Bae SH. Thalidomide for POEMS syndrome. *Ann Hematol* 2006;85:545-6.

INDEX

Printed in the United States
by Baker & Taylor Publisher Services